Comorbidities and Social Complications of Epilepsy and Seizures

Comorbidities and Social Complications of Epilepsy and Seizures

The cognitive, psychological, and psychosocial impact of epilepsy

Edited by

Arjune Sen

Consultant Neurologist, Department of Neurology, John Radcliffe Hospital; Nuffield Department of Clinical Neurosciences, University of Oxford; Centre for Global Epilepsy, Wolfson College, University of Oxford, Oxford, UK

Ian Brown

Consultant Occupational Health Physician and Toxicologist, Department of Neurology, John Radcliffe Hospital; Nuffield Department of Clinical Neurosciences, University of Oxford; Centre for Global Epilepsy, Wolfson College, University of Oxford, Oxford, UK

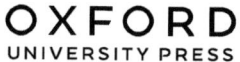

OXFORD
UNIVERSITY PRESS

OXFORD
UNIVERSITY PRESS

Great Clarendon Street, Oxford, OX2 6DP,
United Kingdom

Oxford University Press is a department of the University of Oxford.
It furthers the University's objective of excellence in research, scholarship,
and education by publishing worldwide. Oxford is a registered trade mark of
Oxford University Press in the UK and in certain other countries

Published in the United States of America by Oxford University Press
198 Madison Avenue, New York, NY 10016, United States of America

British Library Cataloguing in Publication Data

Data available

Library of Congress Control Number is on file at the Library of Congress

ISBN 978–0–19–882075–8

DOI: 10.1093/med/9780198820758.001.0001

Printed and bound by
CPI Group (UK) Ltd, Croydon, CR0 4YY

Oxford University Press makes no representation, express or implied, that the
drug dosages in this book are correct. Readers must therefore always check
the product information and clinical procedures with the most up-to-date
published product information and data sheets provided by the manufacturers
and the most recent codes of conduct and safety regulations. The authors and
the publishers do not accept responsibility or legal liability for any errors in the
text or for the misuse or misapplication of material in this work. Except where
otherwise stated, drug dosages and recommendations are for the non-pregnant
adult who is not breast-feeding

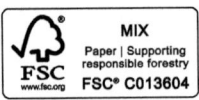

We dedicate this book to Dr Tim Andrews, a close colleague and friend, who always championed thoughtful, holistic care for the most vulnerable in society.

Foreword

This is one of the first books to focus on the topic of *epilepsy comorbidities*—the concept that epilepsy is more than just seizures—and Professors Sen and Brown are to be congratulated in putting this together. This is a topic that has been too often ignored, and yet the comorbidities represent a large component of the epilepsy disease burden. This book, too, is notable for the way in which the consideration of comorbidity is linked to the psychosocial issues in epilepsy, and in doing so the theoretical is translated into the practical in an exemplary fashion. The book succeeds in the task of widening and broadening both the understanding and the practice of epilepsy.

The idea of 'comorbidity' in epilepsy, albeit under a different name, originated in the mid-19th century. Until then, idiopathic epilepsy and epileptic seizures were considered synonymous terms. It was the psychiatrists of the 19th century, particularly in France, who began to see epilepsy as a feature of the broader phenomenon of 'cerebral degeneration', a term which incorporated all sorts of other conditions. 'Degeneration' was manifest by various somatic, psychiatric/psychological, and moral/behavioural symptoms, and epileptic seizures were but one part of this spectrum. By the late 19th century, the prevailing view was that these conditions were all due to an inherited defect in germ plasm—in modern parlance, defective genetic material. Epileptic seizures were a component of this abnormal heredity and so important were the non-seizure aspects of epilepsy that the concept of epilepsy without seizures was also much discussed. The person with epilepsy was assumed to be prone to other features of cerebral degeneration, to have a particular personality (the 'epileptic personality'), and to be someone whose mental capacities deteriorated over time. These ideas were discredited in the early decades of the 20th century and faded over time, perhaps mainly because the underlying causes of epilepsy became more clearly delineated and effective drug therapies for seizures were developed. By the mid-20th century, epilepsy was again in effect seen as a condition in which almost the only core manifestation was the epileptic seizure.

History tends to cycle, and in the last few decades, new interest has grown in the association of seizures with other features—now grouped under the term *comorbidity*. No longer are the comorbid features seen as a symptom of 'degeneration', or a 'moral defect', but they are now much more specifically delineated and their biological mechanisms much more precisely known.

In this book, Section 1 provides an overarching background. The editors have wisely grouped the comorbidities into those caused by treatment (Section 2) and those associated with the causes of the seizures (Section 3). Sections 4 and 5 discuss the effect of comorbidities in specific situations, later life and pregnancy, and the broad impact of epilepsy on the lives those it affects. The result is a fascinating review of current thinking and ideas. Much of the text has been stimulated by the new genetics of epilepsy and much is focused on the psychological and psychosocial consequences; and therein are echoes of previous times. What differentiates current ideas of comorbidity from that of the 19th century, however, is the more rigorous scientific approach and that comorbidity is treated in an objective and non-prejudicial fashion. A sense of humanity shines through the book. It is a text that will appeal to all those interested in a holistic approach to disease. It is aimed primarily at epilepsy specialists, other clinicians, and healthcare professionals, but will also be of value to people with epilepsy, their families, and their carers. This is an excellent, concise, and valuable addition to the epilepsy literature.

Professor Simon Shorvon
Department of Clinical and Experimental Epilepsy
University College London
London, UK
February 2024

Preface

Epilepsy is the most common serious neurological condition and it affects over 600,000 people in the UK alone. Seizures can be dangerous, associating with injuries, including head injuries, and may even associate with mortality owing, for example, to sudden unexpected death in epilepsy (SUDEP). Unlike many neurological conditions, there are several treatments available to help people with epilepsy—both pharmaceutical and surgical. Nonetheless, 30% of individuals with epilepsy continue to experience seizures and the impact of those ongoing seizures contributes to epilepsy causing 1% of the global disease burden worldwide.

However, that is not the whole explanation. Epilepsy represents far more than seizures alone. Indeed, people with epilepsy often cite memory difficulties as their predominant concern, not the epileptic attacks themselves. The pattern of memory impairment seen in those with epilepsy has certain unique features and the intersection of epilepsy and dementia means that clinicians who are appropriately attuned can identify seizures in people with neurodegenerative disease, leading to new treatment options. In addition, one-third of individuals with epilepsy will experience depression during the course of their illness. People with epilepsy are more prone to other psychopathology including anxiety and psychosis and, as might be predicted, epilepsy is over-represented in people with intellectual disabilities. Epilepsy is an episodic condition. Affected individuals can be completely well between seizures. This means that the disease can be 'hidden', something which, coupled with an intrinsic fear of seizures, can contribute to significant stigmatization of those with epilepsy (50% of people with epilepsy do not declare the condition at pre-employment medical screening). Furthermore, epilepsy can significantly affect personal relationships, frequently requires people to stop driving, and can curtail leisure activities.

The comorbidities of epilepsy therefore represent a large component of the disease burden. Yet, this area is frequently ignored or is poorly understood. In clinical practice, many doctors will not enquire about relevant comorbidity or be comfortable in trying to disentangle the contributions that seizures, medication, or disease processes may make to this area in a given individual. Similarly, while there is considerable literature on advances in imaging or epilepsy genomics, for example, practical advice on how to tackle comorbidity in this patient group is difficult to find and a proper understanding of the psychosocial impact of epilepsy also seems lacking.

This book aims to address this gap in the literature and, to a degree, in our understanding. The book is designed to be a practical reference guide, not something taken to clinic, but a book that can be referred to afterwards or indeed beforehand. Chapters provide, within succinct text, a current overview of the relevant area and aim to be short enough, and engaging enough, to be read in a single sitting. While the chapters interlink closely, it is also possible to read each chapter as a stand-alone piece. All of the major comorbidities of epilepsy are reviewed, as well as the impact of antiepileptic medications and other therapies. As epilepsy is more common in older age and demographics are shifting towards an older population in both the developing and developed world, a specific chapter about older people with epilepsy is also included.

The overarching aim of the book is to provide the reader with a deeper understanding of all of the relevant comorbidities in epilepsy as well as providing insights into possible strategies of how best to help in the holistic treatment of people with epilepsy. Although somewhat UK focused, we anticipate that the text will also be of interest to medical/nursing practitioners, including in resource limited settings (developing world also considered pejorative), and to epilepsy charities and to be accessible to people, carers and Families living with epilepsy.

Acknowledgements

It is a great pleasure to complete this book, the idea for which germinated in the joint Epilepsy and Employment Clinic that Ian and I founded in Oxford many years ago. I am very grateful to all of the authors and to the editorial staff at Oxford University Press, in particular Michael Hawkes, Rachel Goldsworthy, and Peter Stevenson, for their belief in the project and for patiently driving this forwards. These endeavours take a lot of time and Ian has been an excellent source of support throughout. I must also thank Dushendree, Prashanti, and Saijayani for providing the time and space to devote to this project. Perhaps our greatest thanks, though, go to the people with epilepsy, their carers, and their families from whom we always learn so much and for whom we strive to deliver optimal care.

Arjune Sen

This book is a summary of one of my greatest interests and would not have been written without the continuous encouragement of my very learned co-editor, Arjune Sen. I am also very grateful to all the eminent neuroscientists and neurologists from all over the globe who gave their time to contribute expert chapters and always remained patient with the editors, as did my wife Sue, who allowed me to complete this work and perhaps neglect her. I would finally like to thank Oxford University Press for their confidence and encouragement in ensuring this work was undertaken and published.

Ian Brown

Contents

Abbreviations

Aβ	amyloid beta		GBP	gabapentin
AD	Alzheimer's disease		HLA	human leucocyte antigen
ADHD	attention deficit hyperactivity disorder		HR	hazard ratio
ALF	accelerated long-term forgetting		HSAWA	Health and Safety at Work etc. Act 1974
ALT	alanine transaminase		ICD	International Classification of Diseases
ANT	anterior nucleus of the thalamus		ID	intellectual disability *or* interictal discharge
ASD	autistic spectrum disorder(s)		ILAE	International League Against Epilepsy
ASM	antiseizure medication		IRR	incident rate ratio
ATL	anterior temporal lobe		LCM	lacosamide
ATLR	anterior temporal lobe resection		LEV	levetiracetam
BMD	bone mineral density		LITT	laser interstitial thermal therapy
BRV	brivaracetam		LMIC	lower- and middle-income countries
CBZ	carbamazepine		LTG	lamotrigine
CI	confidence interval		MCM	major congenital malformation
CNS	central nervous system		MHRA	Medicines and Healthcare products and Regulatory Agency
COVID-19	coronavirus disease 2019		MRI	magnetic resonance imaging
CZP	clonazepam		MTLE	mesial temporal lobe epilepsy
DBS	deep brain stimulation		mTOR	mammalian/mechanistic target of rapamycin
DRESS	drug reaction with eosinophilia and systemic symptoms syndrome		NF1	neurofibromatosis type 1
DSM	*Diagnostic and Statistical Manual of Mental Disorders*		NMDA	*N*-methyl-D-aspartate
EEG	electroencephalography/ electroencephalogram		OR	odds ratio
			OXC	oxcarbazepine
ESL	eslicarbazepine		PB	phenobarbital
ESM	ethosuximide		PER	perampanel
ET	essential tremor		PGB	pregabalin
EU	European Union		PHT	phenytoin
EURAP	International Registry of Antiepileptic Drugs and Pregnancy		PNES	psychogenic non-epileptic seizures
FBM	felbamate		PNS	peripheral nervous system
GABA	gamma-aminobutyric acid			

POLG	polymerase gamma	SWS	Sturge–Weber syndrome
PRM	primidone	T1DM	type 1 diabetes mellitus
QOL	quality of life	TDM	therapeutic drug monitoring
QTc	corrected QT interval	TEA	transient epileptic amnesia
RR	relative risk	TEN	toxic epidermal necrolysis
RUF	rufinamide	TGB	tiagabine
SEEG	stereoelectroencephalography	TIA	transient ischaemic attack
SJS	Stevens–Johnson syndrome	TLE	temporal lobe epilepsy
SLE	systemic lupus erythematosus	TPM	topiramate
SMR	standardized mortality ratio	TSC	tuberous sclerosis complex
SRS	stereotactic radiosurgery	VNS	vagus nerve stimulation
SSRI	selective serotonin reuptake inhibitor	VPA	valproic acid
SUDEP	sudden unexpected death in epilepsy	ZNS	zonisamide

Contributors

Tim Andrews
Chapter 7: Epilepsy and intellectual disabilities
Oxford School of Psychiatry, Oxford, UK

Samantha Ashby
Chapter 9: Epilepsy and mortality
SUDEP Action, Wantage, UK

John Baker
Chapter 5: Epilepsy and cognition
Dementia Research Centre, UCL Queen Square Institute of Neurology, London, UK

Frank M. C. Besag
Chapter 1: Introduction
East London Foundation NHS Trust, University College London, Kings College London, London, UK

Ian Brown
Chapter 12: Epilepsy and the impact on study, learning, and memory; Chapter 13: Epilepsy, employment, and work
Oxford Epilepsy Research Group, Nuffield Department of Clinical Neurosciences, University of Oxford/John Radcliffe Hospital, Oxford UK

Robert M. Brownstone
Chapter 4: The impact of surgery on comorbidities in epilepsy
National Hospital for Neurology and Neurosurgery, London, UK

Chris Butler
Chapter 5: Epilepsy and cognition
Department of Brain Sciences, Imperial College London, London, UK; Department of Neurology, Pontificia Universidad Católica de Chile, Santiago, Chile

John Craig
Chapter 11: Teratogenic risk and aspects of epilepsy relating to women's health
Belfast Health and Social Care Trust, Trust Headquarters, Belfast City Hospital, Belfast, UK

Patricia Dugan
Chapter 8: Epilepsy and Systemic Disease
NYU Grossman School of Medicine, New York, USA

Jane Hanna
Chapter 9: Epilepsy and mortality
SUDEP Action, Wantage, UK

Dale C. Hesdorffer
Chapter 6: Epilepsy and psychopathological comorbidities
Gertrude H. Sergievsky Center and Department of Epidemiology, Columbia
University, New York, USA

Neha Kinariwalla
Chapter 15: Epilepsy, marriage, and other social relationships
Columbia Vagelos College of Physicians & Surgeons in New York,
New York, USA

Michael Kinney
Chapter 11: Teratogenic risk and aspects of epilepsy relating to women's health
Belfast Health and Social Care Trust, Belfast City Hospital, Belfast, UK

Marco Mula
Chapter 6: Epilepsy and psychopathological comorbidities
Institute of Medical and Biomedical Education, St George's University
of London; Atkinson Morley Regional Neuroscience Centre, St George's
University Hospitals NHS Foundation Trust, London, UK

Philip N. Patsalos
Chapter 3: The effects of antiseizure medications on comorbidities
Department of Clinical and Experimental Epilepsy, UCL Queen Square
Institute of Neurology, London, UK

Fergus J. Rugg-Gunn
Chapter 3: The effects of antiseizure medications on comorbidities
Department of Clinical and Experimental Epilepsy, National Hospital for
Neurology and Neurosurgery, Institute of Neurology, UCL, London, UK

Steven C. Schachter
Chapter 10: Epilepsy and comorbidity in later life
Harvard Medical School

Arjune Sen
Chapter 10: Epilepsy and comorbidity in later life;
Chapter 15: Epilepsy, marriage, and other social relationships
Oxford Epilepsy Research Group, Nuffield Department of Clinical
Neurosciences, University of Oxford, UK

Rohit Shankar
Chapter 7: Epilepsy and intellectual disabilities; Chapter 9: Epilepsy and mortality
Peninsula School of Medicine, University of Plymouth, Plymouth; University of Exeter Medical School, Exeter; Falmouth University, Falmouth; Adult LD Services, Cornwall Partnership Foundation Trust, UK

Simon Shorvon
Foreword
Department of Clinical and Experimental Epilepsy, UCL Queen Square Institute of Neurology, London, UK

Ernest Somerville
Chapter 14: Epilepsy and driving
Comprehensive Epilepsy Centre, Prince of Wales Hospital, Sydney, New South Wales, Sydney

Emma Torzillo
Chapter 10: Epilepsy and comorbidity in later life
Department of Clinical and Experimental Epilepsy, UCL Queen Square Institute of Neurology, London, UK

Michael R. Trimble
Chapter 6: Epilepsy and psychopathological comorbidities
Institute of Neurology, University College London, London, UK

Vejay N. Vakharia
Chapter 4: The impact of surgery on comorbidities in epilepsy
UCL Queen Square Institute of Neurology, London, UK

Michael Vasey
Chapter 1: Introduction
University College London, London, UK

Lance Watkins
Chapter 9: Epilepsy and mortality
Neath Port Talbot Community Learning Disability Teams, Morriston, Swansea, UK

Sameer M. Zuberi
Chapter 2: A practical classification of epilepsy with regard to comorbidity
Paediatric Neurosciences Research Group, Institute of Health & Wellbeing, Royal Hospital for Children, Glasgow; University of Glasgow, Glasgow, UK

Section 1

Background to epilepsy and comorbidity

Chapter 1

Introduction

Frank M. C. Besag and Michael Vasey

It could be argued that perhaps one of the greatest advances in the management of epilepsy, alongside the growth of genetics, antiseizure medication (ASM), and surgical options, has been the recognition of the importance of the coexisting cognitive, psychological and psychiatric, and psychosocial conditions. This book brings together leaders in the field to provide an overview of the current evidence and thinking in this area.

The statement 'epilepsy is more than just having seizures' is now widely accepted as being an integral and essential concept in effective epilepsy management. The revised classification of seizure types and epilepsy syndromes acknowledges this from the outset, by including aetiology and comorbidity within the classification.[1] Previous classifications have generated fierce debate. There is a history of classifications being adopted without total agreement or even broad consensus. Some of the terms used in previous classifications could be described as incomprehensible, inappropriate, or both. The new classification uses words that most people will understand and that provide a good description of what actually happens in each respective seizure type.

There has been a remarkable growth in the number of ASMs available to the clinician after a relatively stagnant period of almost no progress in this area.[2,3] The implications are that the clinician has a better opportunity of choosing a medication that matches the life situation of the affected individual including any coexisting conditions that are present with the epilepsy. The situation with regard to cognitive and behavioural comorbidities resulting from epilepsy surgery has been particularly complicated. In terms of the seizures, epilepsy surgery offers a high probability of epilepsy 'cure' in carefully selected cases, for example, anterior temporal lobectomy for hippocampal sclerosis or for another identifiable temporal lobe lesion.[4,5] However, with regard to both cognitive and psychiatric outcomes following epilepsy surgery, some people are worse, some are better, and for the remainder there is relatively little change.[6,7] There is now greater insight into the factors that might predetermine such improvement or deterioration but we have not yet reached the stage where the prognosis of the cognitive and psychiatric outcome of the surgery is predictable. An unexpected consequence of the neuromodulation intervention of vagus nerve stimulation has been the improvement in depression.[8,9] The cognitive and psychiatric outcomes of other forms of neuromodulation surgery remain uncertain.

The issue of cognitive impairment in people with epilepsy covers a wide range of specific situations.[10–12] Epidemiological studies have revealed that the rate of intellectual disability (full-scale IQ less than 70) is around 30% in children with epilepsy.[13,14] The rate in adults with epilepsy is also high. This immediately raises the question of cause and effect. Cognitive impairment is a risk factor for epilepsy[15] but the epilepsy itself can, in some situations, cause either transitory or permanent cognitive impairment.[11,12,16] The obvious example is prolonged status epilepticus causing brain damage with accompanying permanent intellectual impairment.[17,18]

Attention has been drawn to the importance of distinguishing between permanent cognitive impairment and 'state-dependent' cognitive impairment, as may be the result of ASM or the epilepsy itself. The most dramatic example of the latter is the impairment resulting from non-convulsive status epilepticus. This condition can arise *de novo* in the elderly and can sometimes also occur in children with no previous history of epilepsy.[19] Perhaps one of the most important, although rare, clinical situations to recognize is the cognitive impairment that can result from electrical status epilepticus of slow-wave sleep (continuous spike-wave during slow-wave sleep) in children.[20] If this is treated promptly with medication or surgery, permanent cognitive impairment may be avoided or at least minimized.[21,22] The Landau–Kleffner syndrome of acquired epileptic aphasia is the best-known example in this category. The classical work of Morrell showed that surgical intervention with multiple sub-pial transection could reverse the aphasia with dramatic positive clinical effects.[23] Medication can also be effective in this syndrome.[24] The emphasis is on early recognition and treatment, to avoid permanent impairment. Continuous spike-wave during slow-wave sleep can result in profound impairment in other cognitive functions, leaving language relatively intact.[25] Any child with epilepsy who loses cognitive skills for no apparent reason should, therefore, be investigated with overnight electroencephalography monitoring or at least a sleep electroencephalogram.

The range of cognitive impairments associated with epilepsy is very broad. Both attention deficit hyperactivity disorder and autism are common in people with epilepsy and both can be associated with impairments in social cognition.[26–28] Deficits in perception and particularly deficits in memory can also be associated with epilepsy.[29,30] In the past, it was not uncommon for people to complain of memory problems but to have results in the normal range on standard memory testing.[31,32] In recent years, the phenomena of 'transient epileptic amnesia' and 'accelerated long-term forgetting' have been better recognized, pointing to the range of memory problems that can arise in association with epilepsy[29] as well as illustrating how standard neuropsychological testing may not capture the cognitive difficulties experienced by people with epilepsy in their daily lives.

Intellectual disability in the general population is associated with a much higher rate of psychiatric disorder.[33,34] Because intellectual disability is common in people with epilepsy,[35] this implies that the combination of intellectual disability and epilepsy will be associated with a high rate of psychiatric disorder. This has been confirmed in a number of studies.[36-38] Diagnosis of both the epilepsy itself and the psychiatric disorder can be more difficult in a person with intellectual disability. However, the high rate of psychiatric disturbance in this population underlines the importance of ensuring that professionals responsible for the care of people with intellectual disability and epilepsy are able to recognize and manage psychiatric comorbidity.

Several psychiatric disorders have been described as having a 'bidirectional relationship' with epilepsy,[39-42] with the implication that people with these psychiatric disorders have a higher risk of epilepsy and that people with epilepsy have a higher risk of a psychiatric disorder. In many cases this may reflect an underlying cause, either genetic or acquired, for both the epilepsy and psychiatric disorder.[43-45] For the peri-ictal disorders, however, it appears that the transitory brain changes associated with the seizures themselves cause the disorder, perhaps on a background of an underlying predisposition. Postictal psychiatric disorder, including psychosis, depression, and elevated mood states, can all occur after a seizure or, more commonly, after a cluster of seizures.[46] Recognizing the time relationship to the seizures is essential to diagnosis and management; there may be a 'lucid interval' of a few days between the cluster of seizures and postictal psychiatric disorder. These disorders do not usually require long-term treatment whereas some interictal psychoses do require such treatment.[47,48] There has been much discussion about psychiatric states that do not meet the usual threshold for the respective disorder but nevertheless affect the life of the individual significantly and may require treatment.[49,50] Recognition of the spectrum of these disorders and management that is appropriate to the individual patient is the key to correct management.

The risk of suicide is greatly increased in association with epilepsy.[51,52] The suicide rate in people with epilepsy who have a comorbid psychiatric disorder is very high,[52,53] and may be as much as nine times greater than in people with epilepsy without comorbid psychiatric conditions.[54,55] This emphasizes the importance of good psychiatric care of people with epilepsy who also have psychiatric disorders. Identifying individuals who have a personal or family history of psychiatric disorder, especially those who do not also have strong protective factors, and ensuring that they have adequate follow-up arrangements is strongly recommended.

Parents witnessing their child having the first seizure often think that their child is dying. Fortunately, the prevalence of sudden unexpected death in epilepsy (SUDEP) is relatively infrequent in childhood[56] but it is important to emphasize avoidable causes of epilepsy-related death, such as drowning, by ensuring adequate supervision during swimming and avoiding baths, in all age groups.[57] SUDEP becomes much more frequent in young adulthood,[58,59] almost certainly reflecting the decreased supervision that accompanies increased independence. There are, however, steps that can be taken to decrease the risk of SUDEP, without compromising independence, such as achieving the best possible control of tonic–clonic seizures, particularly nocturnal, sleep-associated tonic–clonic seizures. There is a clear association between good epilepsy management and a lower risk of SUDEP.[60]

Some systemic diseases are also associated with an increased rate of both epilepsy and psychiatric disorder. One of the most important of these is tuberous sclerosis, in which the rate of both epilepsy and psychiatric disorder is high.[61] Other examples include neurofibromatosis and systemic lupus erythematosus.[62,63] Increased rates of epilepsy have also been reported in systemic vasculitides such as Wegener granulomatosis and Behçet's disease.[64,65] Reports also suggest an increased risk of epilepsy in other systemic diseases such as diabetes.[66,67] The brain-damaging effects of stroke can lead to motor, cognitive, and psychiatric disorders, as well as increasing the risk of epilepsy.[68]

Women who are pregnant or who are planning a pregnancy have an understandable reluctance to take any medication, on the basis that this might harm the fetus.[69] However, discontinuing ASMs during pregnancy can place both mother and fetus at risk. The risk to the mother of status epilepticus is, perhaps, more obvious than the increased risk of fetal malformation from frequent tonic–clonic seizures during pregnancy.[70,71] Although there does appear to be a small risk of major malformations with the newer ASMs,[72,73] this risk is often outweighed to a major degree by the risks to mother and fetus of discontinuing medication. The risks of major fetal malformation and cognitive impairment/autism in the offspring are, however, considerable with valproate, especially with higher doses.[74,75] There is a very strong case for recommending good specialist care in planning for and managing pregnancy in those with epilepsy.

Although epilepsy can start at any age, most seizures with onset before the middle years begin in childhood or adolescence.[76] However, there is a marked increase in the incidence of epilepsy in older people,[76] resulting in a U-shaped epilepsy-onset curve. With the increased numbers of people surviving into older years, the result is that the prevalence of epilepsy in this age group is now much greater than in other age groups.[76] Although seizures are often responsive to ASMs in older people, the pharmacokinetics are different; lower starting doses, slower escalation, and lower target doses are often appropriate. Accounting for interactions with other medications are very important because older people are typically being treated for more than one medical condition.[77,78]

The impact of the epilepsy on each individual can depend on a number of factors, not necessarily involving identifiable coexisting psychiatric disorders or cognitive impairment. The predicament of each individual will determine, to a large extent, the impact.[79] For example, the impact of having a disorder that can result in unexpected loss of control might be much greater in a barrister than it would be in a retired individual living within a caring family or a child placed in a residential special school with trained staff. Identifying the magnitude of the impact of the epilepsy can typically be best achieved by an experienced multidisciplinary team, including medical, nursing, and psychology staff.[80]

Stigma is still a major issue, not only in resource underprivileged countries but also in so-called developed nations.[81,82] Teachers, employers, friends, and workmates often lack knowledge about epilepsy and how to manage seizures. This can lead to fear of the epilepsy and rejection of the individual with the condition. Against this background it is perhaps not surprising, although very regrettable, that the unemployment rate in people with epilepsy is high[83] even though the individuals concerned may have more than adequate skills to provide a valuable service to employers and to the community. Similar factors of stigma, fear, and lack of confidence can affect other important aspects of the life of the individual with epilepsy. These factors may result in loss of friendships and a decreased prospect of marriage or long-term intimate relationships.[13,84] There is still much to be achieved with regard to education of the general population, so that epilepsy can be accepted without fear and stigma.

Limitations on driving act as a further obstacle to those who have uncontrolled epilepsy.[85,86] Safety considerations dictate that professionals in the epilepsy team must adopt a firm approach to implementing the legal requirements relating to epilepsy and driving. In many countries these regulations are now sensible and balanced. However, the situation is not always straightforward. The diagnosis of tonic–clonic seizures is usually not difficult. In contrast, focal seizures can remain undiagnosed and there are suggestions that absence seizures in adults are underdiagnosed.[87] However, these less obvious seizure types can, nevertheless, present with major risks if they occur in someone driving a vehicle. A meticulous approach to diagnosis and management is particularly important in individuals who are driving or intend to drive, to ensure that risk is kept to a minimum.

There has never been a good time to have epilepsy but the development of so many new ASMs with fewer cognitive and psychiatric adverse effects,[88–90] the availability of new minimally invasive surgical techniques,[91,92] the advances in investigation strategies,[93] the increased understanding from genetics,[94,95] and the acknowledgement that people with epilepsy will often require good management of both the seizures and the comorbidities are all indications that the situation is improving. The prospects for an individual with epilepsy still vary enormously between countries around the world and there is much to be achieved with regard to the global understanding and acceptance of the condition.

Although epilepsy remains a serious neurological condition, potentially associated with many limitations, these factors should be balanced by the knowledge that there are wonderful examples of people with epilepsy who have outstanding achievements. A good example is that of Dame Sheila Sherlock, who was an internationally eminent liver specialist and president of the Royal College of Physicians in the UK. She stated that, after her death, she wanted it to be known that she had epilepsy. Many epileptologists celebrated the fact that she wanted to make her epilepsy public but regretted the fact that she chose to leave the sharing of this diagnosis until after her death. Perhaps, in the future, greater acceptance of the condition will remove any reticence about sharing the diagnosis and will allow people with epilepsy to have all the opportunities that are available to those who happen not to have seizures, without fear or stigma.

References

1. Scheffer IE, Berkovic S, Capovilla G, et al. ILAE classification of the epilepsies: position paper of the ILAE Commission for Classification and Terminology. Epilepsia. 2017;**58**(4):512–21.
2. Perucca E, Brodie MJ, Kwan P, Tomson T. 30 years of second-generation antiseizure medications: impact and future perspectives. Lancet Neurol. 2020;**19**(6):544–56.
3. Rho JM, White HS. Brief history of anti-seizure drug development. Epilepsia Open. 2018;**3**(Suppl 2):114–19.
4. Jobst BC, Cascino GD. Resective epilepsy surgery for drug-resistant focal epilepsy: a review. JAMA. 2015;**313**(3):285–93.
5. Téllez-Zenteno JF, Dhar R, Wiebe S. Long-term seizure outcomes following epilepsy surgery: a systematic review and meta-analysis. Brain. 2005;**128**(5):1188–98.
6. Spencer S, Huh L. Outcomes of epilepsy surgery in adults and children. Lancet Neurol. 2008;**7**(6):525–37.
7. Sherman EMS, Wiebe S, Fay-McClymont TB, et al. Neuropsychological outcomes after epilepsy surgery: systematic review and pooled estimates. Epilepsia.2011;**52**(5):857–69.

8. **Elger G, Hoppe C, Falkai P, Rush AJ, Elger CE.** Vagus nerve stimulation is associated with mood improvements in epilepsy patients. Epilepsy Res. 2000;**42**(2):203–10.

9. **Milby AH, Halpern CH, Baltuch GH.** Vagus nerve stimulation for epilepsy and depression. Neurotherapeutics. 2008;**5**(1):75–85.

10. **Motamedi G, Meador K.** Epilepsy and cognition. Epilepsy Behav. 2003;**4**:25–38.

11. **Berg AT.** Epilepsy, cognition, and behavior: the clinical picture. Epilepsia. 2011;**52**(Suppl 1):7–12.

12. **Meador KJ.** Cognitive outcomes and predictive factors in epilepsy. Neurology. 2002;**58**(8 Suppl 5):S21–26.

13. **Camfield PR, Camfield CS.** What happens to children with epilepsy when they become adults? Some facts and opinions. Pediatr Neurol. 2014;**51**(1):17–23.

14. **Sillanpää M.** Epilepsy in children: prevalence, disability, and handicap. Epilepsia. 1992;**33**(3):444–49.

15. **Robertson J, Hatton C, Emerson E, Baines S.** Prevalence of epilepsy among people with intellectual disabilities: a systematic review. Seizure. 2015;**29**:46–62.

16. **Aarts J, Binnie C, Smit A, Wilkins A.** Selective cognitive impairment during focal and generalized epileptiform EEG activity. Brain. 1984;**107**(1):293–308.

17. **Helmstaedter C.** Cognitive outcome of status epilepticus in adults. Epilepsia. 2007;**48**(Suppl 8):85–90.

18. **Sculier C, Gaínza-Lein M, Sánchez Fernández I, Loddenkemper T.** Long-term outcomes of status epilepticus: a critical assessment. Epilepsia. 2018;**59**(Suppl 2):155–69.

19. **Maganti R, Gerber P, Drees C, Chung S.** Nonconvulsive status epilepticus. Epilepsy Behav. 2008;**12**(4):572–86.

20. **Patry G, Lyagoubi S, Tassinari CA.** Subclinical electrical status epilepticus induced by sleep in children: a clinical and electroencephalographic study of six cases. Arch Neurol. 1971;**24**(3):242–52.

21. **Smith MC, Hoeppner TJ.** Epileptic encephalopathy of late childhood: Landau–Kleffner syndrome and the syndrome of continuous spikes and waves during slow-wave sleep. J Clin Neurophysiol. 2003;**20**(6):462–72.

22. **Loddenkemper T, Fernández IS, Peters JM.** Continuous spike and waves during sleep and electrical status epilepticus in sleep. J Clin Neurophysiol. 2011;**28**(2):154–64.

23. **Morrell F, Whisler WW, Smith MC,** et al. Landau–Kleffner syndrome: treatment with subpial intracortical transection. Brain. 1995;**118**(6):1529–46.

24. **Baumer FM, McNamara NA, Fine AL,** et al. Treatment practices and outcomes in continuous spike and wave during slow wave sleep: a multicenter collaboration. J Pediatr. 2021;**232**:220–28.e3.

25. **Tuchman R.** CSWS-related autistic regression versus autistic regression without CSWS. Epilepsia. 2009;**50**(Suppl 7):18–20.

26. **Reilly CJ.** Attention deficit hyperactivity disorder (ADHD) in childhood epilepsy. Res Dev Disabil. 2011;**32**(3):883–93.

27. **Reilly C, Atkinson P, Das KB,** et al. Neurobehavioral comorbidities in children with active epilepsy: a population-based study. Pediatrics. 2014;**133**(6):e1586–93.

28. **Lukmanji S, Manji SA, Kadhim S,** et al. The co-occurrence of epilepsy and autism: a systematic review. Epilepsy Behav. 2019;**98**:238–48.

29. **Butler CR, Zeman AZ.** Recent insights into the impairment of memory in epilepsy: transient epileptic amnesia, accelerated long-term forgetting and remote memory impairment. Brain. 2008;**131**(9):2243–63.

30. **Helmstaedter C, Kurthen M.** Memory and epilepsy: characteristics, course, and influence of drugs and surgery. Curr Opin Neurol. 2001;**14**(2):211–16.

31. **Hall KE, Isaac CL, Harris P.** Memory complaints in epilepsy: an accurate reflection of memory impairment or an indicator of poor adjustment? A review of the literature. Clin Psychol Rev. 2009;**29**(4):354–67.

32. **Vermeulen J, Aldenkamp AP, Alpherts WCJ.** Memory complaints in epilepsy: correlations with cognitive performance and neuroticism. Epilepsy Res. 1993;**15**(2):157–70.

33. **Buckles J, Luckasson R, Keefe E.** A systematic review of the prevalence of psychiatric disorders in adults with intellectual disability, 2003–2010. J Ment Health Res Intellect Disabil. 2013;**6**(3):181–207.

34. **Emerson E.** Prevalence of psychiatric disorders in children and adolescents with and without intellectual disability. J Intellect Disabil Res. 2003;**47**(1):51–58.

35. **Lhatoo SD, Sander JWAS.** The epidemiology of epilepsy and learning disability. Epilepsia. 2001;**42**(Suppl 1):6–9.

36. **Espie CA, Watkins J, Curtice L, et al.** Psychopathology in people with epilepsy and intellectual disability; an investigation of potential explanatory variables. J Neurol Neurosurg Psychiatry. 2003;**74**(11):1485–92.

37. **van Ool JS, Snoeijen-Schouwenaars FM, Schelhaas HJ, Tan IY, Aldenkamp AP, Hendriksen JGM.** A systematic review of neuropsychiatric comorbidities in patients with both epilepsy and intellectual disability. Epilepsy Behav. 2016;**60**:130–37.

38. **Turky A, Felce D, Jones G, Kerr M.** A prospective case control study of psychiatric disorders in adults with epilepsy and intellectual disability. Epilepsia. 2011;**52**(7):1223–30.

39. **Hesdorffer DC, Ishihara L, Mynepalli L, Webb DJ, Weil J, Hauser WA.** Epilepsy, suicidality, and psychiatric disorders: a bidirectional association. Ann Neurol. 2012;**72**(2):184–91.

40. **Adelöw C, Andersson T, Ahlbom A, Tomson T.** Hospitalization for psychiatric disorders before and after onset of unprovoked seizures/epilepsy. Neurology. 2012;**78**(6):396–401.

41. **Wotton CJ, Goldacre MJ.** Coexistence of schizophrenia and epilepsy: record-linkage studies. Epilepsia. 2012;**53**(4):e71–74.

42. **Bredkjær S, Ensen PBBM, Parnas J.** Epilepsy and non-organic non-affective psychosis: national epidemiologic study. Br J Psychiatry. 1998;**172**(3):235–38.

43. **Campbell C, Cavalleri GL, Delanty N.** Exploring the genetic overlap between psychiatric illness and epilepsy: a review. Epilepsy Behav. 2020;**102**:106669.

44. **Hermann BP, Seidenberg M, Bell B.** Psychiatric comorbidity in chronic epilepsy: identification, consequences, and treatment of major depression. Epilepsia. 2000;**41**(Suppl 2):S31–41.

45. **Swinkels WAM, Kuyk J, van Dyck R, Spinhoven P.** Psychiatric comorbidity in epilepsy. Epilepsy Behav. 2005;**7**(1):37–50.

46. **Trimble M, Kanner A, Schmitz B.** Postictal psychosis. Epilepsy Behav. 2010;**19**(2):159–61.

47. **Kanner AM.** Psychosis of epilepsy: a neurologist's perspective. Epilepsy Behav. 2000;**1**(4):219–27.

48. **Agrawal N, Mula M.** Treatment of psychoses in patients with epilepsy: an update. Ther Adv Psychopharmacol. 2019;**9**:2045125319862968.

49. **Mula M.** The interictal dysphoric disorder of epilepsy: a still open debate. Curr Neurol Neurosci Rep. 2013;**13**(6):355.

50. **Kanner AM.** Depression and epilepsy: a new perspective on two closely related disorders. Epilepsy Curr. 2006;**6**(5):141–46.

51. **Bell GS, Gaitatzis A, Bell CL, Johnson AL, Sander JW.** Suicide in people with epilepsy: how great is the risk? Epilepsia. 2009;**50**(8):1933–42.

52. **Christensen J, Vestergaard M, Mortensen PB, Sidenius P, Agerbo E.** Epilepsy and risk of suicide: a population-based case–control study. Lancet Neurol. 2007;**6**(8):693–98.

53. **Jones JE, Hermann BP, Barry JJ, Gilliam FG, Kanner AM, Meador KJ.** Rates and risk factors for suicide, suicidal ideation, and suicide attempts in chronic epilepsy. Epilepsy Behav. 2003;**4**:31–38.

54. **Nilsson L, Ahlbom A, Farahmand BY, Åsberg M, Tomson T.** Risk factors for suicide in epilepsy: a case control study. Epilepsia. 2002;**43**(6):644–51.

55. **Verrotti A, Cicconetti A, Scorrano B, et al.** Epilepsy and suicide: pathogenesis, risk factors, and prevention. Neuropsychiatr Dis Treat. 2008;**4**(2):365–70.

56. **Abdel-Mannan O, Taylor H, Donner EJ, Sutcliffe AG.** A systematic review of sudden unexpected death in epilepsy (SUDEP) in childhood. Epilepsy Behav. 2019;**90**:99–106.

57. **Mahler B, Carlsson S, Andersson T, Tomson T.** Risk for injuries and accidents in epilepsy. A prospective population-based cohort study. Neurology. 2018;**90**(9):e779–89.

58. **Shankar R, Jalihal V, Walker M, et al.** A community study in Cornwall UK of sudden unexpected death in epilepsy (SUDEP) in a 9-year population sample. Seizure. 2014;**23**(5):382–85.

59. **Tomson T, Nashef L, Ryvlin P.** Sudden unexpected death in epilepsy: current knowledge and future directions. Lancet Neurol. 2008;**7**(11):1021–31.

60. **Shorvon S, Tomson T.** Sudden unexpected death in epilepsy. Lancet. 2011;**378**(9808):2028–38.

61. **Crino PB, Nathanson KL, Henske EP.** The tuberous sclerosis complex. N Engl J Med. 2006;**355**(13):1345–56.

62. **Stafstrom CE, Staedtke V, Comi AM.** Epilepsy mechanisms in neurocutaneous disorders: tuberous sclerosis complex, neurofibromatosis type 1, and Sturge–Weber syndrome. Front Neurol. 2017;**8**:87.

63. **Devinsky O, Schein A, Najjar S.** Epilepsy associated with systemic autoimmune disorders: epilepsy and systemic autoimmune disorders. Epilepsy Curr. 2013;**13**(2):62–68.

64. **Moore BM, Rothman SM, Clark HB, Vehe RK, Laguna TA.** Epilepsy: an anticipatory presentation of pediatric Wegener's granulomatosis. Pediatr Neurol. 2010;**43**(1):49–52.

65. **Kutlu G, Semercioglu S, Ucler S, Erdal A, Inan LE.** Epileptic seizures in neuro-Behcet disease: why some patients develop seizure and others not? Seizure. 2015;**26**:32–35.

66. **Keezer MR, Novy J, Sander JW.** Type 1 diabetes mellitus in people with pharmacoresistant epilepsy: prevalence and clinical characteristics. Epilepsy Res. 2015;**115**:55–57.

67. **Chou IC, Wang C-H, Lin W-D, Tsai F-J, Lin C-C, Kao C-H.** Risk of epilepsy in type 1 diabetes mellitus: a population-based cohort study. Diabetologia. 2016;**59**(6):1196–203.

68. **Myint PK, Staufenberg EFA, Sabanathan K.** Post-stroke seizure and post-stroke epilepsy. Postgrad Med J. 2006;**82**(971):568–72.

69. **Tomson T, Battino D.** Teratogenic effects of antiepileptic drugs. Lancet Neurol. 2012;**11**(9):803–13.

70. **Rajiv KR, Radhakrishnan A.** Status epilepticus in pregnancy: etiology, management, and clinical outcomes. Epilepsy Behav. 2017;**76**:114–19.

71. **Adab N, Kini U, Vinten J, et al.** The longer term outcome of children born to mothers with epilepsy. J Neurol Neurosurg Psychiatry. 2004;**75**(11):1575–83.

72. **Vajda FJE, O'Brien TJ, Lander CM, Graham J, Eadie MJ.** The teratogenicity of the newer antiepileptic drugs—an update. Acta Neurol Scand. 2014;**130**(4):234–38.

73. **Meador K.** Teratogenicity and antiseizure medications. Epilepsy Curr. 2020;**20**(6 Suppl):15S–17S.

74. **Bromley R, Weston J, Adab N, et al.** Treatment for epilepsy in pregnancy: neurodevelopmental outcomes in the child. Cochrane Database Syst Rev. 2014;**2014**(10):CD010236.

75. **Meador KJ, Baker GA, Browning N, et al.** Cognitive function at 3 years of age after fetal exposure to antiepileptic drugs. N Engl J Med. 2009;**360**(16):1597–605.

76. **Beghi E.** The epidemiology of epilepsy. Neuroepidemiology. 2020;**54**(2):185–91.

77. **Ramsay RE, Rowan AJ, Pryor FM.** Special considerations in treating the elderly patient with epilepsy. Neurology. 2004;**62**(5 Suppl 2):S24–29.

78. **Cloyd J, Hauser W, Towne A, et al.** Epidemiological and medical aspects of epilepsy in the elderly. Epilepsy Res. 2006;**68**:39–48.

79. **Taylor D.** The components of sickness: diseases, illnesses, and predicaments. Lancet. 1979;**314**(8150):1008–10.

80. **Kerr MP.** The impact of epilepsy on patients' lives. Acta Neurol Scand. 2012;**126**(Suppl 194):1–9.

81. **Jacoby A, Austin JK.** Social stigma for adults and children with epilepsy. Epilepsia. 2007;**48**(Suppl 9):6–9.

82. **de Boer HM, Mula M, Sander JW.** The global burden and stigma of epilepsy. Epilepsy Behav. 2008;**12**(4):540–46.

83. **Smeets VMJ, van Lierop BAG, Vanhoutvin JPG, Aldenkamp AP, Nijhuis FJN.** Epilepsy and employment: literature review. Epilepsy Behav. 2007;**10**(3):354–62.

84. **Camfield CS, Camfield PR.** Long-term social outcomes for children with epilepsy. Epilepsia. 2007;**48**(Suppl 9):3–5.

85. **Krumholz A.** Driving issues in epilepsy: past, present, and future. Epilepsy Curr. 2009;**9**(2):31–35.

86. **Drazkowski J.** An overview of epilepsy and driving. Epilepsia. 2007;**48**(Suppl 9):10–12.

87. **Trinka E.** Absences in adult seizure disorders. Acta Neurol Scand Suppl. 2005;**112**(182):12–18.

88. **Loring DW, Marino S, Meador KJ.** Neuropsychological and behavioral effects of antiepilepsy drugs. Neuropsychol Rev. 2007;**17**(4):413–25.

89. **Cavanna AE, Ali F, Rickards HE, McCorry D.** Behavioral and cognitive effects of antiepileptic drugs. Discov Med. 2010;**9**(45):138–44.

90. **Moavero R, Santarone ME, Galasso C, Curatolo P.** Cognitive and behavioral effects of new antiepileptic drugs in pediatric epilepsy. Brain Dev. 2017;**39**(6):464–69.

91. **Nowell M, Miserocchi A, McEvoy AW, Duncan JS.** Advances in epilepsy surgery. J Neurol Neurosurg Psychiatry. 2014;**85**(11):1273–79.

92. **Galan FN, Beier AD, Sheth RD.** Advances in epilepsy surgery. Pediatr Neurol. 2021;**122**:89–97.

93. **Moshé SL, Perucca E, Ryvlin P, Tomson T.** Epilepsy: new advances. Lancet. 2015;**385**(9971):884–98.

94. **Orsini A, Zara F, Striano P.** Recent advances in epilepsy genetics. Neurosci Lett. 2018;**667**:4–9.

95. **Ellis CA, Petrovski S, Berkovic SF.** Epilepsy genetics: clinical impacts and biological insights. Lancet Neurol. 2020;**19**(1):93–100.

Chapter 2

A practical classification of epilepsy with regard to comorbidity

Sameer M. Zuberi

Introduction

As epilepsy management has evolved, consequent upon a better understanding of pathophysiology and developments in investigations and therapeutics, so has the classification of epilepsy. The International League Against Epilepsy (ILAE) leads the process of revising the classification of epilepsy through the publication of official ILAE policy documents known as position papers developed by expert groups (Task Forces) following engagement with the wider epilepsy community.[1] The utility of an epilepsy classification should be assessed by its practicality in the clinical management of epilepsy.

Recent drivers for the revision of ILAE position papers on the definition of epilepsy and on classification of the epilepsies have included the need to incorporate the comorbidities of epilepsy and to acknowledge the impact a diagnosis of epilepsy has on a person's relationship with society.[2,3] In any rapidly changing scientific field such as neuroscience there is controversy around new concepts and structures of classifications with active debate at scientific meetings and in the literature.[4] It can take many years before new terminology and concepts find their way into clinical practice and decades before outdated terms such as 'grand mal' or 'petit mal' are finally discarded.

There are epilepsy classifications whose primary purpose differs from those developed by the ILAE. These include versions of the International Classification of Disease and Systematized Nomenclautre of Medicine (SNOMED) Clinical Terms, which guide clinical service management, development of services, public health policy, and billing.[5] Ontologies have been developed for epilepsy surgery programmes which link semiology to anatomy and networks within the nervous system.[6] Revisions of the International Classification of Disease and SNOMED Clinical Terms are now being developed in partnership with the ILAE so there is likely to be closer alignment of these classifications.

The definition of a seizure, epilepsy, and acute symptomatic seizures

An epileptic seizure is a transient occurrence of signs and/or symptoms due to abnormal excessive or synchronous neuronal activity in the brain.[6,7] A seizure or cluster of seizures may occur as a consequence of an acute illness such as infection or trauma or it may be the first sign of the condition, epilepsy, in which there is an enduring predisposition to seizures.

Acute symptomatic seizures are events, occurring in close temporal relationship to an acute central nervous system insult, which may be metabolic, toxic, structural, infectious, or due to inflammation.[8] This implies there is a temporary or reversible factor lowering the threshold for a seizure. The time between the insult and the seizure(s) may vary depending on the underlying cause. Other terms to describe acute symptomatic seizures include provoked and reactive seizures. Seizures within particular clinical contexts, such as in neonates or in the intensive care setting, are more frequently acute symptomatic or provoked. The 2021 ILAE classification of seizures in the neonate prefers the term provoked rather than acute symptomatic.[9]

In 2005, epilepsy was defined as a disorder of the brain characterized by an enduring predisposition to generate epileptic seizures, and by the neurobiological, cognitive, psychological, and social consequences of this condition.[7] This definition acknowledged the comorbidities and social complications of epilepsy. Previously, the diagnosis of an epileptic disorder was made after two unprovoked epileptic seizures. In 2014, there were several important conceptual changes to the definition of epilepsy.[10] The two most important for people with epilepsy were guidance on when an epilepsy diagnosis could be made after a single seizure (see below) and when epilepsy could be said to be resolved (no longer present).

The current ILAE operational (practical) definition of epilepsy is:

1. At least two unprovoked (or reflex) seizures occurring more than 24 hours apart

2. One unprovoked (or reflex) seizure and a probability of further seizures similar to the general recurrence risk (at least 60%) after two unprovoked seizures, occurring over the next 10 years

3. Diagnosis of an epilepsy syndrome.

The general probability of a further seizure after two unprovoked seizures is around 60%. Whether the recurrence risk after one unprovoked seizure reaches the at least 60% or essentially the 'more likely than not' threshold requires an understanding of the likelihood of further seizures when the underlying cause is known. For example, if, following a single seizure, a structural aetiology such as focal cortical dysplasia is identified on magnetic resonance imaging and there are interictal electroencephalographic (EEG) features supportive of the lesion being involved in the epileptogenic network zone, it would be appropriate to diagnose epilepsy. Similarly, if an infant of 6 months presents with a prolonged focal seizure, has a normal magnetic resonance imaging scan, and has a pathogenic variant identified in the *SCN1A* gene, they are almost certainly going to have further epileptic seizures, thereby enabling a diagnosis of epilepsy after a single seizure.

Epilepsy is considered to be resolved for individuals who had an age-dependent epilepsy syndrome but are now past the applicable age or those who have remained seizure-free for the last 10 years, with no antiseizure medicines for the last 5 years.

The diagnosis of epilepsy should be distinguished from the decision whether to treat or not. The new definition supports clinicians in treating people after a single seizure. For the person with epilepsy, or their family, this gives them more choice. If they have been counselled that they have a 60% or greater risk of having another seizure, they may choose early treatment to prevent further seizures. If legislation in their country does not allow driving for a time period after a single seizure, then commencing medication may allow that person to return to driving earlier than if they waited to commence medication until after subsequent events.

An earlier diagnosis of epilepsy supports discussion about risks including seizure-related injury and sudden unexpected death in epilepsy (SUDEP) and ways in which these risks can be reduced. The discussion about SUDEP is one which many clinicians find challenging both in relation to when to first raise the issue and what to say (see Chapter 7). There is evidence from research on the attitudes of people with epilepsy and their families that they prefer SUDEP to be discussed and that they want this discussion early in their management.

An earlier syndromic diagnosis allows specific discussion about the prognosis and comorbidities associated with that syndrome. For example, a teenager with a single generalized tonic seizure and a history elicited at consultation of early morning myoclonus with appropriate EEG findings could have a diagnosis of juvenile myoclonic epilepsy and be counselled on risks related to sleep deprivation, alcohol intake, and the efficacy of medication. If the young person is leaving the parental home, for example, moving into college accommodation, soon after a first generalized tonic–clonic seizure, an early diagnosis might influence the decision on whether to treat or not.

Allowing a diagnosis after a single seizure should encourage early referral to specialist services. The misguided 'everyone is allowed a single seizure' statement frequently heard in Emergency Departments risks people with epilepsy not seeing someone with expertise. The 2014 definition refers to epilepsy as a disease rather than a disorder. This change was made because disease implies a more long-lasting derangement of normal function. The term disorder was not well understood by the public and might minimize the severity of epilepsy.

An early diagnosis of epilepsy may have negative consequences. It may impact employment opportunities, ability to hold a driving licence, access to health insurance, and cultural attitudes to the diagnosis may limit opportunities for marriage (see Chapter 15).

Just as important as making a diagnosis is the ability to say a diagnosis is no longer relevant for an individual. Using previous definitions, it could have been interpreted that epilepsy is a disorder that does not resolve, implying that the enduring predisposition is lifelong. This is incorrect for many well-defined epilepsies of childhood. Self-limited (previously termed benign) neonatal and infantile epilepsies may affect multiple generations but seizures may only occur for days, weeks, or months with only a minority having seizures later in life.[11] Legislation and employment opportunities vary for people with epilepsy around the world and it is important that people with self-limited epilepsy syndromes of childhood can make health declarations stating that they do not have epilepsy because the condition has resolved. For example, children with self-limited epilepsy with centrotemporal spikes (previously known as benign rolandic epilepsy) are not likely to have epilepsy after puberty.

Following successful epilepsy surgery and withdrawal of medication with seizure freedom for 10 years, epilepsy can also be said to have resolved. The term cure might be thought appropriate in the context of surgical intervention in contrast to most other epilepsies where it is the developmental predisposition to epilepsy which is no longer present. Cure is not used in this context as epilepsy may occur later in life due to other causes, many linked to degenerative or vascular diseases of the brain. There is a background general population risk of epilepsy which increases with age and over the age of 70 reaches incidence levels similar to those seen in early childhood (see Chapter 10).[12]

The classification of seizure types

On a superficial basis it may seem that how seizure types are classified has limited relevance to the comorbidities and social consequences of epilepsy; however, one of the main reasons for revising the structure of the classification and nomenclature of seizure types was to make the clinical terminology more easily understandable for people with epilepsy, their families, and wider society. Epilepsy has been in the shadows because of stigma related to loss of personal control and links to mental illness and demonic possession.[13] The ability to better communicate the nature of a seizure and describe what is happening to colleagues and people with epilepsy is critical if the medical and wider community are to better understand epilepsy and accept, as Hippocrates is reported to have said, that: 'The sacred disease is no more sacred than any other disease.' Medical knowledge is now much more easily accessible to people without medical training and medical classifications have developed to meet this need as well as for clinical practice.

The structure of the seizure type classification is shown in Figure 2.1. Focal seizures continue to be divided into those in which there is either retained or

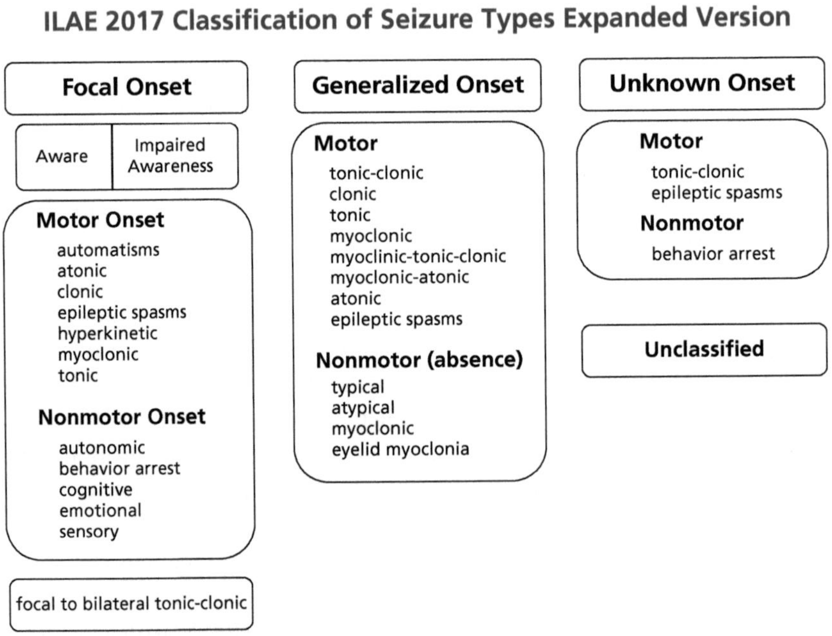

ILAE 2017 Classification of Seizure Types Expanded Version

Figure 2.1 The 2017 ILAE classification of seizure types.
Reproduced with permission from Fisher RS, Cross JH, French JA, et al. Operational classification of seizure types by the International League Against Epilepsy: Position Paper of the ILAE Commission for Classification and Terminology. Epilepsia. 58(4):522–530, 2017.

impaired awareness. Awareness is defined as knowledge of self and environment and is also a surrogate term for consciousness and responsiveness.[14] This important distinction remains, with retained awareness and impaired awareness replacing 'simple partial' and 'complex partial' whose meaning was obscure to people without medical training. For the person with epilepsy, whether a seizure impairs awareness or responsiveness is critical to everyday functioning and interaction with their environment, for example, the ability to work machinery, to drive a car, or understand what is being said in a school lesson.

The 2017 ILAE Classification of the Epilepsies

The framework for the ILAE Classification of the Epilepsies is designed with patient management in mind.[2] Although recognized in previous classifications, incorporating comorbidities and aetiology into the framework emphasizes their importance and directs the clinician to consider both in any individual with epilepsy (Figure 2.2). Considering aetiology at all levels of classification, seizure type, epilepsy type, and syndrome should direct the clinician to relevant investigations and prevent unnecessary investigations. A precise aetiology may

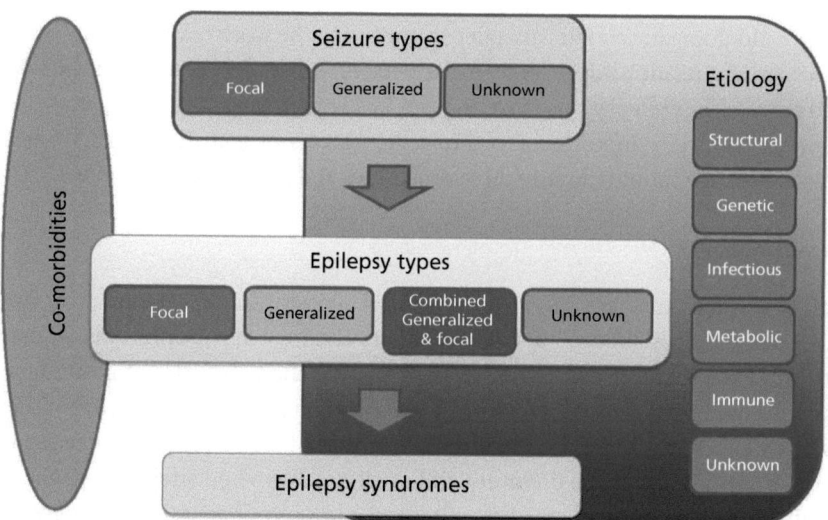

Figure 2.2 The 2017 ILAE framework for the Classification of Seizures and the Epilepsies.
Reproduced with permission from Scheffer IE, Berkovic S, Capovilla G, et al. ILAE classification of the epilepsies: Position paper of the ILAE Commission for Classification and Terminology. Epilepsia. 2017 Apr;58(4):512–521. doi: 10.1111/epi.13709.

suggest a targeted therapy and allow more accurate prognostication. Attention to specific aetiologies should encourage the development of new targeted or precision therapies.[15] The hope is that these therapies will be more effective and have fewer side effects, therefore improving quality of life for the person with epilepsy. A therapy targeting the underlying genetic defect may also ameliorate the other non-seizure-related comorbidities produced by the genetic defect. For example, in the genetic developmental and epileptic encephalopathy Dravet syndrome, an *SCN1A* gene-associated therapy may reduce seizure frequency and prevent or ameliorate the cognitive, behavioural, and motor impairment associated with the syndrome. There are promising data from therapy trials in animal models of Dravet syndrome with human trials of gene-associated technologies having now started.[16]

Epilepsy is a disease of the brain and seizures are frequently associated with other symptoms of neurological disease including learning disability, behaviour problems, neuropsychiatric disease, and motor disorders (see Chapters 6 and 7). This is particularly true in drug-resistant and complex epilepsies.[17] The responsibility of the epileptologist must extend to the health of their patient in the broadest sense. Placing consideration of comorbidities across all levels of the electroclinical classification of seizures and the epilepsies should prompt the clinician to enquire about these aspects. Some of the relevant questions are 'How is the child doing in school?', 'Is epilepsy impacting the work environment?', and 'How are the relationships between the person with epilepsy and their family and peers?' The epilepsy specialist may not be the person best placed to manage neuropsychiatric symptoms or orthopaedic aspects of gait disorders, for example, but they should identify these difficulties and make relevant referrals.

Syndromes

Epilepsy syndromes are the highest level of electroclinical classification. In 2017, the ILAE established a Task Force on Nosology and Definitions whose principal aim was, for the first time, to define the characteristics of individual epilepsy syndromes within a series of ILAE position papers. The concept of the epilepsy syndrome has been established for more than 50 years with descriptions of syndromes in the literature and most notably when after a meeting in Centre St Paul in Marseille the first of several editions of *Epileptic Syndromes in Infancy, Childhood and Adolescence* was published.[18] Syndromes had been listed in ILAE papers since the 1980s but individual syndrome characteristics were not defined.[19] The chapter author is a member of the ILAE Task Force which reported in 2022 their work addressing the cognitive, psychological, and psychosocial aspects of epilepsy syndromes.[20–24]

The Task Force defines an epilepsy syndrome as 'a characteristic cluster of clinical and EEG features, often supported by specific etiological findings (structural, genetic, metabolic, immune and infectious)'. A syndrome diagnosis in an individual with epilepsy carries prognostic and treatment implications. Syndromes often have age-dependent presentations and a range of specific comorbidities.[20] The relationship between the major syndrome groupings of infancy is illustrated in Figure 2.3.

The main goal of the Task Force was to identify criteria to assist with clinical diagnosis. Some proposed developments that seek to encourage early and widespread diagnosis are the development of criteria for epilepsy syndromes in evolution and the recognition that in low-resource regions it may be necessary to define a syndrome without confirmation from investigations, which includes without EEG. These new classifications should make a syndromic diagnosis available to more people with epilepsy and contribute to reducing the treatment gap between high- and low-income regions. The epilepsies are a group of disparate and individually rare diseases with individual experiences differing significantly. Defining epilepsy as a syndrome allows people with epilepsy and their families to communicate with others with shared experiences and build support networks to provide psychological support.

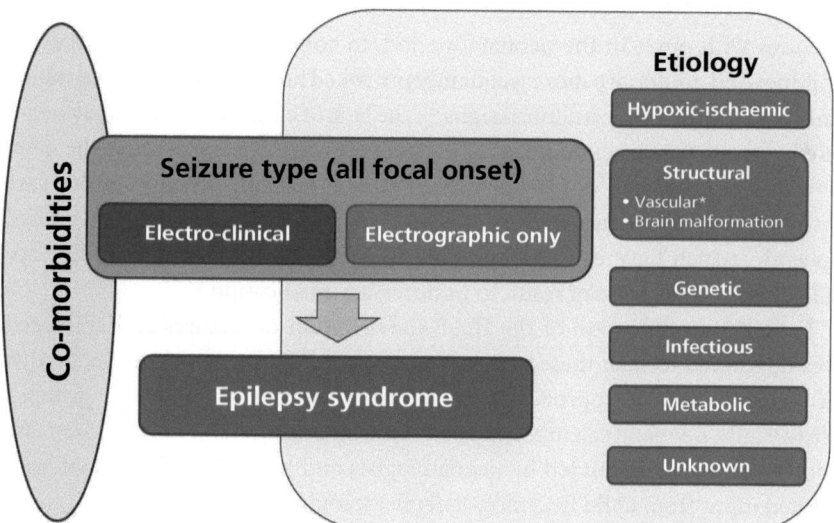

Figure 2.3 The epilepsy syndromes of infancy.
Reproduced with permission from Scheffer IE, Berkovic S, Capovilla G, et al. ILAE classification of the epilepsies: Position paper of the ILAE Commission for Classification and Terminology. Epilepsia. 2017 Apr;58(4):512–521. doi: 10.1111/epi.13709.

Terminology

The adjectives used to describe epilepsy such as 'benign', 'malignant', and 'catastrophic' will inevitably affect the way a person with epilepsy, their family, and wider society perceive the condition. The term benign implies a condition which is mild, not serious, and will not have long-term consequences. Many of the epilepsies described as such, including benign Rolandic epilepsy, are associated in a significant minority with specific learning difficulties and in some people with electrical status epilepticus in slow-wave sleep.[25] Benign as a descriptor in epilepsy has been replaced by self-limited which implies nothing about cognitive or behavioural comorbidities but means that the epilepsy has a typical time course, following which it will resolve. Emotive terms such as catastrophic and malignant are no longer recommended.[26] These had been used to describe severe developmental and epileptic encephalopathies presenting in early childhood. Informing a family that their child has a catastrophic or malignant epilepsy conveys the message that this is a serious diagnosis which may significantly impact life expectancy. While being realistic when discussing prognosis, it is also important not to remove all hope as outcomes vary and new therapies may become available.

Classification of seizures in the neonate

Seizures with onset in the neonatal period, in contrast to those seen in older children and adults, are more frequently provoked and are often electrographic only with minimal or no clinical signs.[27] The lack of clinical correlate may be related to the developmental status of the networks involved or because the newborn infant is sedated or has been given muscle relaxants in an intensive care setting. There are many paroxysmal events in neonates, previously considered epileptic, which have no electrographic correlate. These events, including so-called subtle seizures, can result in unnecessary medication.[28]

The 2021 modification of the ILAE classification of seizures and epilepsies was developed to take these issues into account but also to acknowledge that neonates should be approached in the same manner as other age groups.[9] Historically, neonatal seizures have been classified separately from children and adults and management led by neonatologists and general paediatricians with limited input from child neurologists/epileptologists.

The framework for classification of seizures and epilepsies in neonates (Figure 2.4) includes aetiology, syndrome, and comorbidities with the benefits of considering these factors the same as in other age groups. The neonatal classification emphasizes the key role of EEG with seizures being classified as

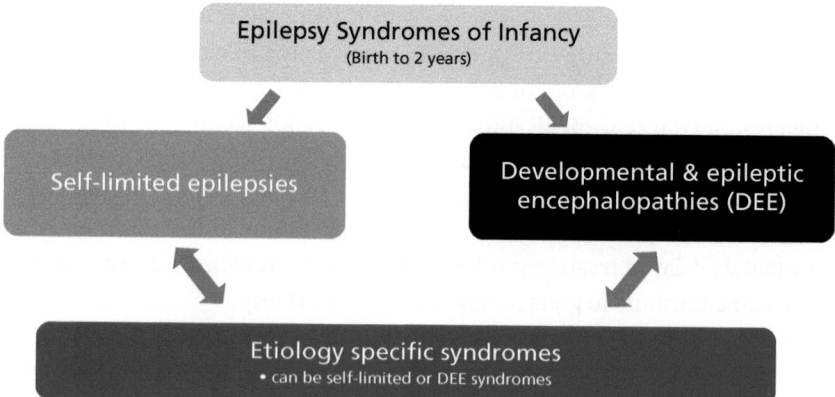

Figure 2.4 Neonatal framework.

electroclinical or electrographic only. Events which are clinical only, and not associated with EEG changes, should not be regarded as epileptic.

When EEG is not available, observation of clinical events, even by specialists in the field, is poor at distinguishing between epileptic and non-epileptic events. The only two types of clinical events where there is most likely to be an EEG correlate are focal clonic and focal tonic and if these are present within the appropriate clinical context it is reasonable to consider them epileptic for treatment purposes.[9,29]

The modification of classification for neonatal seizures encourages more precise treatment and should also reduce the burden of unnecessary treatment including the risks of sedation and subsequent ventilatory support and intensive care unit care.

Classification of status epilepticus

New concepts of status epilepticus impact the psychosocial aspects of epilepsy. The latest conceptual classification of status epilepticus takes into account the time at which normal seizure-terminating mechanisms may not be effective and the time at which the seizure may cause irreversible brain injury.[30] This classification emphasizes the early treatment of status epilepticus and the necessity of rescue medication for people with prolonged seizures.

Status epilepticus is a condition resulting either from the failure of the mechanisms responsible for seizure termination or from the initiation of mechanisms which lead to abnormally prolonged seizures (after time point t_1). It is a condition that can have long-term consequences (after time point t_2), including neuronal death, neuronal injury, and alteration of neuronal networks, depending on the type and duration of seizures.[30]

T_1 for convulsive seizures is 5 minutes with t_2 being 30 minutes. Defining t_1 as the time when a seizure is regarded as abnormally prolonged should result in people with a history of convulsive seizures lasting more than 5 minutes being prescribed rescue medication. For children, adolescents, and adults with learning disability it is important that their families, school, and residential carers should have access to rescue medication and individualized treatment plans. Encouraging early treatment of status epilepticus in the community is important as delayed treatment is less effective in terminating a seizure which in turn can contribute to greater morbidity and mortality.

Non-convulsive seizures such as focal seizures with impairment of awareness or absence seizures can also be prolonged but the evidence for abnormal prolongation causing neuronal death and injury is less certain. T_1 for focal seizures with impairment of awareness and epileptic absences is 10 minutes with t_2 for focal seizures being 60 minutes. There is insufficient evidence to assign a specific t_2 for absence status. The requirement to provide rescue medication in all home and community settings should encourage the use of more socially acceptable routes of administration such as buccal or nasal midazolam rather than rectal preparations.[31]

Conclusion

The classification of seizure types and the epilepsies will continue to evolve as new medical knowledge emerges and the technologies we have to define aetiology improve. Recent developments in classification have emphasized the comorbidities of epilepsy and acknowledged the social implications of epilepsy. Classifications developed to aid the clinician in diagnosis and management should also better serve the needs of people with epilepsy.

References

1. **International League Against Epilepsy**. Process for publishing reports. n. d. Available at: https://www.ilae.org/guidelines/guidelines-and-reports/procedure-for-publishing-reports [accessed 15 December 2020].
2. **Scheffer IE, Berkovic S, Capovilla G**, et al. ILAE classification of the epilepsies: position paper of the ILAE Commission for Classification and Terminology. Epilepsia. 2017;58(4):512–21.
3. **Fisher RS, Cross JH, French JA**, et al. Operational classification of seizure types by the International League Against Epilepsy. Epilepsia. 2017;58(4):522–30.
4. **Shorvon SD**. New terminologies: the downsides. Epilepsia. 2013;54(6):1134.
5. **Jette N, Beghi E, Hesdorffer D**, et al. ICD coding for epilepsy: past, present, and future—a report by the International League Against Epilepsy Task Force on ICD codes in epilepsy. Epilepsia. 2015;56(3):348–55.

6. **Lüders H, Vaca GF, Akamatsu N,** et al. Classification of paroxysmal events and the four-dimensional epilepsy classification system. Epileptic Disord. 2019;**21**(1):1–29.

7. **Beghi E, Carpio A, Forsgren L,** et al. Recommendation for a definition of acute symptomatic seizure. Epilepsia. 2010;**51**(4):671–75.

8. **Pressler RM, Cilio MR, Mizrahi EM,** et al. The ILAE classification of seizures and the epilepsies: modification for seizures in the neonate. Position paper by the ILAE Task Force on Neonatal Seizures. Epilepsia. 2021;**62**(3):615–28.

9. **Fisher RS, van Emde Boas W, Blume W,** et al. Epileptic seizures and epilepsy: definitions proposed by the International League Against Epilepsy (ILAE) and the International Bureau for Epilepsy (IBE). Epilepsia. 2005;**46**(4):470–72.

10. **Fisher RS, Acevedo C, Arzimanoglou A,** et al. ILAE official report: a practical clinical definition of epilepsy. Epilepsia. 2014;**55**(4):475–82.

11. **Grinton BE, Heron SE, Pelekanos JT,** et al. Familial neonatal seizures in 36 families: clinical and genetic features correlate with outcome. Epilepsia. 2015;**56**(7):1071–80.

12. **Hauser WA, Annegers JF, Kurland LT.** Incidence of epilepsy and unprovoked seizures in Rochester, Minnesota: 1935–1984. Epilepsia. 1993;**34**(3):453–68.

13. **Bone I.** Sacred lives: an account of the history, cultural associations and social impact of epilepsy. Kibworth: The Book Guild Ltd; 2020.

14. **Fisher RS, Cross JH, D'Souza C,** et al. Instruction manual for the ILAE 2017 operational classification of seizure types. Epilepsia. 2017;**58**(4):531–42.

15. **Zuberi SM, Brunklaus A.** Epilepsy in 2017: precision medicine drives epilepsy classification and therapy. Nat Rev Neurol. 2018;**14**(2):67–68.

16. **Han Z, Chen C, Christiansen A,** et al. Antisense oligonucleotides increase Scn1a expression and reduce seizures and SUDEP incidence in a mouse model of Dravet syndrome. Sci Transl Med. 2020;**12**(558):eaaz6100.

17. **Nickels KC, Zaccariello MJ, Hamiwka LD, Wirrell EC.** Cognitive and neurodevelopmental comorbidities in paediatric epilepsy. Nat Rev Neurol. 2016;**12**(8):465–76.

18. **Bureau M, Genton P, Delgado-Escueta A,** et al. Epileptic syndromes in infancy, childhood and adolescence, 6th ed. Montrouge: John Libbey Eurotext; 2019.

19. **Commission on Classification and Terminology of the International League Against Epilepsy.** Proposal for classification of epilepsies and epileptic syndromes. Epilepsia. 1985;**26**(3):268–78.

20. **Wirrell EC, Nabbout R, Scheffer IE,** et al. Methodology for classification and definition of epilepsy syndromes with list of syndromes: report of the ILAE Task Force on Nosology and Definitions. Epilepsia. 2022;**63**(6):1333–48.

21. **Zuberi SM, Wirrell E, Yozawitz E,** et al. ILAE classification and definition of epilepsy syndromes with onset in neonates and infants: position statement by the ILAE Task Force on Nosology and Definitions. Epilepsia. 2022;**63**(6):1349–97.

22. **Specchio N, Wirrell EC, Scheffer IE,** et al. International League Against Epilepsy classification and definition of epilepsy syndromes with onset in childhood: position paper by the ILAE Task Force on Nosology and Definitions. Epilepsia. 2022;**63**(6):1398–442.

23. **Riney K, Bogacz A, Somerville E,** et al. International League Against Epilepsy classification and definition of epilepsy syndromes with onset at a variable age: position

statement by the ILAE Task Force on Nosology and Definitions. Epilepsia. 2022;**63**(6):1443–74.

24. **Hirsch E, French J, Scheffer IE**, et al. ILAE definition of the idiopathic generalized epilepsy syndromes: position statement by the ILAE Task Force on Nosology and Definitions. Epilepsia. 2022;**63**(6):1475–99.

25. **van den Munckhof B, van Dee V, Sagi L**, et al. Treatment of electrical status epilepticus in sleep: a pooled analysis of 575 cases. Epilepsia. 2015;**56**(11):1738–46.

26. **Berg AT, Berkovic SF, Brodie MJ**, et al. Revised terminology and concepts for organization of seizures and epilepsies: report of the ILAE Commission on Classification & Terminology, 2005–2009. Epilepsia. 2010;**51**(4):676–85.

27. **Nash KB, Bonifacio SL, Glass HC**, et al. Video-EEG monitoring in newborns with hypoxic-ischemic encephalopathy treated with hypothermia. Neurology. 2011;**76**(6):556–62.

28. **Mizrahi EM, Kellaway P.** Characterization and classification of neonatal seizures. Neurology. 1987;**37**(12):1837–44.

29. **Pellegrin S, Munoz FM, Padula M**, et al. Neonatal seizures: case definition & guidelines for data collection, analysis, and presentation of immunization safety data. Vaccine. 2019;**37**(52):7596–609.

30. **Trinka E, Cock H, Hesdorffer D**, et al. A definition and classification of status epilepticus—report of the ILAE Task Force on Classification of Status Epilepticus. Epilepsia. 2015;**56**(10):1515–23.

31. **O'Regan ME, Brown JK, Clarke M.** Nasal rather than rectal benzodiazepines in the management of acute childhood seizures? Dev Med Child Neurol. 1996;**38**(11):1037–45.

Section 2

The impact of medical and surgical treatment on comorbidity in people with epilepsy

Chapter 3

The effects of antiseizure medications on comorbidities

Fergus J. Rugg-Gunn and Philip N. Patsalos

Introduction

Effective and tolerable antiseizure medications (ASMs) were first introduced over 110 years ago in 1912 with the development of phenobarbital (PB). While this was initially marketed as a nocturnal hypnotic, its effectiveness in reducing seizure activity soon became evident. PB became widely prescribed and continues to be used extensively due to its low cost and proven efficacy. Other ASMs followed, with phenytoin (PHT) obtaining a licence for use in the UK in 1938, carbamazepine (CBZ) in 1963, and sodium valproate in 1974. Similar to PB, CBZ was initially developed for an alternative indication, specifically, trigeminal neuralgia. Over the last 30 years, 25 ASMs have been introduced and novel molecules continue to be developed, with new therapeutic targets and purported modes of action (Table 3.1 and Figures 3.1–3.3).

It is clear, however, both historically and with the newer medications, that the effects of ASMs extend beyond their intended therapeutic benefit on epileptic seizures. As a group, ASMs differ significantly in mode of action, drug–drug interactions, pharmacokinetics, and impact on non-neurological organ systems. The relationship with comorbidities is therefore complex, multidirectional, and varied. This can, however, be summarized as:

1. A therapeutic effect on comorbidities
2. A cause of *de novo* comorbidities
3. An exacerbation of pre-existing comorbidities
4. An indirect influence on comorbidities through interactions with non-ASM medications

Table 3.1 Antiseizure drugs marketed in the UK

Drug	Year introduced
Phenobarbital	1912
Phenytoin	1938
Primidone	1952
Ethosuximide	1960
Carbamazepine	1963
Diazepam	1973
Clonazepam	1974
Valproate	1974
Clobazam	1982
Vigabatrin	1989
Lamotrigine	1991
Gabapentin	1993
Topiramate	1995
Tiagabine	1998
Oxcarbazepine	2000
Levetiracetam	2000
Pregabalin	2004
Zonisamide	2005
Lacosamide	2008
Eslicarbazepine acetate	2009
Perampanel	2012
Brivaracetam	2016
Cannabidiol	2019
Everolimus	2019
Fenfluramine	2020
Cenobamate	2021

5. An effect of comorbidities on antiepileptic medication (this is beyond the scope of this chapter)

6. A teratogenic effect (see Chapter 11).

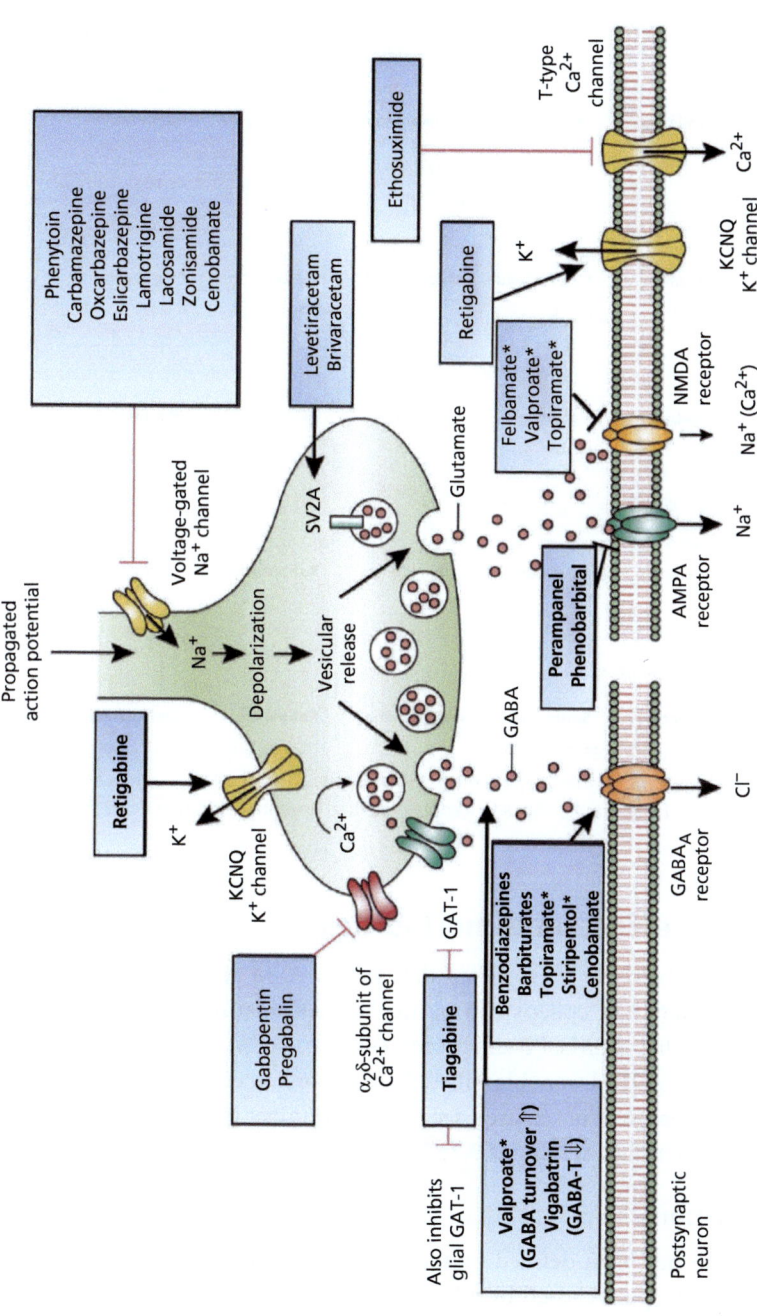

Figure 3.1 Mechanism of action of clinically approved antiseizure medications (ASMs). Asterisks indicate that these compounds act by multiple mechanisms. AMPA, alpha-amino-3-hydroxy-5-methyl-4-isoxazolepropionic acid; GABA, gamma-aminobutyric acid; GABA-T, GABA aminotransferase; GAT-1, GABA transporter 1; KCNQ, Kv7 potassium channel family; NMDA, N-methyl-D-aspartate; SV2A, synaptic vesicle protein 2A. Reproduced with permission from Löscher, W., Klein, P. The Pharmacology and Clinical Efficacy of Antiseizure Medications: From Bromide Salts to Cenobamate and Beyond. CNS Drugs 35, 935–963 (2021).

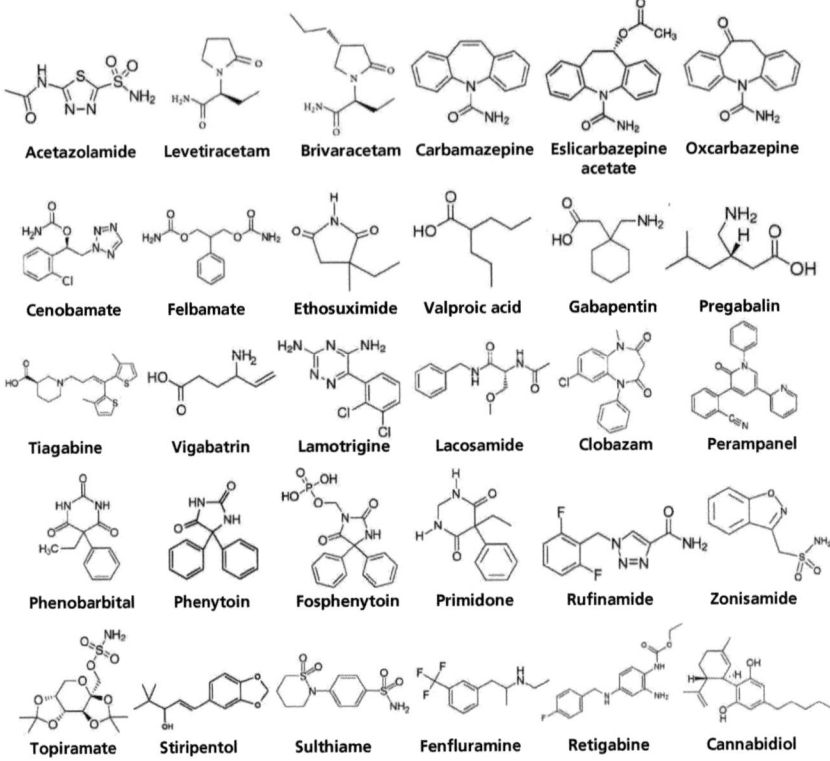

Figure 3.2 Chemical structures of ASMs.
Reproduced with permission from Löscher, W., Klein, P. The Pharmacology and Clinical Efficacy of Antiseizure Medications: From Bromide Salts to Cenobamate and Beyond. CNS Drugs 35, 935–963 (2021).

A therapeutic effect on comorbidities

In 2003, neurologists in the US reported that 45% of ASM prescriptions were for conditions other than epilepsy, in particular, neuropathic pain and migraine. Notably, the first ASMs, PB and bromides, were used as hypnotics before their antiseizure properties were identified. While more recent ASMs are used primarily for the treatment of seizures, a significant number of medications are also effective in other illnesses (Table 3.2).

Neuropathic pain

Neuropathic pain has been defined by the 2011 International Association of the Study of Pain as 'pain caused by a lesion or disease of the somatosensory system'.[1] The causes are wide ranging and include peripheral neuropathies,

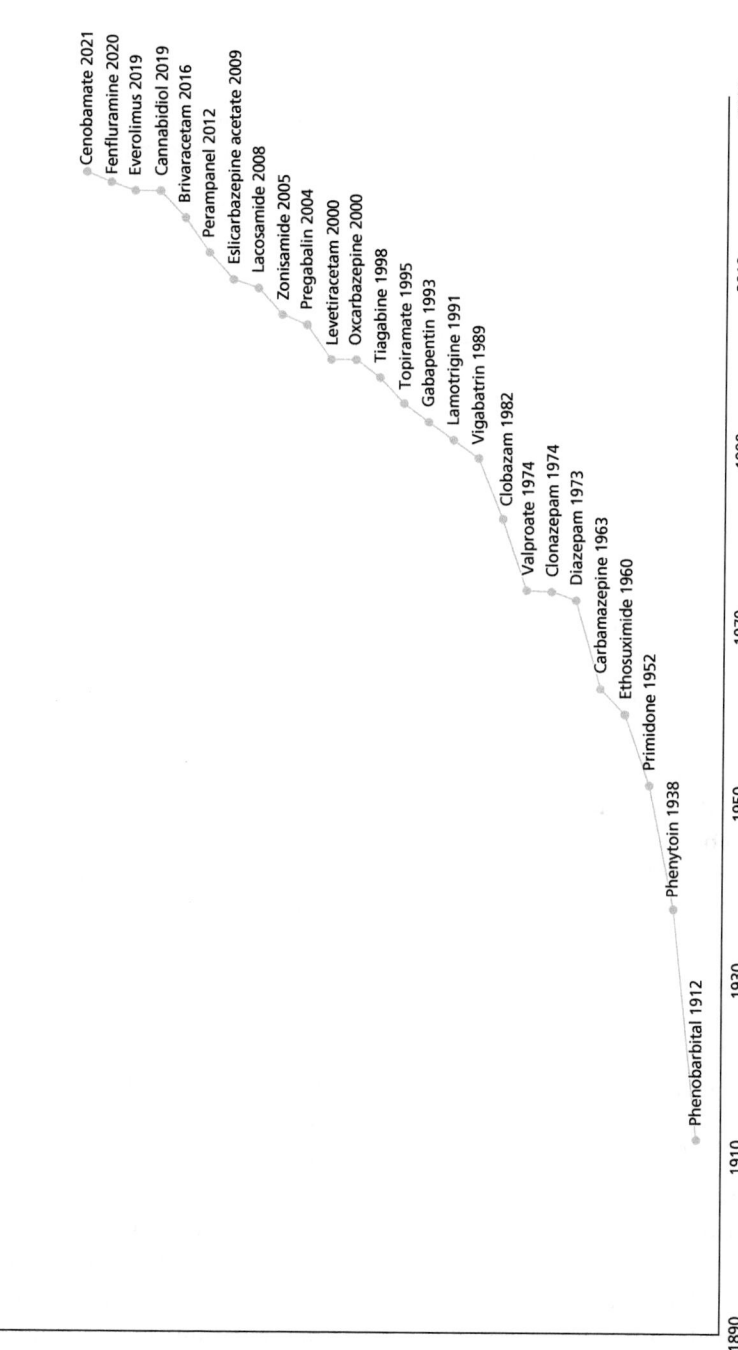

Figure 3.3 Timeline for the introduction of ASMs in the UK.

Table 3.2 A summary of medical disorders which undergo treatment with antiseizure medications

Comorbidity	ASMs (in alphabetical order)
Neuropathic pain	Carbamazepine, clonazepam, gabapentin, lacosamide, lamotrigine, levetiracetam, pregabalin, oxcarbazepine, phenytoin, tiagabine, topiramate, valproic acid, zonisamide
Bipolar disorder	Carbamazepine, lamotrigine, oxcarbazepine, topiramate, valproic acid, zonisamide
Migraine	Lamotrigine, topiramate, valproic acid, zonisamide
Trigeminal neuralgia	Carbamazepine, lamotrigine, oxcarbazepine
Obesity	Topiramate, zonisamide
Essential tremor	Gabapentin, levetiracetam, tiagabine, valproic acid
Anxiety disorders	Clobazam, pregabalin, tiagabine

especially those due to diabetes, chemotherapy, excess alcohol intake, and HIV infection, in addition to phantom limb pain, compression neuropathies, central pain, peripheral nerve trauma, and postherpetic neuralgia. In primary care in the UK, the incidences per 100,000 person years have been reported as 28 for postherpetic neuralgia, 27 for trigeminal neuralgia, 0.8 for phantom limb pain, and 21 for painful diabetic neuropathy.[2] There is therefore a significant number of affected individuals, often on long-term medication. Neuropathic pain arises from chronic injury to sensory neurons leading to axonal sprouting and the formation of neuroma. Subsequently, there are changes in the genes encoding both sodium and calcium channels resulting in altered distribution and composition. Specifically, sodium channels accumulate in nociceptors and changes in gene expression prime these cells to fire spontaneously at high frequencies.[3] The hyperexcitable mechanisms underlying neuropathic pain may be similar to those in epilepsy and this underpins the therapeutic effect of ion channel-blocking ASMs.

Typical first-line treatment includes antidepressant medications such as duloxetine and amitriptyline.[4] ASMs have, however, been used in the management of pain since the 1960s[5] and it is commonplace for new ASMs to be trialled for analgesic properties on a routine basis. In the UK, CBZ and PHT are licensed for the treatment of trigeminal neuralgia, and gabapentin (GBP) and pregabalin (PGB) for the treatment of neuropathic pain. The rationale for the use of ASMs is the ability of these drugs to reduce both central and peripheral rapid neuronal firing through a potentiation of gamma-aminobutyric acid (GABA) inhibition (such as valproic acid (VPA), PGB, and clonazepam

(CZP)), the modulation of ion channels and the stabilization of neuronal cell membranes (such as lamotrigine (LTG), CBZ, GBP, PGB, and lacosamide (LCM)), and the blockade of N-methyl-D-aspartate (NMDA) receptor sites (such as topiramate (TPM)). The most studied of the ASMs in the management of pain are PGB, GBP, CBZ, and LTG.[4] There is good evidence for the modest effectiveness of PGB and GBP in painful diabetic neuropathy and trigeminal neuralgia, and for PGB in central neuropathic pain,[6,7] but a paucity of high-quality data confirming efficacy for other, traditional, ASMs such as CBZ,[8] oxcarbazepine (OXC),[9] LTG,[10] levetiracetam (LEV),[11] and VPA.[4] Newer ASMs including LCM are currently being evaluated and results of a randomized double-blind placebo-controlled trial in peripheral neuropathic pain are awaited.[12] A study of postherpetic neuralgia showed that brivaracetam (BRV) up to doses of 400 mg per day was not significantly different from placebo in reducing pain intensity scores (https://clinicaltrials.gov/ct2/show/results/NCT00160667).

Migraine

People with epilepsy are 2.4-fold more likely to develop migraine than family members without epilepsy.[13] Migraine pain results from activation of the trigeminovascular afferents from the meninges by cortical spreading depression, in turn due to neocortical hyperexcitability. Both migraine and epilepsy are therefore linked pathophysiologically and, often, semiologically. The sodium and calcium channel active ASMs most likely exert their therapeutic effect by reducing excessive activity in sensitized trigeminal sensory fibres. Additionally, ASMs may inhibit the release of inflammatory mediators, such as calcitonin gene-related peptide, that are involved in pain generation and are now an immunological target for a novel class of migraine preventative.[14] They may also reduce cortical hyperexcitability through mechanisms such as inhibition of glutamate-mediated postsynaptic excitation or enhanced GABA inhibition, leading to attenuation of cortical spreading depression. ASMs are therefore particularly useful with coexisting migraine and epilepsy due to similar neurobiological mechanisms and genetic and molecular substrates.[15] Regarding migraine, VPA, GBP, and TPM have been shown to be effective preventatives in placebo-controlled trials, but only TPM has been licensed for migraine prophylaxis in the UK.[16-20]

VPA reduces both migraine severity and frequency by 50% in 40–50% of treated individuals at dose of between 500 and 1000 mg/day and can be of particular value in people with epilepsy and coexisting depression or bipolar disease.[21] The teratogenic risk of VPA precludes its use in women of childbearing potential without a clear discussion of the risks and, in the UK, participation in the Medicines and Healthcare products Regulatory Agency pregnancy prevention programme (see Chapter 11).

TPM has been shown to be similarly effective in reducing monthly migraine days and migraine rescue medication use at lower doses than are typically used for epilepsy, at between 50 and 200 mg per day.[22] Common side effects include acral paraesthesia, mood disturbance, and cognitive issues including word finding and memory difficulties. There is a two- to fourfold increased risk of nephrolithiasis and TPM may precipitate acute closed-angle glaucoma. TPM may be particularly useful in people with epilepsy, migraine, and obesity due to the commonly seen weight loss, but also in intracranial hypertension and type 2 diabetes.

Conflicting evidence for the efficacy of GBP in migraine has prevented its widespread use as a first-line therapy. A randomized, double-blind, placebo-controlled study showed no significant difference between GBP up to 2400 mg/day and placebo[23] but an earlier study showed a 50% reduction in migraine frequency in 46.4% of patients compared to 16.1% in the placebo arm.[24] However, in clinical practice, GBP appears to be less effective than both VPA and TPM, a situation paralleled by the experience in treating seizures in epilepsy clinics. In view of its beneficial effect on neuropathic pain, GBP may be advantageous in patients with coexisting painful neuropathy or trigeminal neuralgia.

Other, newer, ASMs have been evaluated but less conclusive evidence exists for their use. Zonisamide (ZNS) has shown similar efficacy to TPM in migraine with improved tolerability and may be therefore a suitable alternative.[25] LEV has shown similar efficacy to TPM and VPA in a number of small studies[26] but this has not been a universal finding[27] and large-scale studies are required to establish unequivocal evidence for its effectiveness. LTG blocks sodium channels possibly involved in the process of neuronal excitability and cortical spreading depression, and therefore may be effective for migrainous auras[28] but it does not appear to be effective in headaches.[29] There is no clear evidence for the effectiveness of CBZ or OXC in the management of migraine.[19]

Metabolic

The weight loss reported as an adverse effect of TPM in epilepsy and migraine has been explored further in interventional studies in obesity, type 1 diabetes, and hypertension.[30] A mean weight loss of 6–8 kg was shown with combination therapy of phentermine/TPM, at a dose of up to 15/92 mg/day.[31] In contrast to the US, where the Food and Drug Administration approved phentermine/TPM for the pharmacological treatment of obesity in 2012, the European Medicines Agency refused approval in Europe due to safety concerns and the potential for long-term adverse psychiatric and cognitive effects.

Movement disorders

The modulation of GABAergic transmission in basal ganglia may underpin the neuronal hyperexcitability that characterizes some forms of hyperkinetic movement disorders, such as tremor, paroxysmal dyskinesias, subcortical myoclonus, and restless legs syndrome. Accordingly, it was postulated that ASMs able to increase GABAergic neurotransmission may offer novel therapeutic avenues.[32]

Essential tremor (ET) is characterized by alternate contraction of agonist and antagonist muscles causing involuntary oscillatory movements and is thought to be due to dysfunction in the GABAergic system with loss of inhibitory neurotransmission by cerebellar Purkinje cells. On this basis, ASMs that may be effective treatment for ET include CZP, primidone (PRM), tiagabine (TGB), PGB, GBP, TPM, LEV, and ZNS. Of these, PRM is the most effective, with the therapeutic effect attributed to the parent compound rather than the metabolites, such as PB, but it is limited by sedative and other adverse effects.[33] The evidence is less robust for GBP and PGB, but studies of the efficacy of TPM and ZNS on ET are more promising.[34] The predominant site of action of LEV is the synaptic vesicle protein 2A but LEV also enhances the chloride currents in $GABA_A$ receptors and has been shown to be partially effective in ET[35] but this has not been a universal finding.[36] Larger studies need to be undertaken to explore this further.

Neuronal ion channelopathies are considered to be implicated in paroxysmal kinesigenic dyskinesias, and as such respond to sodium channel-blocking medications such as CBZ, OXC, and LCM. Non-kinesigenic and tardive dyskinesias can also be suppressed by LEV but through an alternative mechanism such as by reducing neuronal hypersynchrony in the basal ganglia.[37,38] ASMs can also be efficacious in choreiform movements, through the stabilization of the inactivated state of voltage-gated sodium channels (CBZ[39]) or by modulating potassium channels (VPA[40]). Newer ASMs such as GBP, TPM, and LEV have been shown in individual cases or small-series studies to be effective in choreoathetosis and hemichorea/hemiballismus.[41]

While cortical myoclonus is seen frequently in epilepsy, typically in the genetic generalized epilepsy syndromes such as juvenile myoclonic epilepsy or progressive myoclonic disorders, such as Unverricht–Lundborg disease, myoclonus can arise from subcortical, brainstem, and spinal generators. The dysfunction of fast inhibitory mechanisms, mediated by GABA may be implicated, and medications such as VPA (indirect effect on GABA levels) and CZP (direct $GABA_A$ receptor agonist) are first-line treatments. LEV is not only helpful in cortical but also spinal myoclonus[42,43] and medications which reduce the overactivity of postsynaptic excitatory neurotransmission, such as TPM, are also effective.[44]

Psychiatric disorders

While there is an increased lifetime prevalence of psychiatric disorders, such as depression, anxiety, and bipolar disorder, in epilepsy, due to a multitude of direct and indirect factors[45] (see Chapter 6), ASMs are often used to treat psychiatric symptoms in the absence of a diagnosis of epilepsy. Despite a wide range of disorders purported to be helped by ASMs, the approved and licensed psychiatric indications for ASMs are relatively narrow and comprise only bipolar and generalized anxiety disorder.[46] The molecular basis for a number of psychiatric illnesses, such as bipolar disorder, is uncertain and the therapeutic target for ASMs remains obscure. There is some evidence, however, that the mood-stabilizing actions of VPA and CBZ may be due to inositol depletion—a shared mechanism with lithium.[3] Lithium, LTG, and VPA also inhibit glycogen synthase kinase, and CBZ exerts a similar, functional, effect by influencing upstream signalling mechanisms.

CBZ, at doses between 400 and 2000 mg per day, has been shown to be effective in the treatment of both acute mania and maintenance bipolar disorder in approximately 50–60% of patients and is often used in combination with lithium for refractory patients.[47] Studies on the use of CBZ and schizophrenia showed mixed results and in the absence of clear efficacy data from larger, well-conducted trials, it cannot be recommended for routine clinical use.[48] CBZ has also been evaluated, and found effective, in post-traumatic stress disorder, benzodiazepine and alcohol withdrawal, impulsive aggression, and pathological gambling.[46]

VPA has a similar, beneficial impact in bipolar disorder, particularly with depressive symptoms and for the treatment of acute mania where approximately 60% of patients experience marked improvement.[49] VPA possibly exerts an antipsychotic effect through an action on histone deacetylases leading to a reduced downregulation of reelin and glutamate decarboxylase,[67] an enzyme involved in GABA synthesis. Reduced glutamate decarboxylase[67] has been identified in prefrontal cortices of patients with schizophrenia and this may contribute to the therapeutic effect of VPA in patients with positive psychotic symptoms.[3,50] VPA has also been found to be effective, typically in small series studies, in obsessive–compulsive disorders, social anxiety, impulsive aggression, and borderline personality among others.[46]

LTG is effective in bipolar disorders, particularly as prophylaxis against depressive rather than manic symptomatology and in patients with rapid cycling bipolar II, with doses ranging between 50 and 200 mg per day.[51,52] It has been reported to be as equally effective as lithium, the current standard treatment for bipolar disorder but better tolerated and with more favourable teratogenicity data.[53] Due to the risk of rash, LTG needs to be titrated slowly and this makes it more suitable as maintenance rather than acute therapy.

PGB is structurally similar to GABA but its anxiolytic and antiseizure effect is mediated through the specific binding to the voltage-gated calcium channels of the presynaptic neurons, reducing the release of excitatory neurotransmitters glutamate and substance P. PGB is effective, and licensed for use, in patients with generalized anxiety disorder,[54] and has been shown to have a lower drop-out rate than benzodiazepines.[55] For other ASMs such as GBP, TPM,[56] ZNS,[57] and LEV, sufficient efficacy from large, well-conducted trials has not been demonstrated for bipolar or other psychiatric disorders.

Antiseizure medications as a cause of, or exacerbation of pre-existing, comorbidities

Population-based studies have reported an eightfold increased prevalence of some comorbid conditions in people with epilepsy compared to the general population.[58] While these may be causative, such as cerebrovascular disease, or resultant, such as a seizure-related injury, or share common risk factors, ASMs may also contribute to either the *de novo* development of a comorbidity or an exacerbation of a pre-existing condition.

Cardiac

ASMs may influence cardiac electrophysiology via similar mechanisms to their antiseizure effect, principally via ion channel modulation. This results in, typically, prolongation of the PR interval (>200 ms) and either lengthening or shortening of the corrected QT interval (QTc). Prolongation of the PR interval, due to atrioventricular (AV) conduction delay either at the AV node (voltage-gated calcium channel mediated) or within the infra-Hisian bundles (voltage-gated sodium channel mediated) leads to first-degree AV block. Although this is typically benign and asymptomatic, it can progress to type 2 AV block which is associated with complete heart block, symptomatic bradycardia, and cardiac arrest.[59] Predictably, therefore, the sodium and calcium channel active ASMs are most likely to influence cardiac conduction. Prolongation of the PR interval has been reported with PHT, CBZ, OXC, LCM, LTG, eslicarbazepine (ESL), and PGB.[60,61] Typically, the magnitude of prolongation is small, but these effects can be additive and the potential impact of ASM polypharmacy in susceptible individuals needs to be carefully considered.

Prolongation of the QT interval—the period of time required for ventricular depolarization and repolarization—is a reliable biomarker of fatal arrhythmias.[62] Long QT syndrome can be acquired or genetic. A number of medications, such as antimicrobials, antipsychotics, and antihistamines but also ASMs including PB, PHT, and CBZ have the potential to prolong the QT interval. There are conflicting data regarding LTG. While a carefully conducted QT/QTc double-blind, placebo- and active-controlled crossover study showed no significant prolongation of QT interval at doses between 100 and 400 mg/day,[63] other small series and experimental studies have suggested an impact from either prolongation or shortening the QT interval in susceptible individuals.[64] Interestingly, other sodium channel-blocking ASMs such as LCM and ESL have shown no effect on the QT interval, suggesting that this is not necessarily a class effect.[65] No alterations in PR or QTc intervals have been seen with perampanel (PER) or TPM which are ASMs without a predominantly ion channel modulatory effect. There are similarly reassuring data regarding LEV, other than a single case report of an individual with an occult KCNH2 potassium channel mutation who developed torsade de pointes after treatment with LEV.[66,67] ASMs that shorten the QTc interval include PRM and rufinamide (RUF)[64] and, similar to the genetic short QT syndromes, this may indicate a potential arrhythmogenic risk but, to date, this is unproven.

Beyond the well-recognized effect on PR and QTc intervals, a recent US Food and Drug Administration safety warning has been issued highlighting the potential effect of LTG on ventricular conduction leading to widening of the QRS interval and an increased risk of a cardiac arrhythmia and sudden death. This is based on *in vitro* data and remains to be confirmed in studies on people with epilepsy.[68] The effect is thought to be mediated via a class IB antiarrhythmic effect at therapeutically relevant concentrations and may only be relevant in those with pre-existing cardiac disease. Ideally, therefore, in patients with pre-existing heart disease, especially those with abnormal cardiac electrophysiology, advancing age, electrolyte disturbance, and concomitant medications, ASMs with the least impact on the heart should be selected, and electrocardiographic monitoring should be undertaken when indicated.

Enzyme-inducing ASMs may also contribute to an adverse cardiovascular risk profile, and possibly accelerated atherosclerosis, due to elevated serological vascular risk markers such as total cholesterol, low-density lipoprotein, and homocysteine.[69] In a study of 320 children with epilepsy, low-density lipoprotein cholesterol was elevated in 27.9% of patients taking CBZ and in 31.8% of patients taking PB, but only in 7% taking VPA and 11% of control subjects.[70] Switching from enzyme-inducing ASMs to either LTG or LEV is associated with a decline in total cholesterol, atherogenic cholesterol, triglycerides, and

C-reactive protein.[71] Furthermore, the use of enzyme-inducing ASMs, and VPA, has been shown to increase common carotid artery intima–media thickness, a marker of atherosclerosis. There was no change noted with LTG.[72]

Finally, some ASMs, for example, VPA, PGB, and PER, also cause weight gain and increase the risk of non-alcoholic fatty liver disease and metabolic syndrome.

Dermatological

The cutaneous adverse drug reactions to ASMs, seen in approximately 75 per 100,000 patients per year, are idiosyncratic immune-activated responses and range from a mild maculopapular exanthema to the potentially fatal toxic epidermal necrolysis (TEN), Stevens–Johnson syndrome (SJS), and drug reaction with eosinophilia and systemic symptoms syndrome (DRESS). They usually emerge within the first 2–3 months of use and are most commonly associated with the use of aromatic ASMs such as PB, PHT, CBZ, LTG, and OXC or sulphonamide-derived ASMs such as ZNS. The aromatic ASMs are metabolized by cytochrome P450 isoenzymes to arene oxide and then detoxified by an epoxide hydrolase enzyme. Individuals with decreased epoxide hydrolases, due to a genetic predisposition, accumulate arene oxides that bind to macromolecules and trigger an immunological response, resulting in a cutaneous reaction.

The risk of drug-induced hypersensitivity syndrome of TEN and SJS with LTG is 5–10%, 5–17% with CBZ, and 5–7% with PHT. There is a high risk of cross-reactivity, up to 70%, with another aromatic ASM.[73] Although a rash is seen in up to 10% of patients, the risk of a severe cutaneous reaction is much lower, but not eliminated completely, with the non-aromatic ASMs such as VPA,[74] TPM, LEV,[75] GBP, PER, and benzodiazepines. Interestingly, some aromatic ASMs such as LCM do not appear to be associated with an increased risk, with 2.9% of patients experiencing a rash compared to 3% in the placebo group in the pivotal, licensing trials. No cases of SJS or TEN were seen.[76]

The idiosyncratic nature of the skin reaction prompted a search for a genetic predisposition. The first report of an association between the human leucocyte antigen (HLA)-B*15:02 allele, found in 8% of the Han Chinese population and CBZ-induced SJS/TEN was published in 2004.[77] Since then, additional associations have been identified, including HLA-A*24:02, HLA-B*44:03, HLA-B*15:11, and HLA-B*38:01.[78] The HLA-A*31:01 allele is seen in 2–5% of Northern Europeans; the presence of the allele increases the risk of a CBZ hypersensitivity reaction from 5% to 26% whereas the absence reduces the risk from 5% to 3.8%.[79] While it is mandatory that the offending ASM is withdrawn immediately in the context of a severe skin hypersensitivity reaction, milder forms of skin eruption without systemic symptoms or abnormal haematological, inflammatory, or hepatic parameters may respond to a dose reduction, slower titration schedule, or desensitization programme.[80]

Hepatic

ASM-induced hepatotoxicity is a rare adverse effect. Nevertheless, in patients undergoing liver transplantation for non-paracetamol-related drug toxicity in the US between 1990 and 2002, ASMs (VPA and PHT) were the third most common cause.[81] The risk of hepatotoxicity is approximately 1 in 10,000–50,000 for PHT, and 1 in 45,000 for VPA. Drug-induced hepatoxicity is defined as an increase in the alanine transaminase (ALT) level of at least three times the upper limit of normal and total bilirubin levels of at least two times the upper limit of normal, or an increase in the ALT level of at least five times the upper limit of normal with an increase in the alkaline phosphatase level of at least two times the upper limit of normal. Drug withdrawal is mandatory in this setting to avoid fulminant liver failure.

Asymptomatic elevations of liver enzymes are common, however, with increased gamma-glutamyl transferase levels in up to 95% of patients taking enzyme-inducing medication.[82] The cause of ASM-induced hepatotoxicity is uncertain, but it is likely that hypersensitivity is implicated, particularly with aromatic ASMs. The hepatotoxic potential of a non-aromatic ASM, VPA, is well documented, however; it is the third most common cause of drug-induced fatalities reported by the World Health Organization. The mechanism of injury is likely to be related to interference of mitochondrial beta oxidation of fatty acids and this is influenced by acquired and genetic factors. A markedly increased risk of hepatic failure is seen in patients with mutations of the *POLG* gene which encodes the catalytic subunit of mitochondrial DNA polymerase gamma.[83]

Asymptomatic hyperammonaemia is common with VPA and does not require discontinuation but marked hyperammonaemia may result in encephalopathy, with behavioural change, confusional state, and obtundation, and requires dose reduction. This is more likely to occur with concomitant use of TPM and ZNS.[84] PHT induces an asymptomatic increase in ALT in approximately 25% of patients. Severe hepatic injury can occur rarely and is, most likely, a hypersensitivity reaction related to elevated arene oxide production in liver microsomes. CBZ causes a transient elevation in hepatic enzymes in 10% of patients, but severe toxicity, which typically occurs in the first 12 months is rare. Again, this is often due to arene oxide accumulation and hypersensitivity, but this is less common than with PHT (30% vs 70%). Other hepatic injuries associated with CBZ include granulomatous hepatitis and ductopenia, a rare condition characterized by loss of small bile ducts which is also seen with VPA, LTG, and ZNS.[85] Felbamate (FBM) was initially widely used until reports of aplastic anaemia and hepatic failure emerged, typically within the first 6–12 months of use. The risk of fulminant liver failure is between 1 in 26,000 and 1 in 34,000, and, as a result, FBM is now used only rarely.[86] Other ASMs such as OXC, TPM, PB, LTG, LEV, LCM, ZNS, GBP, benzodiazepines, PGB, and ESL are associated only infrequently with liver injury. There is no evidence of hepatotoxicity with TGB, PER, and BRV. Hepatotoxicity is challenging to predict despite the known associations and regular monitoring of liver enzymes is recommended, especially with enzyme-inducing ASMs. Enhanced vigilance is warranted if there is a two- to threefold increase in liver function tests from baseline and if this is surpassed, medication withdrawal is recommended. If required, there are treatments for hepatotoxicity associated with specific drugs, for example, levocarnitine for VPA, N-acetylcysteine for CBZ and PHT, and steroids for CBZ, PHT, and LTG. Haemodialysis and liver transplantation are treatment modalities of last resort.[82]

Most of the available ASMs may precipitate an acute attack of porphyria, characterized by abdominal pain, symmetrical motor neuropathy, confusion, and seizures. Treatment with CBZ, PB, PHT, PRM, TPM, VPA, LTG, ethosuximide (ESM), and ZNS should be avoided. It is therefore challenging to select an ASM to manage pre-existing or emergent seizures. ASMs with minimal hepatic metabolism, such as LEV, PGB, and GBP should be first-line treatments.[87] OXC (low hepatic induction of hepatic microsomes) and benzodiazepines have been used successfully, although at high doses, CZP may exacerbate symptoms.

Valproate-induced acute pancreatitis was first reported in 1979[88] and has subsequently been recognized as the ASM most likely to cause pancreatitis, with an incidence of 0.2–0.5% of exposed individuals.[89,90] Pancreatitis typically occurs within the first year of treatment, and the risk increases with higher doses and in children.[89,91] The proposed mechanisms of action of valproate-induced acute pancreatitis are a direct toxic effect of free radicals on the pancreatic tissue and a depletion of superoxide dismutase, catalase, and glutathione peroxidase.[91] Other ASM medications have also been implicated, typically as isolated case reports, including CBZ, PHT, PGB, LEV, FBM, LTG, TPM, and LCM.[92]

Haematological

ASMs may induce changes in haematological parameters, from mild thrombocytopenia seen commonly with VPA, to fulminant aplastic anaemia with CBZ, VPA, or FBM. In addition to a low platelet count, VPA may induce cytopenia in other cell lines and a coagulopathy.[93] CBZ also causes thrombocytopenia and, in 12% of patients, transient leucopenia. This typically emerges in the first 3 months of treatment and becomes persistent in 2% of cases, remitting only with medication withdrawal. More recently, thrombocytopenia has been seen with LEV therapy, with platelet counts 14% lower than the control group.[94] Idiosyncratic aplastic anaemia is the most serious haematological complication. Exposure to ASM therapy is associated with a ninefold increase in risk of aplastic anaemia, and is most commonly seen with CBZ, VPA, and, to a lesser extent, PHT.[95] The risk of aplastic anaemia with FBM is 20 times higher than with CBZ, which contributed to its discontinuation. Other ASMs, such as LCM, LTG, ZNS, TPM, OXC, and GBP cause haematological adverse events only rarely.

Bone

There is accumulating evidence that patients on ASMs are at increased risk of metabolic bone disease and fractures are seen two to three times more commonly in people with epilepsy than in the general population.[96] Up to one-third of this risk is related to seizure-related injuries, but metabolic bone disease, possibly secondary to ASM use, has been implicated. This was explored in a large case–control study which accounted for potential confounds such as seizure severity and comorbidities. The risk of fractures increased with cumulative duration of exposure, with a relative risk of 4.15 (95% confidence interval (CI) 2.71–6.34) compared to matched controls, for longer than 12 years of use.[97] In a similar population-based case–control study, enzyme-inducing ASMs conferred a relative increased risk of 1.38 (95% CI 1.31–1.45), compared to non-enzyme-inducing ASMs of 1.19 (95% CI 1.11–1.27), and there was a clear dose–response relationship.[98] Enzyme-inducing ASMs increase hepatic vitamin D catabolism, and there may be additional effects on sex hormones and osteoblast function resulting in reduced bone mineral density and, accordingly, an increased risk of fractures. While most of the evidence relates to the older ASMs, the majority of which are enzyme inducers but include VPA, there is insufficient evidence regarding the newer ASMs. Animal studies suggest multiple mechanisms are involved, many independent of enzyme inhibition, and newer drugs may prove to be equally culpable. On this basis, vitamin D supplementation at a minimum dose of 400 IU/day is recommended for all patients with borderline vitamin D serum levels of between 30 and 50 nmol/L and this should be in the context of offering advice on regular exercise, diet, smoking, and alcohol.

Renal

The incidence of ASM-related nephrotoxicity is rare, typically less than 0.1%. CBZ, PHT, PB, and PRM may cause renal impairment as part of the hypersensitivity reaction, DRESS. Non-hypersensitivity kidney-related adverse reactions have also been seen with CBZ (hyponatraemia), GBP (haematuria, cystitis), LTG (hyponatraemia, hyperkalaemia), ESM (haematuria, nephrotic syndrome), PER (haematuria), and LEV/BRV (hyponatraemia, acute kidney injury).[99] The direct effect of VPA on mitochondria in the proximal renal tubules can cause Fanconi syndrome, characterized by excessive urinary excretion of glucose, bicarbonate, phosphates, uric acid, potassium, and amino acids.

Hyponatraemia is commonly seen with CBZ, OXC, and ESL but has also been reported with VPA, LEV, and LTG.[100] The mechanism is uncertain but may be related to the syndrome of inappropriate antidiuretic hormone secretion, changes in hypothalamic osmoreceptor sensitivity, and enhanced renal tubular responsiveness to antidiuretic hormone. Typically, the hyponatraemia is chronic, asymptomatic, and of no clinical significance. However, in the context of symptomatic hyponatraemia such as dizziness and somnolence, or a persistent serum sodium level less than 125 mmol/L (reference range: 135–145 mmol/L), fluid restriction and dose reduction are indicated.

Nephrolithiasis is associated with the use of acetazolamide, ZNS, and TPM due to the inhibition of carbonic anhydrase activity. In the kidneys, carbonic anhydrase inhibitors act on the proximal convoluted tubule and block the reabsorption of bicarbonate and inhibit the excretion of hydrogen ions. This causes intracellular acidosis and enhanced tubular reabsorption of citrate ions, resulting in hypocitraturia, an elevated urinary pH, and hypercalciuria which increases the risk of calcium oxalate and calcium phosphate stone formation.[101] Nephrolithiasis has been reported to occur in up to 10% of patients on acetazolamide, 1–3% of patients on TPM, although up to 10.7% has been reported,[102] and only 1.4% of patients taking ZNS.[103] It is likely that there is a greater number of asymptomatic cases, for example, in one series, asymptomatic calculi were detected by computed tomography scan in 20% of patients taking TPM at a mean daily dose of 300 mg/day.[102] ASM-induced renal calculi are more prevalent with concomitant use of other lithogenic ASM and non-ASMs and in the context of dehydration.

Psychiatric

While a number of ASMs have a therapeutic effect on psychiatric comorbidities, others have a negative impact and an exacerbation of, or the emergence of novel, psychiatric symptomatology will adversely affect quality of life, independent of seizure control, and lead to drug withdrawal (see Chapter 6). Psychiatric and behavioural side effects were seen in 17% of individuals in a large retrospective case-note review, and these led to discontinuation in 13%. LEV and ZNS were the ASMs most likely to be associated with psychiatric and behavioural side effects, whereas CBZ, CLB, GBP, LTG, OXC, PHT, and VPA had more favourable profiles.[104] In a series of audits from 1996 to 2014, it was noted that, in general, patients receiving sodium channel-blocking ASMs were less likely to develop significant psychiatric symptoms than patients on medications with alternative modes of action. Depression was the most common psychiatric adverse effect, leading to discontinuation in 2.8% of patients.[105] Overall, there is evidence that PB, PHT, PRM, TGB, TPM, and PER may cause depression, while LEV is associated with anxiety and irritability. The development of psychotic symptoms has been seen with ESM, LEV, TPM, ZNS, and PER. Pre-existing psychiatric symptoms and intellectual disability are risk factors for the development of ASM-related psychiatric or behavioural side effects.[104,106] Furthermore, enzyme-inducing ASMs may lower the serum levels of psychotropic medications such as selective serotonin reuptake inhibitors and tricyclic antidepressants, and some neuroleptics resulting in loss of symptom control.

Intellectual disability

The efficacy of ASMs is similar in people with intellectual disability (see Chapter 7) but those with intellectual disability are more susceptible to the sedative and cognitive adverse effects of ASMs.[105,107] These and other side effects are more likely to be exhibited as behavioural disturbance, and in the context of polypharmacy, assessment of the benefit and negative impact of an individual ASM can be challenging. ASMs with a low rate of cognitive adverse effects such as LEV, LTG, OXC, VPA, and GBP as monotherapy should therefore be used whenever possible.[108] Sodium channel-blocking ASMs should be used cautiously in people with impaired motor skills and incoordination, and those with severe behavioural issues should avoid LEV, TPM, ZNS, and PER.[109-111] Patients with intellectual disability are also at particular risk of experiencing ASM paradoxical effects, such as hyperactivity with benzodiazepines such as clobazam.

Antiseizure medications may indirectly influence comorbidities through interactions with non-antiseizure drugs

ASM versus non-ASM interactions are prevalent in epilepsy and present a therapeutic challenge, particularly since many ASMs can affect the pharmacokinetics of various non-ASM drugs and in turn influence the management of concurrent comorbidities. Typically, the most substantial mechanism of interaction is that of inhibition or induction of non-ASM drug metabolism by ASMs. However, pharmacodynamic interactions can also occur, for example, the delirium that is observed in some patients when quetiapine is co-administered with VPA is considered to be the consequence of a pharmacodynamic interaction.[112] Additionally, the combination of lithium and CBZ has been associated with a syndrome characterized by somnolence, confusion, disorientation, and ataxia and other cerebellar symptoms consequent to a pharmacodynamic interaction.[113,114]

Most pharmacokinetic interactions can be attributable to just four ASMs, namely CBZ, PHT, PB, and PRM. These ASMs are potent hepatic enzyme inducers and enhance the metabolism of many drugs that are prescribed for the management of various comorbidities and thus reduce their efficacy. ASMs, such as VPA, that can inhibit metabolism can result in non-ASM drug toxicity. It is not unreasonable in these circumstances to increase or decrease non-ASM drug dosage, respectively. Table 3.3 highlights examples of drug interactions in which ASMs can affect the pharmacokinetics of various non-ASM drugs.

Table 3.3 Examples of drug interactions in which antiseizure medications affect the pharmacokinetics of various non-antiseizure drugs

Antiseizure medication	Therapeutic class
	Antineoplastic agents (mechanism of interaction: induction of hepatic metabolism)
Carbamazepine and phenytoin	9-aminocamptothecin, cyclophosphamide, glufosfamide, imatinib, methotrexate, paclitaxel, procarbazine, temozolomide, temsirolimus, teniposide, thiotepa, vincristine
Phenobarbital	9-aminocamptothecin, etoposide, glufosfamide, irinotecan, methotrexate, paclitaxel, procarbazine, teniposide
	Cardiovascular drugs (mechanism of interaction: induction of hepatic metabolism)
Carbamazepine	Ivabradine, felodipine, nilvadipine, warfarin, simvastatin
Phenytoin	Amiodarone, diazoxide, dicoumarol, digoxin, disopyramide, felodipine, ivabradine, mexiletine, nimodipine, nisoldipine, propranolol, quinidine, verapamil, simvastatin
	Psychoactive drugs (mechanism of interaction: induction of hepatic metabolism)
Carbamazepine	Amitriptyline, aripiprazole, bromperidol, chlorpromazine, citalopram, clomipramine, clozapine, desipramine, doxepin, fluphenazine, haloperidol, imipramine, mianserin, mirtazapine, moclobemide, nefazodone, nortriptyline, olanzapine, paliperidone, quetiapine, risperidone, sertraline, thioridazine, trazodone, ziprasidone
Phenytoin	Clozapine, desipramine, haloperidol, mianserin, mirtazapine, nortriptyline, quetiapine, risperidone, sertraline, thioridazine,
Phenobarbital	Chlorpromazine, clozapine, desipramine, haloperidol, imipramine, mianserin, nortriptyline, paroxetine, thioridazine
	Psychoactive drugs (mechanism of interaction: inhibition of hepatic metabolism)
Valproic acid	Amitriptyline, clomipramine, doxepin, moclobemide, nortriptyline, quetiapine, venlafaxine

Source: Patsalos PN. Antiepileptic drug interactions: a clinical guide, 3rd ed. Switzerland: Springer International Publishing; 2016.

Conclusion

It is clear that the effects of ASMs often extend beyond their therapeutic benefit on seizure activity. The exploration of a clinical benefit beyond improved seizure control is an important therapeutic strategy and this approach has yielded novel treatment paradigms for other conditions such as pain, migraine, movement disorders, and psychiatric illness.

While the introduction of an ASM provides novel treatment strategies for individuals with epilepsy and non-seizure disorders, it is noteworthy that there may be unintended consequences ranging from minor adverse effects such as a self-limiting rash to potentially harmful cardiac conduction changes or major haematological or hepatic complications. The idiosyncratic nature of some of these effects warrants enhanced vigilance and a low threshold for reporting unexpected changes following the introduction of a novel ASM, particularly as these effects can be summative in the context of ASM polytherapy.

The degree of interaction between different ASMs and between ASM and non-ASM has diminished more recently with the almost universal development of non-enzyme-inducing ASMs. Nevertheless, important pharmacokinetic and pharmacodynamic interactions still exist and should be considered carefully.

To conclude, the relationship between ASMs and comorbidities can be summarized as complex, multidirectional, and varied. Accordingly, the use of ASMs is challenging and possibly harmful. Knowledge of the potential benefits, adverse effects, and interactions is important in the effective and safe prescribing of ASMs to manage both epilepsy and non-seizure disorders.

References

1. Jensen TS, Baron R, Haanpaa M, et al. A new definition of neuropathic pain. Pain. 2011;152(10):2204–205.
2. Hall GC, Carroll D, McQuay HJ. Primary care incidence and treatment of four neuropathic pain conditions: a descriptive study, 2002–2005. BMC Fam Pract. 2008;9:26.
3. Rogawski MA, Loscher W. The neurobiology of antiepileptic drugs for the treatment of nonepileptic conditions. Nat Med. 2004;10(7):685–92.
4. Wiffen PJ, Derry S, Moore RA, et al. Antiepileptic drugs for neuropathic pain and fibromyalgia—an overview of Cochrane reviews. Cochrane Database Syst Rev. 2013;11:CD010567.
5. Blom S. Trigeminal neuralgia: its treatment with a new anticonvulsant drug (G-32883). Lancet. 1962;1(7234):839–40.
6. Derry S, Bell RF, Straube S, Wiffen PJ, Aldington D, Moore RA. Pregabalin for neuropathic pain in adults. Cochrane Database Syst Rev. 2019;1:CD007076.

7. **Wiffen PJ, Derry S, Bell RF, et al.** Gabapentin for chronic neuropathic pain in adults. Cochrane Database Syst Rev. 2017;**6**:CD007938.

8. **Wiffen PJ, Derry S, Moore RA, Kalso EA.** Carbamazepine for chronic neuropathic pain and fibromyalgia in adults. Cochrane Database Syst Rev. 2014;**4**:CD005451.

9. **Zhou M, Chen N, He L, Yang M, Zhu C, Wu F.** Oxcarbazepine for neuropathic pain. Cochrane Database Syst Rev. 2017;**12**:CD007963.

10. **Wiffen PJ, Derry S, Moore RA.** Lamotrigine for chronic neuropathic pain and fibromyalgia in adults. Cochrane Database Syst Rev. 2013;**12**:CD006044.

11. **Wiffen PJ, Derry S, Moore RA, Lunn MP.** Levetiracetam for neuropathic pain in adults. Cochrane Database Syst Rev. 2014;**7**:CD010943.

12. **Carmland ME, Kreutzfeldt M, Holbech JV, et al.** Effect of lacosamide in peripheral neuropathic pain: study protocol for a randomized, placebo-controlled, phenotype-stratified trial. Trials. 2019;**20**(1):588.

13. **Ottman R, Lipton RB.** Comorbidity of migraine and epilepsy. Neurology. 1994;**44**(11):2105–10.

14. **Zobdeh F, Ben Kraiem A, Attwood MM, et al.** Pharmacological treatment of migraine: drug classes, mechanisms of action, clinical trials and new treatments. Br J Pharmacol. 2021;**178**(23):4588–607.

15. **Bianchin MM, Londero RG, Lima JE, Bigal ME.** Migraine and epilepsy: a focus on overlapping clinical, pathophysiological, molecular, and therapeutic aspects. Curr Pain Headache Rep. 2010;**14**(4):276–83.

16. **Linde M, Mulleners WM, Chronicle EP, McCrory DC.** Valproate (valproic acid or sodium valproate or a combination of the two) for the prophylaxis of episodic migraine in adults. Cochrane Database Syst Rev. 2013;**6**:CD010611.

17. **Linde M, Mulleners WM, Chronicle EP, McCrory DC.** Topiramate for the prophylaxis of episodic migraine in adults. Cochrane Database Syst Rev. 2013;**6**:CD010610.

18. **Linde M, Mulleners WM, Chronicle EP, McCrory DC.** Gabapentin or pregabalin for the prophylaxis of episodic migraine in adults. Cochrane Database Syst Rev. 2013;**6**:CD010609.

19. **Linde M, Mulleners WM, Chronicle EP, McCrory DC.** Antiepileptics other than gabapentin, pregabalin, topiramate, and valproate for the prophylaxis of episodic migraine in adults. Cochrane Database Syst Rev. 2013;**6**:CD010608.

20. **Parikh SK, Silberstein SD.** Current status of antiepileptic drugs as preventive migraine therapy. Curr Treat Options Neurol. 2019;**21**(4):16.

21. **Freitag FG, Collins SD, Carlson HA, et al.** A randomized trial of divalproex sodium extended-release tablets in migraine prophylaxis. Neurology. 2002;**58**(11):1652–59.

22. **Brandes JL, Saper JR, Diamond M, et al.** Topiramate for migraine prevention: a randomized controlled trial. JAMA. 2004;**291**(8):965–73.

23. **Silberstein S, Goode-Sellers S, Twomey C, Saiers J, Ascher J.** Randomized, double-blind, placebo-controlled, phase II trial of gabapentin enacarbil for migraine prophylaxis. Cephalalgia. 2013;**33**(2):101–11.

24. **Mathew NT, Rapoport A, Saper J, et al.** Efficacy of gabapentin in migraine prophylaxis. Headache. 2001;**41**(2):119–28.

25. **Mohammadianinejad SE, Abbasi V, Sajedi SA, et al.** Zonisamide versus topiramate in migraine prophylaxis: a double-blind randomized clinical trial. Clin Neuropharmacol. 2011;**34**(4):174–77.

26. de Tommaso M, Guido M, Sardaro M, et al. Effects of topiramate and levetiracetam vs placebo on habituation of contingent negative variation in migraine patients. Neurosci Lett. 2008;**442**(2):81–85.

27. Beran RG, Spira PJ. Levetiracetam in chronic daily headache: a double-blind, randomised placebo-controlled study. (The Australian KEPPRA Headache Trial [AUS-KHT]). Cephalalgia. 2011;**31**(5):530–36.

28. Bogdanov VB, Multon S, Chauvel V, et al. Migraine preventive drugs differentially affect cortical spreading depression in rat. Neurobiol Dis. 2011;**41**(2):430–35.

29. Steiner TJ, Findley LJ, Yuen AW. Lamotrigine versus placebo in the prophylaxis of migraine with and without aura. Cephalalgia. 1997;**17**(2):109–12.

30. Siebenhofer A, Winterholer S, Jeitler K, et al. Long-term effects of weight-reducing drugs in people with hypertension. Cochrane Database Syst Rev. 2021;**1**:CD007654.

31. Gadde KM, Allison DB, Ryan DH, et al. Effects of low-dose, controlled-release, phentermine plus topiramate combination on weight and associated comorbidities in overweight and obese adults (CONQUER): a randomised, placebo-controlled, phase 3 trial. Lancet. 2011;**377**(9774):1341–52.

32. Siniscalchi A, Gallelli L, De Sarro G. Use of antiepileptic drugs for hyperkinetic movement disorders. Curr Neuropharmacol. 2010;**8**(4):359–66.

33. Zesiewicz TA, Elble R, Louis ED, et al. Practice parameter: therapies for essential tremor: report of the Quality Standards Subcommittee of the American Academy of Neurology. Neurology. 2005;**64**(12):2008–20.

34. Handforth A, Martin FC, Kang GA, Vanek Z. Zonisamide for essential tremor: an evaluator-blinded study. Mov Disord. 2009;**24**(3):437–40.

35. Bushara KO, Malik T, Exconde RE. The effect of levetiracetam on essential tremor. Neurology. 2005;**64**(6):1078–80.

36. Elble RJ, Lyons KE, Pahwa R. Levetiracetam is not effective for essential tremor. Clin Neuropharmacol. 2007;**30**(6):350–56.

37. Alemdar M, Iseri P, Selekler M, Komsuoglu SS. Levetiracetam-responding paroxysmal nonkinesigenic dyskinesia. Clin Neuropharmacol. 2007;**30**(4):241–44.

38. Woods SW, Saksa JR, Baker CB, Cohen SJ, Tek C. Effects of levetiracetam on tardive dyskinesia: a randomized, double-blind, placebo-controlled study. J Clin Psychiatry. 2008;**69**(4):546–54.

39. Tschopp L, Raina G, Salazar Z, Micheli F. Neuroacanthocytosis and carbamazepine responsive paroxysmal dyskinesias. Parkinsonism Relat Disord. 2008;**14**(5):440–42.

40. Genel F, Arslanoglu S, Uran N, Saylan B. Sydenham's chorea: clinical findings and comparison of the efficacies of sodium valproate and carbamazepine regimens. Brain Dev. 2002;**24**(2):73–76.

41. Vles GF, Hendriksen JG, Visschers A, Speth L, Nicolai J, Vles JS. Levetiracetam therapy for treatment of choreoathetosis in dyskinetic cerebral palsy. Dev Med Child Neurol. 2009;**51**(6):487–90.

42. Keswani SC, Kossoff EH, Krauss GL, Hagerty C. Amelioration of spinal myoclonus with levetiracetam. J Neurol Neurosurg Psychiatry. 2002;**73**(4):457–58.

43. Schauer R, Singer M, Saltuari L, Kofler M. Suppression of cortical myoclonus by levetiracetam. Mov Disord. 2002;**17**(2):411–15.

44. Siniscalchi A, Mancuso F, Russo E, Ibbadu GF, De Sarro G. Spinal myoclonus responsive to topiramate. Mov Disord. 2004;**19**(11):1380–81.

45. Christensen J, Vestergaard M, Mortensen PB, Sidenius P, Agerbo E. Epilepsy and risk of suicide: a population-based case-control study. Lancet Neurol. 2007;**6**(8):693–98.

46. Kaufman KR. Antiepileptic drugs in the treatment of psychiatric disorders. Epilepsy Behav. 2011;**21**(1):1–11.

47. Peselow ED, Clevenger S, IsHak WW. Prophylactic efficacy of lithium, valproic acid, and carbamazepine in the maintenance phase of bipolar disorder: a naturalistic study. Int Clin Psychopharmacol. 2016;**31**(4):218–23.

48. Leucht S, Helfer B, Dold M, Kissling W, McGrath J. Carbamazepine for schizophrenia. Cochrane Database Syst Rev. 2014;**5**:CD001258.

49. Jochim J, Rifkin-Zybutz RP, Geddes J, Cipriani A. Valproate for acute mania. Cochrane Database Syst Rev. 2019;**10**:CD004052.

50. Hosak L, Libiger J. Antiepileptic drugs in schizophrenia: a review. Eur Psychiatry. 2002;**17**(7):371–78.

51. Oya K, Sakuma K, Esumi S, et al. Efficacy and safety of lithium and lamotrigine for the maintenance treatment of clinically stable patients with bipolar disorder: a systematic review and meta-analysis of double-blind, randomized, placebo-controlled trials with an enrichment design. Neuropsychopharmacol Rep. 2019;**39**(3):241–46.

52. Calabrese JR, Suppes T, Bowden CL, et al. A double-blind, placebo-controlled, prophylaxis study of lamotrigine in rapid-cycling bipolar disorder. Lamictal 614 Study Group. J Clin Psychiatry. 2000;**61**(11):841–50.

53. Pariente G, Leibson T, Shulman T, Adams-Webber T, Barzilay E, Nulman I. Pregnancy outcomes following in utero exposure to lamotrigine: a systematic review and meta-analysis. CNS Drugs. 2017;**31**(6):439–50.

54. Slee A, Nazareth I, Bondaronek P, Liu Y, Cheng Z, Freemantle N. Pharmacological treatments for generalised anxiety disorder: a systematic review and network meta-analysis. Lancet. 2019;**393**(10173):768–77.

55. Generoso MB, Trevizol AP, Kasper S, Cho HJ, Cordeiro Q, Shiozawa P. Pregabalin for generalized anxiety disorder: an updated systematic review and meta-analysis. Int Clin Psychopharmacol. 2017;**32**(1):49–55.

56. Pigott K, Galizia I, Vasudev K, Watson S, Geddes J, Young AH. Topiramate for acute affective episodes in bipolar disorder in adults. Cochrane Database Syst Rev. 2016;**9**:CD003384.

57. Dauphinais D, Knable M, Rosenthal J, Polanski M, Rosenthal N. Zonisamide for bipolar depression: a randomized, double blind, placebo-controlled, adjunctive trial. Psychopharmacol Bull. 2011;**44**(2):73–84.

58. Gaitatzis A, Sisodiya SM, Sander JW. The somatic comorbidity of epilepsy: a weighty but often unrecognized burden. Epilepsia. 2012;**53**(8):1282–93.

59. Nizam A, Mylavarapu K, Thomas D, et al. Lacosamide-induced second-degree atrioventricular block in a patient with partial epilepsy. Epilepsia. 2011;**52**(10):e153–55.

60. Zaccara G, Lattanzi S. Comorbidity between epilepsy and cardiac arrhythmias: implication for treatment. Epilepsy Behav. 2019;**97**:304–12.

61. Aksakal E, Bakirci EM, Emet M, Uzkeser M. Complete atrioventricular block due to overdose of pregabalin. Am J Emerg Med. 2012;**30**(9):2101.e1–4.

62. Feldman AE, Gidal BE. QTc prolongation by antiepileptic drugs and the risk of torsade de pointes in patients with epilepsy. Epilepsy Behav. 2013;**26**(3):421–26.

63. Dixon R, Job S, Oliver R, et al. Lamotrigine does not prolong QTc in a thorough QT/QTc study in healthy subjects. Br J Clin Pharmacol. 2008;**66**(3):396–404.

64. Schimpf R, Veltmann C, Papavassiliu T, et al. Drug-induced QT-interval shortening following antiepileptic treatment with oral rufinamide. Heart Rhythm. 2012;**9**(5):776–81.

65. Kropeit D, Johnson M, Cawello W, Rudd GD, Horstmann R. Lacosamide cardiac safety: a thorough QT/QTc trial in healthy volunteers. Acta Neurol Scand. 2015;**132**(5):346–54.

66. Issa NP, Fisher WG, Narayanan JT. QT interval prolongation in a patient with LQT2 on levetiracetam. Seizure. 2015;**29**:134–36.

67. Hulhoven R, Rosillon D, Bridson WE, Meeus MA, Salas E, Stockis A. Effect of levetiracetam on cardiac repolarization in healthy subjects: a single-dose, randomized, placebo- and active-controlled, four-way crossover study. Clin Ther. 2008;**30**(2):260–70.

68. Harmer AR, Valentin JP, Pollard CE. On the relationship between block of the cardiac Na(+) channel and drug-induced prolongation of the QRS complex. Br J Pharmacol. 2011;**164**(2):260–73.

69. Mintzer S, Yi M, Hegarty S, Maio V, Keith S. Hyperlipidemia in patients newly treated with anticonvulsants: a population study. Epilepsia. 2020;**61**(2):259–66.

70. Eiris J, Novo-Rodriguez MI, Del Rio M, Meseguer P, Del Rio MC, Castro-Gago M. The effects on lipid and apolipoprotein serum levels of long-term carbamazepine, valproic acid and phenobarbital therapy in children with epilepsy. Epilepsy Res. 2000;**41**(1):1–7.

71. Mintzer S, Skidmore CT, Abidin CJ, et al. Effects of antiepileptic drugs on lipids, homocysteine, and C-reactive protein. Ann Neurol. 2009;**65**(4):448–56.

72. Chuang YC, Chuang HY, Lin TK, et al. Effects of long-term antiepileptic drug monotherapy on vascular risk factors and atherosclerosis. Epilepsia. 2012;**53**(1):120–28.

73. Hirsch LJ, Arif H, Nahm EA, Buchsbaum R, Resor SR Jr, Bazil CW. Cross-sensitivity of skin rashes with antiepileptic drug use. Neurology. 2008;**71**(19):1527–34.

74. Wu XT, Hong PW, Suolang DJ, Zhou D, Stefan H. Drug-induced hypersensitivity syndrome caused by valproic acid as a monotherapy for epilepsy: first case report in Asian population. Epilepsy Behav Case Rep. 2017;**8**:108–10.

75. Rashid M, Rajan AK, Chhabra M, Kashyap A. Levetiracetam and cutaneous adverse reactions: a systematic review of descriptive studies. Seizure. 2020;**75**:101–109.

76. Biton V, Gil-Nagel A, Isojarvi J, Doty P, Hebert D, Fountain NB. Safety and tolerability of lacosamide as adjunctive therapy for adults with partial-onset seizures: analysis of data pooled from three randomized, double-blind, placebo-controlled clinical trials. Epilepsy Behav. 2015;**52**(Pt A):119–27.

77. Chung WH, Hung SI, Hong HS, et al. Medical genetics: a marker for Stevens–Johnson syndrome. Nature. 2004;**428**(6982):486.

78. Shi YW, Min FL, Zhou D, et al. HLA-A*24:02 as a common risk factor for antiepileptic drug-induced cutaneous adverse reactions. Neurology. 2017;**88**(23):2183–91.

79. McCormack M, Alfirevic A, Bourgeois S, et al. HLA-A*3101 and carbamazepine-induced hypersensitivity reactions in Europeans. N Engl J Med. 2011;**364**(12):1134–43.

80. Fowler T, Bansal AS, Lozsadi D. Risks and management of antiepileptic drug induced skin reactions in the adult out-patient setting. Seizure. 2019;**72**:61–70.

81. **Russo MW, Galanko JA, Shrestha R, Fried MW, Watkins P.** Liver transplantation for acute liver failure from drug induced liver injury in the United States. Liver Transpl. 2004;**10**(8):1018–23.

82. **Vidaurre J, Gedela S, Yarosz S.** Antiepileptic drugs and liver disease. Pediatr Neurol. 2017;**77**:23–36.

83. **Rajakulendran S, Pitceathly RD, Taanman JW, et al.** A clinical, neuropathological and genetic study of homozygous A467T POLG-related mitochondrial disease. PLoS One. 2016;**11**(1):e0145500.

84. **Nicolai J, Carr RB.** The measurement of ammonia blood levels in patients taking valproic acid: looking for problems where they do not exist? Epilepsy Behav. 2008;**12**(3):494–96.

85. **Gokce S, Durmaz O, Celtik C, Aydogan A, Gulluoglu M, Sokucu S.** Valproic acid-associated vanishing bile duct syndrome. J Child Neurol. 2010;**25**(7):909–11.

86. **Pellock JM.** Felbamate in epilepsy therapy: evaluating the risks. Drug Saf. 1999;**21**(3):225–39.

87. **Solinas C, Vajda FJ.** Epilepsy and porphyria: new perspectives. J Clin Neurosci. 2004;**11**(4):356–61.

88. **Camfield PR, Bagnell P, Camfield CS, Tibbles JA.** Pancreatitis due to valproic acid. Lancet. 1979;**1**(8127):1198–99.

89. **Pellock JM, Wilder BJ, Deaton R, Sommerville KW.** Acute pancreatitis coincident with valproate use: a critical review. Epilepsia. 2002;**43**(11):1421–24.

90. **Norgaard M, Jacobsen J, Ratanajamit C, et al.** Valproic acid and risk of acute pancreatitis: a population-based case-control study. Am J Ther. 2006;**13**(2):113–17.

91. **Gerstner T, Busing D, Bell N, et al.** Valproic acid-induced pancreatitis: 16 new cases and a review of the literature. J Gastroenterol. 2007;**42**(1):39–48.

92. **Wolfe D, Kanji S, Yazdi F, et al.** Drug induced pancreatitis: a systematic review of case reports to determine potential drug associations. PLoS One. 2020;**15**(4):e0231883.

93. **Kumar R, Vidaurre J, Gedela S.** Valproic acid-induced coagulopathy. Pediatr Neurol. 2019;**98**:25–30.

94. **Bachmann T, Bertheussen KH, Svalheim S, et al.** Haematological side effects of antiepileptic drug treatment in patients with epilepsy. Acta Neurol Scand Suppl. 2011;**191**:23–27.

95. **Handoko KB, Souverein PC, van Staa TP, et al.** Risk of aplastic anemia in patients using antiepileptic drugs. Epilepsia. 2006;**47**(7):1232–36.

96. **Souverein PC, Webb DJ, Petri H, Weil J, Van Staa TP, Egberts T.** Incidence of fractures among epilepsy patients: a population-based retrospective cohort study in the General Practice Research Database. Epilepsia. 2005;**46**(2):304–10.

97. **Souverein PC, Webb DJ, Weil JG, Van Staa TP, Egberts AC.** Use of antiepileptic drugs and risk of fractures: case-control study among patients with epilepsy. Neurology. 2006;**66**(9):1318–24.

98. **Vestergaard P, Rejnmark L, Mosekilde L.** Fracture risk associated with use of antiepileptic drugs. Epilepsia. 2004;**45**(11):1330–37.

99. **Mahmoud SH, Zhou XY, Ahmed SN.** Managing the patient with epilepsy and renal impairment. Seizure. 2020;**76**:143–52.

100. **Lu X, Wang X.** Hyponatremia induced by antiepileptic drugs in patients with epilepsy. Expert Opin Drug Saf. 2017;**16**(1):77–87.

101. **Daudon M, Frochot V, Bazin D, Jungers P.** Drug-induced kidney stones and crystalline nephropathy: pathophysiology, prevention and treatment. Drugs. 2018;**78**(2):163–201.

102. **Maalouf NM, Langston JP, Van Ness PC, Moe OW, Sakhaee K.** Nephrolithiasis in topiramate users. Urol Res. 2011;**39**(4):303–307.

103. **Wroe S.** Zonisamide and renal calculi in patients with epilepsy: how big an issue? Curr Med Res Opin. 2007;**23**(8):1765–73.

104. **Chen B, Choi H, Hirsch LJ, et al.** Psychiatric and behavioral side effects of antiepileptic drugs in adults with epilepsy. Epilepsy Behav. 2017;**76**:24–31.

105. **Stephen LJ, Wishart A, Brodie MJ.** Psychiatric side effects and antiepileptic drugs: observations from prospective audits. Epilepsy Behav. 2017;**71**(Pt A):73–78.

106. **Hamed SA.** Psychiatric symptomatologies and disorders related to epilepsy and antiepileptic medications. Expert Opin Drug Saf. 2011;**10**(6):913–34.

107. **Jackson CF, Makin SM, Marson AG, Kerr M.** Pharmacological interventions for epilepsy in people with intellectual disabilities. Cochrane Database Syst Rev. 2015;**9**:CD005399.

108. **Huber B, Bommel W, Hauser I, et al.** Efficacy and tolerability of levetiracetam in patients with therapy-resistant epilepsy and learning disabilities. Seizure. 2004;**13**(3):168–75.

109. **Huber B.** [Effects of topiramate in patients with epilepsy and intellectual deficits]. Nervenarzt. 2002;**73**(6):525–32.

110. **Hansen CC, Ljung H, Brodtkorb E, Reimers A.** Mechanisms underlying aggressive behavior induced by antiepileptic drugs: focus on topiramate, levetiracetam, and perampanel. Behav Neurol. 2018;**2018**:2064027.

111. **Mula M, Trimble MR, Sander JW.** Psychiatric adverse events in patients with epilepsy and learning disabilities taking levetiracetam. Seizure. 2004;**13**(1):55–57.

112. **Huang CC, Wei IH.** Unexpected interaction between quetiapine and valproate in patients with bipolar disorder. Gen Hosp Psychiatry. 2010;**32**(4):446.e1–2.

113. **Shukla S, Godwin CD, Long LE, Miller MG.** Lithium-carbamazepine neurotoxicity and risk factors. Am J Psychiatry. 1984;**141**(12):1604–606.

114. **McGinness J, Kishimoto A, Hollister LE.** Avoiding neurotoxicity with lithium-carbamazepine combinations. Psychopharmacol Bull. 1990;**26**(2):181–84.

115. **Loscher W, Klein P.** The pharmacology and clinical efficacy of antiseizure medications: from bromide salts to cenobamate and beyond. CNS Drugs. 2021;**35**(9):935–63.

Chapter 4

The impact of surgery on comorbidities in epilepsy

Vejay N. Vakharia and Robert M. Brownstone

Introduction

As can be seen throughout this book, epilepsy is associated with wide-ranging neurological, neuropsychological, psychiatric, and social comorbidities. Surgery can provide sustained and durable seizure remission in people with drug-resistant focal epilepsy.[1] While early studies of epilepsy surgery focused on seizure outcome, it is equally important to consider the effects of surgery on these comorbidities.

The relationship of surgery to comorbidities in epilepsy is somewhat unique. On the one hand, surgery can cause comorbidities through its complications. And on the other hand, it can reduce comorbidities either directly through the elimination of seizures, or indirectly through, for example, the reduced requirement for medications.

The surgical armamentarium includes resective, ablative, disconnective, and neuromodulatory procedures.[2] Optimal outcomes are heavily dependent on patient selection, but in those with mesial temporal sclerosis, seizure-free rates at 2 years are as high as 85% following surgery compared to close to 0% with medical therapy; furthermore, these improvements are associated with significant enhancements in quality of life.[3]

To achieve seizure remission, the surgical aim is to resect, ablate, or disconnect the entire epileptogenic zone. In some situations, however, these goals may not be achievable without resultant neurological or neuropsychological sequelae. In these people, palliative procedures may be offered to reduce the seizure frequency, as the reduction in seizure frequency by surgical intervention has been found to improve the person's quality of life as well as reduce caregiver burden.[4]

Surgery carries risks that are more acute than those posed by medical therapies. These risks, which can lead to an increase in comorbidities, depend on the anatomical site of the surgical resection, ablation, or disconnection, and the chosen surgical intervention. An understanding of the functional cortical and subcortical anatomy is critical to avoiding associated comorbidities. Resective and ablative procedures return the greatest chance of achieving seizure remission, but also carry the greatest risks. To reduce postoperative morbidity and to predict positive outcomes, preoperative multidisciplinary team assessments are critical.[5]

In considering the effects of epilepsy surgery on comorbidities, we will focus on comorbidities with a causative relationship to surgery[6]: those in which surgery increases their prevalence or severity (e.g. surgical complications), and those in which surgery leads to their reduction. We will focus on non-tumour-related epilepsy, in particular on resections for temporal lobe epilepsy (TLE). We will also briefly examine frontal lobe and other epilepsies. In addition to discussing resections, we will address other forms of ablative surgery as well as neuromodulatory therapies such as deep brain stimulation (DBS) and vagus nerve stimulation (VNS).

Resective and ablative procedures

Mesial temporal lobe epilepsy

Mesial temporal lobe epilepsy (MTLE) is the most common drug-resistant focal epilepsy in adults, accounting for approximately 60% of cases; mesial temporal sclerosis is the most frequent histological finding.[7] Surgical resection or ablation has shown superior outcomes compared to medical therapy, and is associated with significant improvements in quality of life.[3] In contrast to these benefits, however, there can also be negative impacts on comorbidities: the neurological complications associated with mesial temporal lobe resections include visual field defects, cranial nerve injury (most commonly oculomotor and abducens nerve), and brainstem injury.[8] Furthermore, people can have deleterious psychological or psychiatric effects resulting from surgery. By contrast, some psychological manifestations may improve following resection.

Anatomical considerations

The goal of surgery for MTLE is to remove or disconnect the epileptogenic zone (typically hippocampus and amygdala), and prevent seizure propagation to other cortical or deep grey matter structures. The mesial temporal lobe structures are surrounded by several white matter fibre tracts critical for vision (optic radiation), language (inferior fronto-occipital fasciculus, middle longitudinal fasciculus, arcuate fasciculus, inferior longitudinal fasciculus, and uncinate fasciculus), and neuropsychological functions including memory (Figure 4.1). The outflow of the hippocampus is through the fimbria/fornix, a building block of the limbic system. The fimbria/fornix must be disconnected to prevent seizure propagation along the circuit of Papez, a critical brain pathway involved in memory and emotion. The proximity of these tracts to the hippocampus, however, puts them at risk for surgical harm that can cause complications (Table 4.1).[9-11] That is,

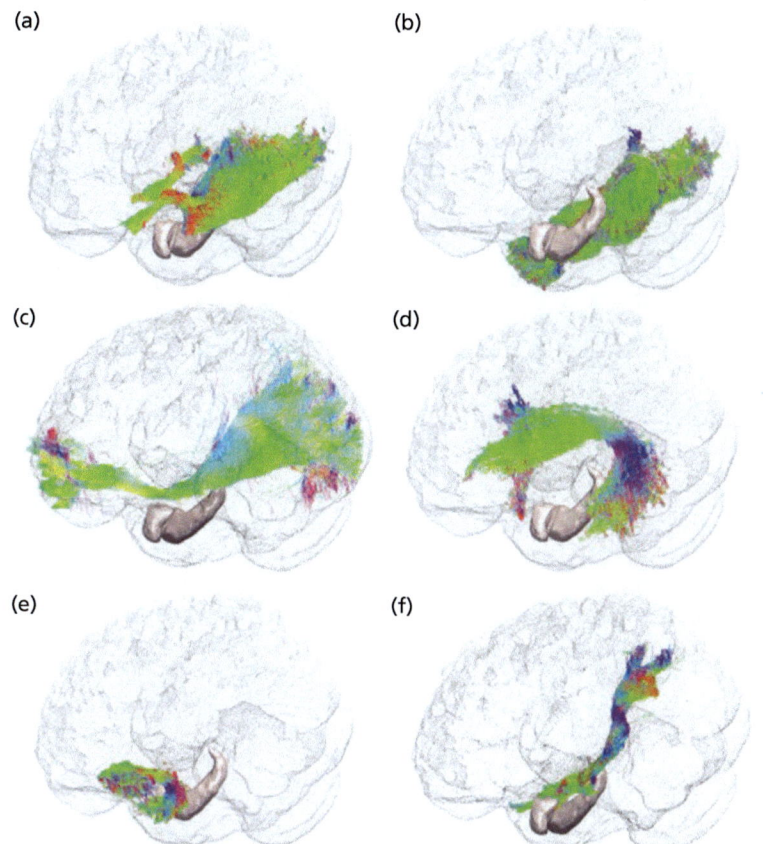

Figure 4.1 Tractographic reconstructions of the white fibre tracts in the dominant temporal lobe in relation to the amygdalohippocampal complex. Probabilistic tractography reconstructions with left–right fibre orientations shown in red, anterior–posterior in green, and superior–inferior in blue. Superior lateral view of the left hemisphere (transparent) depicting the amygdalohippocampal complex (solid). (a) The optic chiasm, optic tract, and optic radiation (Meyer's loop) fibre reconstructions, depicted as transversely orientated red fibres (arrow), can be seen overlying the hippocampus and thus are most likely to be damaged during transcortical and transsylvian approaches. (b) The inferior longitudinal fasciculus extends from the temporal pole to the occipital pole. The fibre tract runs below the amygdalohippocampal complex and would therefore be disrupted by surgical approaches from below, such as the subtemporal approach. (c) The inferior fronto-occipital fasciculus connects the frontal pole and orbitofrontal cortex with the parietal and occipital cortices. This fibre tract is thus at high risk in resections that pass more than 5 mm through the anterior temporal stem, such as the transsylvian approach. (d) The arcuate fasciculus extending between the frontal and temporal opercula. Resections through the middle or posterior portion of the superior temporal gyrus, such as the transcortical approach, may damage this fibre tract. (e) The uncinate fasciculus extends from the frontal pole and orbitofrontal cortices to the temporal pole. Resections transgressing the anterior temporal stem, such as the transsylvian approach, are associated with a risk of damage to this fibre tract. (f) The middle longitudinal fasciculus connects the superior temporal gyrus and the inferior parietal lobule. Surgical access through the middle or posterior portion of the superior temporal gyrus, such as the transcortical approach, may damage this fibre tract.

Table 4.1 Summary of white matter tracts at risk during temporal lobe resections

Tract	Function	Anatomy	Associated deficit	Surgical approach transgressing tract
Optic radiation (Figure 4.1a)	Vision	Between lateral geniculate nucleus and primary visual cortex	Contralateral superior homonymous quadrantanopia	ATLR Transcortical selective amygdalohippocampectomy
Inferior longitudinal fasciculus (Figure 4.1b)	Object recognition Parallel connectivity in the ventral language steam	Between the frontal and occipital lobes	Dysfunction of object recognition and discrimination[9]	Subtemporal selective amygdalohippocampectomy Supracerebellar transtentorial selective amygdalohippocampectomy
Inferior fronto-occipital fasciculus (Figure 4.1c)	Functional roles in the semantic aspects of language	Between frontal and parieto-occipital lobes passing through the temporal stem	Reduction in verbal fluency and naming resulting in semantic paraphasias[10]	Transsylvian selective amygdalohippocampectomy
Arcuate fasciculus (Figure 4.1d)	Functional roles in the phonemic aspects of language	Between frontal operculum and temporal opercula and posteroinferior temporal lobe via the inferior parietal lobule	Phenomic (sound) paraphasias Conduction aphasia	Transcortical selective amygdalohippocampectomy
Uncinate fasciculus (Figure 4.1e)	Social and emotional processing	Between frontal and temporal lobes	Changes in decision-making and behaviour[11]	ATLR Transsylvian selective amygdalohippocampectomy
Middle longitudinal fasciculus (Figure 4.1f)	Suggested roles in both semantic and phenomic language Multimodal visual-auditory integration	Between the temporal pole and inferior parietal lobule within the superior temporal gyrus	Not defined	Transcortical selective amygdalohippocampectomy involving the superior temporal gyrus ATLR

comorbidities can result from resection of the epileptogenic region of the brain, or from damaging nearby structures en route to the intended resection. It is thus crucial to understand these structures and the different surgical approaches designed to minimize their damage.

Surgical procedures

In MTLE, numerous surgical procedures have been described, including standardized and selective resections, and minimally invasive ablative procedures such as laser interstitial thermal therapy (LITT), radiofrequency ablation, and stereotactic radiosurgery (SRS).[12–14]

Compared to best medical therapy, anteromesial temporal lobe resections result in an absolute increase in seizure remission of 58%,[15] and with early surgical intervention (within 2 years of the onset of disabling seizures), this reduction increases to 85%.[3] Seizure remission rates are similar between standardized and selective approaches, but various modifications have been described to prevent disruption of the surrounding white fibre tracts and the resulting neurological and psychological comorbidities. Here, we first describe these different approaches to demonstrate how surrounding structures are implicated, and then discuss the related comorbidities (Figure 4.2).

Early descriptions of anterior mesial temporal lobe resections involved neocortical resections extending to approximately 4 cm from the temporal lobe tip in the dominant hemisphere and up to approximately 6 cm in the non-dominant hemisphere. The 4 cm limit was to prevent postoperative receptive language deficits. Neocortical resection facilitated direct access to the amygdalohippocampal complex, facilitating resection of the hippocampus to the level of the mesencephalic sulcus or tectal plate. As both knowledge and microsurgical techniques improved, the extent of lateral neocortical resection was commonly reduced to approximately 3.5 cm bilaterally. The amygdala could then be resected, allowing access to the temporal horn of the lateral ventricle.

To reduce neocortical resection even further, various selective approaches to the amygdalohippocampal complex were described. While these procedures may have had some theoretical advantages, a meta-analysis revealed that people undergoing selective approaches for amygdalohippocampectomies may be less likely to achieve seizure remission compared to anterior temporal lobe resections (ATLRs).[16,17] Some centres consider selective approaches may be associated with improved neuropsychological outcomes, but this remains contentious.[18]

Transcortical selective amygdalohippocampectomy approaches the temporal horn of the lateral ventricle through the middle temporal gyrus and in doing so transgresses the temporal white matter containing the optic radiation, arcuate

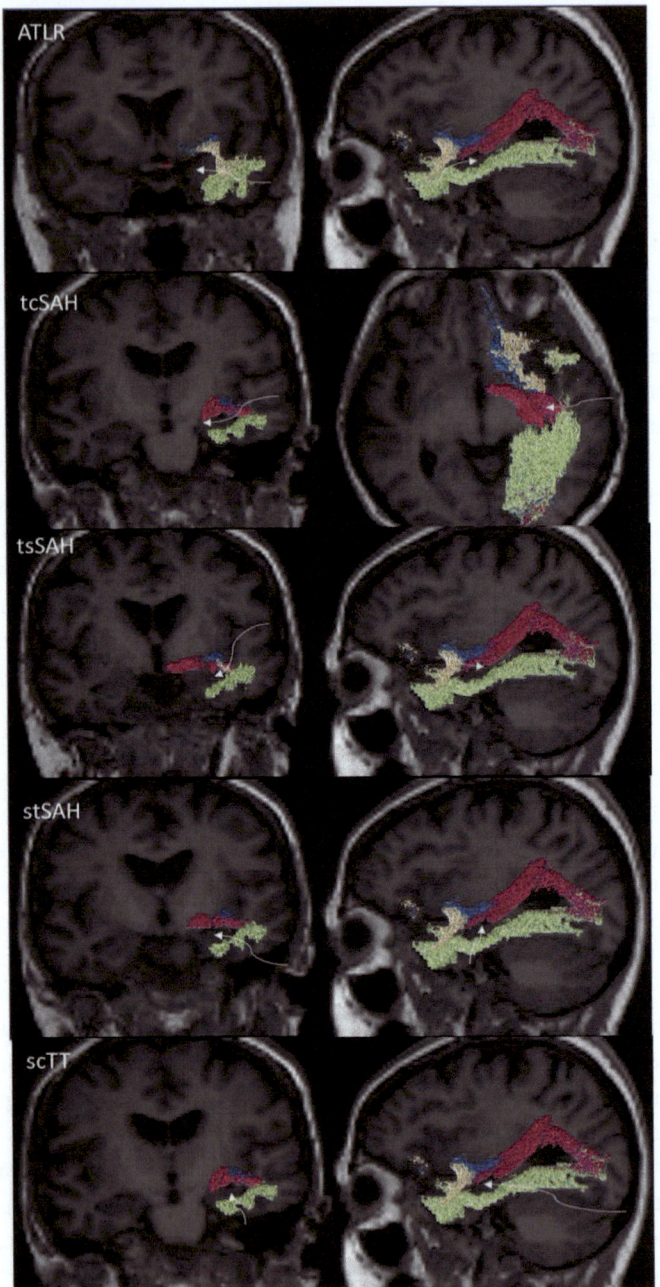

Figure 4.2 Coronal and sagittal T1 MRI sections with overlaid representations of the uncinate fasciculus (yellow), inferior fronto-occipital fasciculus (green), inferior fronto-occipital fasciculus (blue), and optic radiation (magenta). Different surgical approaches to the amygdalohippocampal complex are represented with a white arrow for the anterior temporal lobe resection (ATLR), transcortical (tcSAH), transsylvian (tsSAH), subtemporal (stSAH), and supracerebellar transtentorial (ssTT) selective amygdalohippocampectomies.

fasciculus, and inferior longitudinal fasciculus, but spares the inferior fronto-occipital fasciculus in the temporal stem.[19]

Transsylvian selective amygdalohippocampectomy involves access to the mesial temporal structures through the anterior-most aspect of the temporal stem,[20] typically through a 2 cm incision through the limen insulae.[20] The amygdala and hippocampus are then resected through the temporal horn of the lateral ventricle. The surgical corridor through the temporal stem requires frontal lobe retraction and risks transgression of the uncinate fasciculus, inferior fronto-occipital fasciculus, and optic radiation.[21] This approach has a comparatively higher rate of ischaemic complications due to manipulation of the middle cerebral artery branches in the Sylvian fissure. A prospective randomized controlled trial comparing transcortical and transsylvian selective amygdalohippocampectomy revealed no difference in seizure-free or cognitive outcomes.[18] The transsylvian approach, however, resulted in worse postoperative phenomic fluency which may result from damage to both the uncinate and inferior fronto-occipital fasciculus, or from cortical injury secondary to frontal lobe retraction.

To reduce the need for both temporal neocortical and temporal stem resections, subtemporal[22] and supracerebellar transtentorial selective amygdalohippocampectomy approaches were described.[23] Both approaches involve resecting the amygdala and hippocampus from the underside of the temporal lobe while sparing the structures at risk in the transcortical and transsylvian approaches. These approaches transgress the inferior longitudinal fasciculus (Figure 4.2), which may result in impairments of object discrimination and recognition.[24]

The main limitation of the subtemporal approach is the potential retraction injury during the elevation of the temporal lobe and subsequent limitations imposed by bridging veins.[25] The supracerebellar approach involves a posterior fossa craniectomy and transtentorial approach to the mesial temporal lobe, which is technically demanding due to the long operative working distances. The approach, however, does allow access to the mesial temporal lobe structures without significant retraction. It has also been shown to prevent postoperative visual field deficits.[26]

Another way to minimize white matter tract disruption is via minimally invasive techniques, such as radiofrequency ablation or SRS.

Stereotactic radiofrequency ablation is a technique that is now rarely used as isolated primary procedure.[27] Historically, electric current was passed to heat the tip of the electrode and thus generate a thermal lesion.[28] In contemporary practice, this is most commonly performed following stereoelectroencephalography recordings where current is passed between the electrode contacts in an attempt to disrupt the ictal network. While the likelihood of this technique resulting in long-term seizure freedom is low,[17] transient reductions in seizure freedom are predictive of improved seizure freedom following subsequent resective surgery.[29]

SRS for MTLE involves the delivery of focused radiation to the amygdala, anterior 2 cm of the hippocampus, and adjacent parahippocampal gyrus. The efficacy of SRS for the treatment of MTLE in people with hippocampal sclerosis was assessed in a recently published randomized controlled radiosurgery versus open surgery for mesial temporal lobe epilepsy (ROSE) trial.[12] Seizure remission was reported in 52% (16/31) of people following SRS, compared to 78% (21/27) after ATLR. The onset of effectiveness following SRS was also delayed by up to 2–3 years following surgery.

LITT is a novel minimally invasive ablative therapy where a 1.65 mm laser fibre and cooling catheter are inserted through a small (3.2 mm) burr hole. The trajectory is critical to achieve seizure remission and aims to ablate the length of the amygdalohippocampal complex, while minimizing collateral damage to surrounding white matter fibre tracts.[30,31] Studies have shown that failure to ablate the mesial hippocampal head may be related to poorer seizure-free outcome.[32] Simulation studies recommend an optimal entry point at the confluence of the middle temporal, inferior, and middle occipital gyri and an optimal target point at the anterior and mesial border of the amygdala.[33] Seizure remission rates have been reported to be approximately 58% at 24 months.[14]

Complications and comorbidities

Following temporal lobe surgery for epilepsy, there can be improvement or deterioration in comorbidities (Table 4.2).

Visual field defects

Studies have reported that every 1 mm of Meyer's loop that is transgressed during surgery corresponds to a 5-degree loss in the opposite upper outer quadrant of the visual field.[34] Surgical series of ATLRs have shown that the risk of developing a postoperative visual field defect is 3.5 times higher with left-sided compared to right-sided resections,[35] which corresponds to magnetic resonance imaging (MRI) studies that have revealed that Meyer's loop extends more anteriorly in the language dominant hemisphere.[36]

Historically, ATLRs were carried posteriorly to 4 cm in the language-dominant and 6 cm in the non-language-dominant hemispheres.[37] The subsequent contralateral superior temporal quadrantanopia was considered an expected complication. Selective approaches, such as transcortical[38] and transsylvian selective amygdalohippocampectomy,[20] also led to similar rates of visual field defects. As the proportion of people achieving seizure remission

Table 4.2 Differential effects of left and right temporal lobe surgery on postoperative comorbidities

Comorbidities	Overall	Left TLE	Right TLE
Visual field defects	Overall risk ranges from 4% to 13% with anterior temporal lobectomy and 33% to 88% with selective approaches. The supracerebellar transtentorial approach and use of intraoperative MRI with anterior temporal lobectomy have been reported to prevent significant visual field defects	3.5-fold higher relative risk of significant visual field defect following surgery due to anterior projection of Meyer's loop in the language-dominant hemisphere	
Cranial neuropathies	Most series report rates of <1%. Higher rates of transient oculomotor nerve palsy were reported following transcisternal modifications of the transsylvian approach	No difference in rates between left and right TLE	
Language defects	Verbal fluency remains stable or improves in the majority of patients Bilateral hemispheric language activations during functional MRI studies are associated with improved outcomes Improvements were greater following transcortical compared to transsylvian approaches; independent of seizure remission SRS does not have any lateralizing effects on naming function	Associated with higher rates of decline in verbal fluency and naming function following surgery Improved phenomic and semantic fluency outcomes reported following transsylvian approaches	Improved phenomic and semantic fluency outcomes reported following subtemporal approaches
Neuropsychology	Outcomes are based on the duration of epilepsy, seizure burden, preoperative functioning, and drug side effects Memory function is affected by antiepileptic drugs, which may be weaned following successful surgery No difference in outcome reported between transcortical and transsylvian approach	Verbal memory decline Improved memory outcomes reported following ATLRs	Non-verbal memory decline Improved memory outcomes reported following transsylvian approaches
Psychiatric outcomes	Following successful surgery, depression rates fall to those of the unaffected population Paranoia has been reported to be lower following the transcortical approach	Associated with higher rates of anxiety	Slightly higher rates of depression

increased, it became more evident that those undergoing neocortical resections to these posterior extents were subsequently disqualified from driving—thus obviating one common goal of surgery—owing to the degree of visual loss.[39] In most countries, driving authorities stipulate that the field of vision along the horizontal meridian should subtend an angle of at least 120 degrees and there should be no defects present within a radius of the central 30 degrees.[40]

Limiting the lateral neocortical resection to less than 3.5 cm has been reported to reduce the incidence of field deficits that preclude driving to 4–13%.[35] A single study of 21 people describing the use of intraoperative MRI with continuous tractography overlays projected onto the surgical field reported no visual field deficits that could preclude driving.[41] In the same study, the use of brain shift correction through the use of intraoperative MRI was shown to reduce the incidence of small visual field deficits from 89% to 67%. Each of these defects were asymptomatic, so the clinical utility of this has yet to be proven.

Selective approaches still have high rates of visual field deficits, with one study reporting a rate of 89% (16/18) following a transcortical approach,[42] while with transsylvian selective amygdalohippocampectomy, rates of visual field deficit range widely from 37% to 88%.[43,44] A randomized controlled trial comparing transsylvian and subtemporal approaches resulted in 33% and 66% of patients who achieved seizure remission being eligible to apply for a driving licence.[44] Modifications of the transsylvian approach, such as transsylvian-transcisternal approaches, have been described to limit the transgression of the temporal stem to 5 mm, but this is technically more demanding, limits the posterior extent of the hippocampal resection, and has a high rate of double vision (due to transient oculomotor nerve palsies).[45]

Regarding minimally invasive techniques, the ROSE trial (see above) reported visual field deficits in 88% of people undergoing SRS, but driving eligibility was not formally assessed. Based on the extent of central field involvement reported, it is likely that the visual field deficit was sufficiently severe to affect driving in one-quarter of patients.[46] Visual field deficit rates from early series of LITT range from 5% to 20%[47,48] and have been ascribed to either heat dissipating across the choroidal fissure to the lateral geniculate nucleus or damage to the optic radiation during posterior hippocampal ablation.[49] In summary, visual field deficits remain a significant comorbidity that can directly result from surgery, whether resective (ATLR or selective), or ablative.

Cranial nerve injury

Damage to cranial nerves following temporal lobe surgery ranges from 0.3% to 14%,[45,50,51] with deficits in the majority of cases being transient. Cranial nerve palsies are restricted to the oculomotor and trochlear nerves. The oculomotor nerve exits the midbrain in the interpeduncular cistern and runs medial to the free edge of the tentorium. Resection of the mesial temporal structures that violate the pial boundaries may lead to nerve injury. Similarly, transcisternal modifications of the transsylvian amygdalohippocampectomy utilize a transuncal resection of the amygdala to facilitate hippocampectomy and, therefore, result in higher rates of oculomotor nerve paresis.[45] The trochlear nerve exits the midbrain posteriorly under the inferior colliculus running through the ambient cistern to lie under the free end of the tentorium. Damage to these nerves results in double vision.

Language deficits

Preoperative nomograms have been developed to predict the extent of naming decline following temporal lobe surgery, and reveal that the most important prognostic factors include older age at seizure onset and left hemisphere resections. Other factors include higher levels of education, older age at surgery, and female sex.

Functional MRI analyses have revealed that frontotemporal connectivity on the same side of surgery decreases following both right and left mesial temporal resections; these declines are associated with deficits in verbal fluency and naming function. Over 40% of people undergoing left ATLR have a decline in naming compared to 5% with right-sided resection.[52] The mechanism underlying naming dysfunction is thought to be associated with the temporal pole and superior temporal gyrus.[53] Right or bilateral hemispheric language representation reduced the postoperative decline in verbal fluency and naming in surgery for left MTLE. Similarly, in people with right MTLE, left hemispheric dominance correlated with retained verbal fluency and naming postoperatively, highlighting the importance of the dominant temporal lobe for naming.[54]

Diffusion imaging has also been used to correlate white matter fibre tract demyelination with neuropsychological outcomes postoperatively. Compared to those with right MTLE, individuals with left MTLE had more extensive demyelination preoperatively affecting more bilateral fibre tracts.[55] Conversely, postoperative changes in white matter structure were found in the contralateral uncinate fasciculus and superior longitudinal fasciculus following left compared to right ATLR. These correlated with improved phonemic fluency postoperatively (i.e. the ability to generate words starting with a specific letter). This suggests plasticity in the contralateral language function.[55]

A comparative study of subtemporal and transsylvian approaches revealed that fluency was best preserved following a transsylvian approach in the left hemisphere and subtemporal amygdalohippocampectomy in the right hemisphere.[56] This is most likely due to preservation of the lateral temporal neocortex and dorsal language streams in the language-dominant hermisphere.[57]

Similarly, with regard to semantic fluency (i.e. the ability to name objects), improved outcomes were found when transsylvian approaches were undertaken in the left hemisphere. A left subtemporal selective amygdalohippocampectomy carried a sixfold higher risk of decline in semantic fluency compared to the transsylvian approach. These findings may be explained by the associated transgression of the inferior longitudinal fasciculus and the fusiform gyrus, which represent the basal temporal language areas.[58-60]

Studies comparing the transcortical and transsylvian approaches have revealed postoperative improvement in verbal fluency in 30% of people undergoing transcortical selective amygdalohippocampectomy compared to 5% with transsylvian selective amygdalohippocampectomy—these results were independent of seizure remission.[18] Verbal fluency tasks are considered a test of executive processing requiring frontal lobe function. The transsylvian approach requires retraction of the frontal lobe as well as transection of the inferior fronto-occipital fasciculus, both of which are spared with transcortical amygdalohippocampectomy. Studies have also shown that the extent of collateral damage following transsylvian selective amygdalohippocampectomy are more extensive than expected.[61]

Studies of language outcomes following SRS report no change in naming function following treatment for right or left MTLE.[62]

Neuropsychological comorbidities

Epilepsy affects cognition, learning, and memory (see Chapters 5 and 12). The severity of deficits is dependent on the localization and lateralization of the ictal network, duration of epilepsy, seizure burden, psychiatric comorbidities, and drug side effects. In addition to language deficits, dominant temporal lobe dysfunction is associated with verbal memory decline while seizure onset in the non-dominant temporal lobe typically affects non-verbal memory. TLE primarily affects declarative memory (the recall of facts and events), while the learning of procedural tasks (learning complex movements) remains mostly unaffected. Additionally, lateral temporal neocortical dysfunction is associated with impaired learning while mesial temporal pathologies affect long-term memory and recall.[63] Antiseizure medications also have significant effects on memory through influences on cognition and attention. Overall, people with epilepsy have similar memory function to healthy people who are 20 years older.[64]

Epilepsy surgery results in a decline in memory in 30–40% of people. Individuals with good preoperative neuropsychological function are most vulnerable to memory deficits resulting from epilepsy surgery, and these deficits are compounded if they fail to achieve seizure remission.

While several studies have compared the differential effect of the varied surgical approaches on memory, the results are not consistent, leaving the question of optimal approach unresolved. While not definitive, comparative results are presented in Table 4.3.[65–68]

The neuropsychological outcomes following SRS are similar to open surgery.[62] In comparison to open ATLRs, however, LITT has been reported to reduce the postoperative decline in recognizing famous faces and common nouns in the dominant hemisphere, and famous faces alone in the non-dominant hemisphere.[69] This may be due to the sparing of the temporal pole and inferior longitudinal fasciculus.

In summary, the neuropsychological comorbidities following mesial temporal resections include verbal and non-verbal memory deficits and are dependent on whether the resection is in the dominant or non-dominant hemisphere. The lateral neocortex is important for short-term memory, while the hippocampus is critical for consolidation into long-term memory. The key predicative factor is the person's preoperative function. There is currently no consensus regarding the optimal surgical approach for memory preservation. Studies have suggested that selective approaches that transgress the temporal

Table 4.3 Comparison of reported neuropsychological outcomes between anterior temporal lobe resections and selective approaches

	Right	**Left**
Anterior temporal lobe resection	Decline in non-verbal memory	Decline in verbal memory
Transsylvian	Less non-verbal memory decline compared to ATLR[65] Improvement in delayed recall compared to ATLR Worse immediate recall and recognition compared to ATLR	Worse verbal memory outcomes compared to ATLR[65] Greater decline in word recognition compared to ATLR Improved immediate recall compared to ATLR[66]
Transcortical	No difference in verbal memory, IQ, or attention compared to ATLR[67] No difference in cognitive and memory outcomes compared to transsylvian approach[18]	
Subtemporal	Postoperative improvement in verbal IQ, performance IQ, and full-scale IQ[68]	

stem, such as the transsylvian approach, may result in greater memory decline when performed in the dominant hemisphere. High-functioning individuals preoperatively, are most likely to suffer from greater postoperative decline irrespective of the laterality or approach taken.[64]

Psychiatric comorbidities

Preoperative psychiatric comorbidities are common in people with both temporal and extratemporal epilepsy and include depression, anxiety disorders, personality disorders, substance abuse, and a 'schizophrenia-like' psychosis (see Chapter 6).[70] The baseline rates of depression in people with epilepsy are estimated to be between 35% and 65% with a trend towards a slightly higher predominance in individuals with right TLE. In contrast, preoperative anxiety was more common in people with left TLE, with an overall prevalence of 48%.[71]

The severity of psychiatric symptoms as a whole was found to be lower 6 months following surgery, with psychiatric diagnoses resolving entirely in around 15% of people undergoing temporal lobe resections.[71] Specifically, depression rates have been shown to fall postoperatively.[72]

De novo onset of depression, assessed 2 years postoperatively, was reported to occur in around 6% of patients, and was associated with ongoing seizure activity. People with a previous history of psychiatric comorbidities, even if not active in the 6 months before surgery, were at risk of psychiatric complications following surgery, with peak onset in the first 1–4 weeks.[73]

A prospective control study compared depression and anxiety in people with MTLE who underwent presurgical evaluation at a single centre.[74] Eighty per cent (76/94) chose to undergo surgery (46/76 transsylvian approach, 11/76 anterior temporal resection, and 19/76 extended temporal lesionectomy) compared to the remaining 20% (18/96) who opted to continue with best medical management. The selection between surgery and medical management was based on individual choice rather than suitability for surgery, consequently minimizing selection bias. Preoperatively, incidence and severity of depression were not significantly different between the groups. Postoperatively, however, the depression rate in those undergoing surgery had fallen to what would be expected in a healthy control population, whereas in the medically treated group depression rates continued to be significantly elevated. The improvement in depression was found to correlate with the degree of seizure improvement and not with changes in antidepressant medications. People with worse Beck Depression Inventory scores preoperatively achieved the greatest improvements in their symptoms. Other predictive factors for depression and anxiety include worse baseline cognitive measures of frontal lobe dysfunction.[75] Conversely, there was no difference between the two groups in postoperative anxiety levels. Overall, anxiety appeared to be more refractory to surgery compared to depression, with some studies also reporting a correlation with ongoing seizure activity.[72]

Despite the improvements seen in depression, suicidality appears refractory to surgical intervention. A meta-analysis of suicidality in people with epilepsy found a 3.3-fold higher rate compared to the average population, which rises to 6.6-fold in those with TLE and 13.9-fold following temporal lobe resections.[76] This finding may be related to the increased prevalence of psychosis and behavioural changes seen in MTLE, which is at risk of increasing after surgery. It should be noted, however, that this rate is heavily outweighed by a reduction in all-cause mortality following surgery.[77]

A longitudinal series of postoperative people with hippocampal sclerosis undergoing anterior temporal resections with a 6-year follow-up period revealed that the incidence of preoperative anxiety and personality disorders correlated with Engel outcome 1B (persisting auras).[78] The implication of this is that the persistent aura arises from parts of the epileptogenic zone outside of the temporal lobe, such as 'temporal-plus' areas including the orbitofrontal, mesial frontal, and anterior insular regions.[79]

De novo 'schizophrenia-like' psychosis is rare following surgery, with an incidence of new-onset psychosis estimated to be 1–3%[70,73] in those undergoing anterior temporal lobectomy. The onset of *de novo* psychosis was not related to seizure remission rates. Preoperative risk factors for *de novo* psychosis following temporal lobe surgery included bilateral electroencephalogram (EEG) abnormalities, a small-volume contralateral amygdala, and non-mesial temporal sclerosis diagnosis.[70]

A comparison of the neuropsychiatric outcomes revealed a lower rate of postoperative paranoia in the transcortical amygdalohippocampectomy group compared to the ATLR group,[67] which may be due to sparing of the uncinate fasciculus.[11] Damage to the uncinate fasciculus has been associated with psychiatric sequelae including schizotypal traits.[80] Minimally invasive techniques, such as LITT when performed through an occipital entry point, also tend to spare the uncinate fasciculus more than conventional surgical approaches. Further clinical studies are needed, however, to determine if these techniques are associated with lower rates or degrees of neuropsychiatric morbidity.

In summary, worsening neuropsychiatric comorbidities are relatively rare following resective surgery. Preoperative psychiatric evaluation is essential to predict and treat psychiatric relapse. Higher rates and severity of depression are associated with failure to achieve seizure remission. Postoperative paranoia may be related to damage to the uncinate fasciculus, but further studies are needed to confirm this correlation.

Frontal lobe epilepsy

The frontal lobe is the second most common focus of focal epilepsy, accounting for up to 30% of cases.[81] Unlike MTLE, frontal lobe epilepsies are typically less well localized anatomically and involve a larger ictal network. The consequence is that postoperative seizure remission rates are lower than in TLE, being approximately 45%. In addition, there is less long-term durability, with most relapses occurring within the first year.[82] As in all epilepsies, defining the epileptogenic zone is crucial, but can be more challenging in frontal lobe epilepsy. The epileptogenic zone is often more extensive than the epileptogenic lesion identified on MRI; an invasive stereoelectroencephalography (SEEG) investigation can lead to better definition and thus guide tailored resections that lead to improved seizure remission rates.[83] Furthermore, bilateral SEEG implantations may be required due to the widespread ictal network and rapid propagation to the contralateral frontal lobe. Of note, even in the absence of an MRI lesion, SEEG can delineate the seizure onset; in these cases, histological analysis identifies an underlying focal cortical dysplasia in around 40% of cases.[84]

The dominant frontal lobe subserves language, motor, cognitive, and executive functions. The neural circuits underlying these functions are complex and incompletely understood, but key white matter fibre tracts include the superior longitudinal fasciculi I–III, inferior fronto-occipital fasciculus, uncinate fasciculus, arcuate fasciculus, frontal tract of Aslant, cingulum bundle, and motor corticofugal (including corticospinal) tracts.[85] The superior longitudinal fasciculi I–III are long-association fibre tracts found deep to the superior, middle, and inferior frontal gyri, respectively, connecting the frontal lobe to the parietal, occipital, and temporal lobes. The frontal tract of Aslant connects the supplementary motor area to the ventral premotor cortex and to the pars opercularis and triangularis (Broca's area) of the inferior frontal gyrus, with a role in speech generation. The corticofugal tracts emanating from the motor cortex play an important role in motor control.

Resections, particularly in the dominant frontal lobe, are therefore bound by these functionally relevant subcortical fibre tracts with the degree of postoperative neurological and neuropsychological deficits being inversely dependent on their preservation.[86] When affected, postoperative complications can include hemiparesis, dysphasia, psychosis, cognitive decline, and personality change. The roles of these fibre tracts in the non-dominant hemisphere are less well known, but in general, their preservation is thought to be important to maintain postoperative neuropsychological function.[87]

A series of individuals undergoing resections of the supplementary motor area revealed that 90% of people had a transient neurological deficit (weakness and/or speech impairment) immediately following surgery, the extent of which correlated with the size of resection. In this series, the neurological deficit recovered in all cases except for a decline in fine dexterity during complex motor tasks involving the contralateral upper limb.[88] Also, people with greater cognitive and intellectual abilities preoperatively, in the absence of focal cortical dysplasia, were more likely to suffer from decline. Improvements in non-verbal intelligence and memory were associated with seizure remission rates, even when controlling for drug reduction.[89]

Insular lobe epilepsy

The insular lobe is less commonly recognized as the primary ictal onset zone but is often associated in the ictal network of seizures arising in adjacent brain regions. The symptomatogenic features of spread to the insula include throat tightening, somatic pain, dysphagia, and autonomic manifestations.[90] Due to its deep location, scalp EEG has limited sensitivity in localizing insular onset, and SEEG studies are usually required. Depending on the location of the epileptogenic zone and involvement of the frontal or parietal operculum, surgical approaches may be transsylvian, transopercular, or increasingly through LITT.[91] Seizure remission rates following insular resections are reported to be between 60% and 70%.[91] Due to the proximity of insular perforating vessels to the internal capsule, some series report transient hemiparesis rates of around 50%.[92] Studies reporting neuropsychological outcomes in individuals undergoing insular resections are limited, but findings suggest that there are minimal changes, with one study reporting a decline in colour naming, suggesting a deficit in oromotor speed and lexical access.[93]

Parietal lobe epilepsy

Parietal lobe epilepsies are rarer entities and account for only 2–6% of surgical cases.[94] Diagnosis can be particularly challenging as parietal lobe epilepsies tend to be clinically 'silent', producing semiological features only when they spread to adjacent cortical regions such as the frontal or temporal lobes, causing hypermotor signs and automatisms, or auditory hallucinations, respectively. Nevertheless, early semiological features of sensory disturbances, complex visual hallucinations, disturbances of body image, vertigo, and language dysfunction may point to the parietal lobe, which is vital for higher-order sensory perception and integration. Scalp EEG findings are poorly localized and invasive EEG investigations are usually required.[95] The presence of an MRI lesion correlated well with outcome, with postoperative seizure remission rates reported to be 45–78%.[94]

Subcortical fibre tracts include the superior longitudinal fasciculus I–III tracts, arcuate fasciculus, inferior fronto-occipital fasciculus, and U-fibres connecting adjacent gyri such as the supramarginal and angular gyri to temporal and occipital regions. The dominant inferior parietal lobule is commonly termed Geschwind's territory and has important roles in language, mathematical operations, and body image.[96] Resections in the parietal lobe have not been found to cause impairments in general cognition but may lead to deficits in visuospatial and visual perception tasks. In one series, half of the patients were found to have visual field deficits (mainly hemianopia) due to disruption of the optic radiation.[97]

Occipital lobe epilepsy

Occipital lobe epilepsy is another rare entity. Semiologically, occipital involvement results in visual auras, visual hallucinations, blindness, mental state disturbances, and more frequent secondary generalization. Scalp EEG tends to reveal interictal spike discharges in the temporal lobe, most likely due to propagation along fibre tracts such as the inferior longitudinal fasciculus.[98] Seizure remission rates vary widely and are dependent on the presence of an MRI lesion and the underlying histological substrate.[99] Resections involving the occipital lobe are almost uniformly associated with visual field defects due to the proximity to the primary visual cortex and optic radiations. Language deficits and visual neglect may also be seen.

Disconnective procedures

Disconnective procedures are palliative procedures that are undertaken when the region of seizure onset is too extensive for resection but still confined to a single hemisphere or quadrant. These are considered palliative procedures as the chance of achieving seizure remission rates is low. These procedures aim to prevent secondary generalization or disabling drop attacks.

Corpus callosotomy

Corpus callosotomy is a procedure in which the major commissural fibre pathway between the two hemispheres is disconnected. Corpus callosotomy is most commonly undertaken for Lennox–Gastaut syndrome, which is associated with debilitating drop attacks and commonly results in severe injuries. Callosotomies are traditionally performed through a midline craniotomy

and interhemispheric disconnection, although endoscopic and laser ablation techniques have also been described.[100] Differences in surgical practices
range from performing anterior two-thirds, posterior one-third, or complete
callosotomies.[101]

A debilitating complication associated with corpus callosotomy is disconnection syndromes. Although rarely seen with anterior two-thirds disconnections, these syndromes have been reported in 12% of complete callosotomies.
Other complications include mutism and urinary incontinence; these are usually transient.[102] In adults, an anterior two-thirds callosotomy is performed as
an initial procedure, with a completion callosotomy performed only if drop
attacks remain. In contrast, a complete callosotomy is typically performed in
children as case series report worthwhile seizure reduction in 33% of anterior
two-thirds disconnections compared to 82% following total callosotomy.[103]
Children undergoing callosotomy are able to perform as well as their peers in
cognitive tasks suggesting that under the age of 12 years, neuroplasticity allows
for compensatory mechanisms.

Hemispherotomy

Functional hemispherotomies are performed to completely disconnect the
cerebral hemispheres. The most common indications include Rasmussen's encephalitis, hemimegalencephaly, Sturge–Weber syndrome, hemiconvulsion-
hemiplegia epilepsy, and large perinatal strokes.[104] Historically,
procedures involved hemispherectomy, but high rates of hydrocephalus
and haemosiderosis led to the development of hemispherotomy techniques.
Transventricular and transsylvian approaches as well as endoscopic techniques have also been described.[105] In addition to a corpus callosotomy,
frontobasal, subinsular, hippocampal, and suprasylvian disconnections are
also performed. Hemispherotomy can be very effective in these patients, resulting in seizure remission rates of up to 90%. Postoperative outcomes are
better when performed in younger patients.[106] Homonymous hemianopia
and hemiparesis are expected complications, but most patients who are ambulatory before surgery remain so, albeit often with the aid of ankle orthoses
as a result of limitations in ankle dorsiflexion. In younger people, language
function tends to reorganize to the contralateral hemisphere, but fine dexterity in the contralateral upper limb remains impaired. Long-term studies
of cognitive outcomes following hemispherotomy showed an intellectual recovery in approximately 75%, highlighting the detrimental effect of the ongoing seizure burden.

Neuromodulation

Neuromodulation procedures involve the implantation of electrodes connected to a pulse generator (pacemaker) to provide constant, intermittent, or on-demand stimulation to nerves or brain regions to modulate seizure activity. These procedures are an alternative to disconnection procedures, and in contrast to the above-mentioned procedures, are also sometimes performed for generalized epilepsies.

Vagus nerve stimulation

VNS is an extracranial procedure. The vagus nerve is identified within the carotid sheath through a left transverse neck incision. Electrodes are then deployed around the nerve and connected to an implantable pulse generator, which is usually sited on the anterior chest wall. Despite over 30 years of human use, the mechanisms of action of VNS are poorly understood.[101] Seizure reduction rates have been found to increase with duration of use. The left vagus nerve is preferentially stimulated to avoid cardiac side effects, such as bradycardia or, rarely, asystole. Other side effects include cough and abnormal throat sensations, which may be attributable to stimulation spread to the superior laryngeal nerve, as well as hoarse voice and shortness of breath. In a series of people with epilepsy who failed frontal or temporal lobe resections, VNS was shown to have positive psychotropic effects in patients with postictal psychosis, depression, and behavioural disorders beyond that expected from reduction in seizure frequency alone. Overall, VNS has a low complication rate and may, in time, reduce seizure frequency by greater than 50% in more than 50% of patients.[109]

Deep brain stimulation

DBS involves the modulation of neural circuits through electrodes stereotactically implanted in target nuclei and connected to implanted pulse generators. Unlike resective or ablative techniques, the effects are reversible and can be titrated by adjusting stimulation parameters. DBS is most commonly performed for movement disorders, but has been used for a range of psychiatric and neurological conditions, including drug-resistant epilepsy. The two most common implantation targets for epilepsy include the anterior nucleus of the thalamus (ANT) and the centromedian nucleus of the thalamus. A third, less common target is the hippocampus, which is now reserved for cases of bilateral hippocampal seizure onset[110] (Figure 4.3).

The ANT is a key component of the circuit of Papez with afferent connections from the fornix/mammillary bodies and efferent connections to cingulate cortices. The stimulation of the ANT for epilepsy (SANTE) double-blinded

(a)   (b)

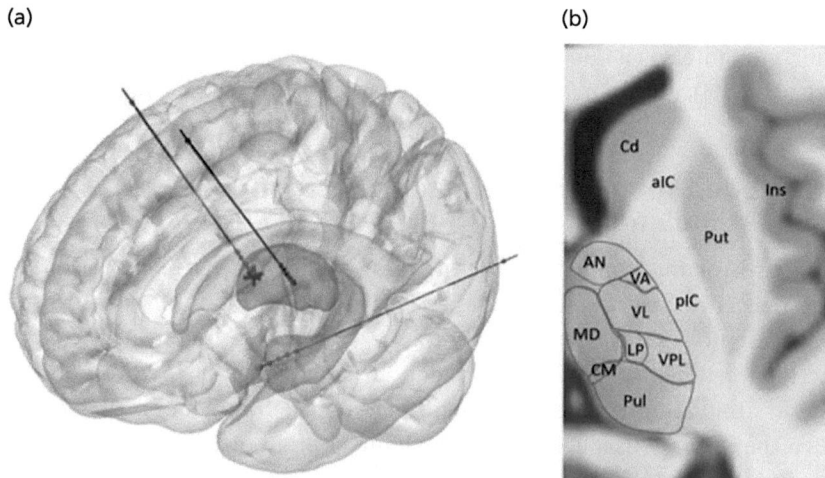

Figure 4.3 DBS trajectories to the anterior nucleus of the thalamus, centromedian nucleus, and hippocampus. Left: 3D cortical model with left lateral ventricle (cyan), thalamus (magenta), and hippocampus (yellow) with representative electrode trajectories to anterior nucleus of the thalamus (green), centromedian nucleus (black), and hippocampus (red). Right: axial image through the left thalamus at the level of the foramen of Monroe showing surrounding anatomical structures: caudate (Cd), putamen (Put), insula (Ins), anterior (aIC) and posterior (pIC) limbs of the internal capsule, and thalamic nuclei—anterior (AN), ventral anterior (VA), ventrolateral (VL), lateral posterior (LP), ventral posterior lateral (VPL), pulvinar (Pul), centromedial (CM), and mediodorsal (MD) nuclei. The thalamus acts as a relay projecting to the prefrontal (MD), premotor (VA), motor (VL), sensory (VPL), parietal (LP and Pul), and temporal (AN) cortices.

randomized controlled trial revealed a median reduction in seizure frequency of 56% at 2 years and 68% at 3 years in people with focal seizures with altered awareness.[111] Those with temporal lobe seizures showed the greatest benefit. ANT stimulation has also been shown to improve quality of life with improvement in executive function and attention, and no decline in cognitive domains or depression scores at 7-year follow-up.[112]

The centromedian nucleus of the thalamus is connected to the ascending reticular system and projects to the dorsolateral putamen and the motor and premotor cortices. Stimulation of the centromedian nucleus appears most efficacious for absence and generalized seizures as well as Lennox–Gastaut syndrome, but not dialeptic focal seizures.[101] Centromedian thalamic nucleus stimulation alone has been shown to be as effective as when combined with simultaneous ANT stimulation with regard to seizure frequency, severity, and life satisfaction.[113]

Other complications associated with DBS for epilepsy are uncommon, and similar to those when undertaken for movement disorders, and include haemorrhage (<5%), infection (<2%), lead malposition (2%), and hardware discomfort (1%).[114]

Other brain stimulation techniques: responsive neural stimulation

Responsive neural stimulation is an emerging technology that involves closed-loop delivery of electrical stimulation in which electrodes are placed over epileptogenic regions. These electrodes are used to detect epileptic activity, and then automatically deliver stimulation to abort the seizure. Responsive neural stimulation has replaced multiple subpial transections performed when the seizure onset zone is within eloquent brain regions that cannot be resected.[115] Given that it is an emerging technology, comorbidities are not yet well defined.

Conclusion

The vast majority of medical complications occur gradually over a sustained period of time. On the other hand, surgical complications are most often acute or subacute, and as such can be very clear. In this chapter, we have reviewed how surgery can contribute to the comorbidities associated with epilepsy in either a positive or negative way.

Surgery for epilepsy can be efficacious for drug-resistant focal epilepsy, but remains significantly underutilized, with patients often subjected to years of ineffective medical therapies before referral to epilepsy surgery centres.[116] Patient selection through a comprehensive multidisciplinary approach remains key to achieving optimal seizure remission rates and minimizing postoperative complications.

TLE is the most amenable to surgery, achieving long-term seizure remission rates in over two-thirds of appropriate individuals. Comorbidities following surgery include visual field defects, cranial neuropathies, language defects, neuropsychological decline, and psychiatric disorders. On the other hand, some comorbidities can improve, including language and neuropsychological function. These improvements are due to reductions in both seizure burden and side effects of antiepileptic medications.[5]

Modified operative approaches have been described to minimize collateral damage to nearby cortical and subcortical white matter fibre tracts to minimize new comorbidities. For example, visual field defects following transection of Meyer's loop, once considered an inevitable consequence of temporal lobe surgery, have significantly been reduced such that the majority of people can expect to regain a driving licence if they achieve seizure remission.[117,118]

Improvements in SEEG technology and increased adoption in epilepsy centres has been particularly useful to improve outcomes and minimize complications in extratemporal lobe surgery: resection margins can be safely tailored to be more extensive to cover the epileptogenic zone while avoiding nearby eloquent areas.

Finally, if resective surgery is not appropriate then disconnective and neuromodulatory therapies have been shown to reduce the seizure burden and improve the quality of life for people with epilepsy and caregivers, even in the absence of complete seizure remission.

In summary, as with any treatment, surgery can lead to complications that increase comorbidities. Surgery for epilepsy, however, can be very effective in eliminating or significantly reducing seizures and the associated risks of injury and mortality. In so doing, epilepsy surgery can also reduce certain pre-existing comorbidities. As such, epilepsy surgery can lead to significant improvements in quality of life for those with seizures which are refractory to medical therapy.

References

1. Wiebe S, Blume WT, Girvin JP, Eliasziw M. A randomized, controlled trial of surgery for temporal-lobe epilepsy. N Engl J Med. 2001;**345**(5):311–18.
2. Vakharia VN, Duncan JS, Witt J-A, Elger CE, Staba R, Engel JJ. Getting the best outcomes from epilepsy surgery. Ann Neurol. 2018;**83**(4):676–90.
3. Engel JJ, McDermott MP, Wiebe S, et al. Early surgical therapy for drug-resistant temporal lobe epilepsy. JAMA. 2012;**307**(9):922–30.
4. Karakis I, Montouris GD, Piperidou C, Luciano MS, Meador KJ, Cole AJ. The effect of epilepsy surgery on caregiver quality of life. Epilepsy Res. 2013;**107**(1–2):181–89.
5. Vakharia VN, Duncan JS, Witt J-AA, Elger CE, Staba R, Engel JJ. Getting the best outcomes from epilepsy surgery. Ann Neurol. 2018;**83**(4):676–90.
6. Keezer MR, Sisodiya SM, Sander JW. Comorbidities of epilepsy: current concepts and future perspectives. Lancet Neurol. 2016;**15**(1):106–15.
7. Blumcke I, Spreafico R, Haaker G, et al. Histopathological findings in brain tissue obtained during epilepsy surgery. N Engl J Med. 2017;**377**(17):1648–56.
8. Gooneratne IK, Mannan S, de Tisi J, et al. Somatic complications of epilepsy surgery over 25 years at a single center. Epilepsy Res. 2017;**132**:70–77.
9. Yagmurlu K, Vlasak AL, Rhoton AL Jr. Three-dimensional topographic fiber tract anatomy of the cerebrum. Neurosurgery. 2015;**11**(Suppl 2):274–305.
10. De Benedictis A, Duffau H, Paradiso B, et al. Anatomo-functional study of the temporo-parieto-occipital region: dissection, tractographic and brain mapping evidence from a neurosurgical perspective. J Anat. 2014;**225**(2):132–51.
11. Von Der Heide RJ, Skipper LM, Klobusicky E, Olson IR. Dissecting the uncinate fasciculus: disorders, controversies and a hypothesis. Brain. 2013;**136**(6):1692–707.

12. Barbaro N, Quigg M, Ward M, et al. Radiosurgery versus open surgery for mesial temporal lobe epilepsy: the randomized, controlled ROSE trial. Epilepsia. 2018;**59**(6):1198–207.

13. Josephson CB, Dykeman J, Fiest KM, et al. Systematic review and meta-analysis of standard vs selective temporal lobe epilepsy surgery. Neurology. 2013;**80**(18):1669–76.

14. Wu C, Jermakowicz WJ, Chakravorti S, et al. Effects of surgical targeting in laser interstitial thermal therapy for mesial temporal lobe epilepsy: a multicenter study of 234 patients. Epilepsia. 2019;**60**(6):1171–83.

15. Wiebe S, Blume WT, Girvin JP, et al. A randomized, controlled trial of surgery for temporal-lobe epilepsy. N Engl J Med. 2001;**345**(5):311–18.

16. Josephson CB, Dykeman J, Fiest KM, et al. Systematic review and meta-analysis of standard vs selective temporal lobe epilepsy surgery. Neurology. 2013;**80**(18):1669–76.

17. Marathe K, Alim-Marvasti A, Dahele K, Xiao F, Buck S. Resective, ablative and radiosurgical interventions for drug resistant mesial temporal lobe epilepsy: a systematic review and meta-analysis of outcomes. 2021;**12**:777845.

18. Lutz MT, Clusmann H, Elger CE, Schramm J, Helmstaedter C. Neuropsychological outcome after selective amygdalohippocampectomy with transsylvian versus transcortical approach: a randomized prospective clinical trial of surgery for temporal lobe epilepsy. Epilepsia. 2004;**45**(7):809–16.

19. Bozkurt B, da Silva Centeno R, Chaddad-Neto F, et al. Transcortical selective amygdalohippocampectomy technique through the middle temporal gyrus revisited: an anatomical study laboratory investigation. J Clin Neurosci. 2016;**34**:237–45.

20. Wieser HG, Yasargil MG. Selective amygdalohippocampectomy as a surgical treatment of mesiobasal limbic epilepsy. Surg Neurol. 1982;**17**(6):445–57.

21. Ribas EC, Yagmurlu K, Wen HT, Rhoton AL Jr. Microsurgical anatomy of the inferior limiting insular sulcus and the temporal stem. J Neurosurg. 2015;**122**(6):1263–73.

22. Hori T, Yamane F, Takenobu A. Microanatomy of medial temporal area and subtemporal amygdalohippocampectomy. Stereotact Funct Neurosurg. 2002;**77**(1–4):208–12.

23. Türe U, Harput MV, Kaya AH, et al. The paramedian supracerebellar-transtentorial approach to the entire length of the mediobasal temporal region: an anatomical and clinical study. Laboratory investigation. J Neurosurg. 2012;**116**(4):773–91.

24. Ortibus E, Verhoeven J, Sunaert S, Casteels I, de Cock P, Lagae L. Integrity of the inferior longitudinal fasciculus and impaired object recognition in children: a diffusion tensor imaging study. Dev Med Child Neurol. 2012;**54**(1):38–43.

25. Delev D, Schramm J, Clusmann H. How I do it—selective amygdalohippocampectomy via a navigated temporobasal approach, when veins forbid elevation of the temporal lobe. Acta Neurochir (Wien). 2018;**160**(3):597–601.

26. Serra C, Akeret K, Staartjes VE, et al. Safety of the paramedian supracerebellar-transtentorial approach for selective amygdalohippocampectomy. Neurosurg Focus. 2020;**48**(4):E4.

27. Bai J, Zhou W, Wang H, et al. Value of stereoelectroencephalography (SEEG)-guided radiofrequency thermocoagulation in treating drug-resistant focal epilepsy. Brain Sci Adv. 2019;**5**(3):189–202.

28. Parrent AG, Blume WT. Stereotactic amygdalohippocampotomy for the treatment of medial temporal lobe epilepsy. Epilepsia. 1999;**40**(10):1408–16.

29. **Bourdillon P, Isnard J, Catenoix H, et al.** Stereo electroencephalography-guided radiofrequency thermocoagulation (SEEG-guided RF-TC) in drug-resistant focal epilepsy: results from a 10-year experience. Epilepsia. 2017;**58**(1):85–93.

30. **Vakharia VN, Sparks RE, Li K, et al.** Multicenter validation of automated trajectories for selective laser amygdalohippocampectomy. Epilepsia. 2019;**60**(9):1949–59.

31. **Vakharia VN, Sparks R, Li K, et al.** Automated trajectory planning for laser interstitial thermal therapy in mesial temporal lobe epilepsy. Epilepsia. 2018;**59**(4):814–24.

32. **Jermakowicz WJ, Kanner AM, Sur S, et al.** Laser thermal ablation for mesiotemporal epilepsy: analysis of ablation volumes and trajectories. Epilepsia. 2017;**58**(5):801–10.

33. **Li K, Vakharia VN, Sparks R, et al.** Optimizing trajectories for cranial laser interstitial thermal therapy using computer-assisted planning: a machine learning approach. Neurotherapeutics. 2019;**16**(1):182–91.

34. **Winston GP, Daga P, Stretton J, et al.** Optic radiation tractography and vision in anterior temporal lobe resection. Ann Neurol. 2012;**71**(3):334–41.

35. **Jeelani NUO, Jindahra P, Tamber MS, et al.** 'Hemispherical asymmetry in the Meyer's Loop': a prospective study of visual-field deficits in 105 cases undergoing anterior temporal lobe resection for epilepsy. J Neurol Neurosurg Psychiatry. 2010;**81**(9):985–91.

36. **Nowell M, Vos SB, Sidhu M, et al.** Meyer's loop asymmetry and language lateralisation in epilepsy. J Neurol Neurosurg Psychiatry. 2016;**87**(8):836–42.

37. **Taylor DC, Falconer MA.** Clinical, socio-economic, and psychological changes after temporal lobectomy for epilepsy. Br J Psychiatry. 1968;**114**(515):1247–61.

38. **Niemeyer P.** The transventricular amygdalo-hippocampectomy in temporal lobe epilepsy. In: **Baldwin M, Bailey P,** eds. Temporal lobe epilepsy. Springfield, IL: CC Thomas; 1958:461–82.

39. **Manji H, Plant GT.** Epilepsy surgery, visual fields, and driving: a study of the visual field criteria for driving in patients after temporal lobe epilepsy surgery with a comparison of Goldmann and Esterman perimetry. J Neurol Neurosurg Psychiatry. 2000;**68**(1):80–82.

40. **Pathak-Ray V, Ray A, Walters R, Hatfield R.** Detection of visual field defects in patients after anterior temporal lobectomy for mesial temporal sclerosis—establishing eligibility to drive. Eye (Lond). 2002;**16**(6):744–48.

41. **Winston GP, Daga P, White MJ, et al.** Preventing visual field deficits from neurosurgery. Neurology. 2014;**83**(7):604–11.

42. **Mengesha T, Abu-Ata M, Haas KF, et al.** Visual field defects after selective amygdalohippocampectomy and standard temporal lobectomy. J Neuro-Ophthalmology. 2009;**29**(3):208–13.

43. **Yeni SN, Tanriover N, Uyanik Ö, et al.** Visual field defects in selective amygdalohippocampectomy for hippocampal sclerosis: the fate of Meyer's loop during the transsylvian approach to the temporal horn. Neurosurgery. 2008;**63**(3):507–13.

44. **Delev D, Wabbels B, Schramm J, et al.** Vision after trans-sylvian or temporobasal selective amygdalohippocampectomy: a prospective randomised trial. Acta Neurochir (Wien). 2016;**158**(9):1757–65.

45. **Vajkoczy P, Krakow K, Stodieck S, Pohlmann-Eden B, Schmiedek P.** Modified approach for the selective treatment of temporal lobe epilepsy: transsylvian-transcisternal mesial en bloc resection. J Neurosurg. 1998;**88**(5):855–62.

46. Quigg M, Barbaro NM, Ward MM, et al. Visual field defects after radiosurgery versus temporal lobectomy for mesial temporal lobe epilepsy: findings of the ROSE trial. Seizure. 2018;63:62–67.

47. Jermakowicz WJ, Ivan ME, Cajigas I, et al. Visual deficit from laser interstitial thermal therapy for temporal lobe epilepsy: anatomical considerations. Oper Neurosurg. 2017;13(5):627–33.

48. Yin D, Thompson JA, Drees C, et al. Optic radiation tractography and visual field deficits in laser interstitial thermal therapy for amygdalohippocampectomy in patients with mesial temporal lobe epilepsy. Stereotact Funct Neurosurg. 2017;95(2):107–13.

49. Voets NL, Alvarez I, Qiu D, et al. Mechanisms and risk factors contributing to visual field deficits following stereotactic laser amygdalohippocampotomy. Stereotact Funct Neurosurg. 2019;97(4):255–65.

50. Tanriverdi T, Ajlan A, Poulin N, Olivier A. Morbidity in epilepsy surgery: an experience based on 2449 epilepsy surgery procedures from a single institution. J Neurosurg. 2009;110(6):1111–23.

51. Jacobson DM, Warner JJ, Ruggles KH. Transient trochlear nerve palsy following anterior temporal lobectomy for epilepsy. Neurology. 1995;45(8):1465–68.

52. Busch RM, Floden DP, Prayson B, et al. Estimating risk of word-finding problems in adults undergoing epilepsy surgery. Neurology. 2016;87(22):2363–69.

53. Wilmskoetter J, Fridriksson J, Gleichgerrcht E, et al. Neuroanatomical structures supporting lexical diversity, sophistication, and phonological word features during discourse. NeuroImage Clin. 2019;24:101961.

54. Balter S, Lin G, Leyden KM, Paul BM, McDonald CR. Neuroimaging correlates of language network impairment and reorganization in temporal lobe epilepsy. Brain Lang. 2019;193:31–44.

55. Pustina D, Doucet G, Evans J, et al. Distinct types of white matter changes are observed after anterior temporal lobectomy in epilepsy. PLoS One. 2014;9(8):e104211.

56. Von Rhein B, Nelles M, Urbach H, Von Lehe M, Schramm J, Helmstaedter C. Neuropsychological outcome after selective amygdalohippocampectomy: subtemporal versus transsylvian approach. J Neurol Neurosurg Psychiatry. 2012;83(9):887–93.

57. Duffau H, Thiebaut De Schotten M, Mandonnet E. White matter functional connectivity as an additional landmark for dominant temporal lobectomy. J Neurol Neurosurg Psychiatry. 2008;79(5):492–95.

58. Duffau H. Stimulation mapping of white matter tracts to study brain functional connectivity. Nat Rev Neurol. 2015;11(5):255–65.

59. Mandonnet E, Nouet A, Gatignol P, Capelle L, Duffau H. Does the left inferior longitudinal fasciculus play a role in language? A brain stimulation study. Brain. 2007;130(3):623–29.

60. Duffau H, Moritz-Gasser S, Mandonnet E. A re-examination of neural basis of language processing: proposal of a dynamic hodotopical model from data provided by brain stimulation mapping during picture naming. Brain Lang. 2014;131:1–10.

61. Giacomini L, de Souza JPSA, Formentin C, et al. Temporal lobe structural evaluation after transsylvian selective amygdalohippocampectomy. Neurosurg Focus. 2020;48(4):E14.

62. Quigg M, Broshek DK, Barbaro NM, et al. Neuropsychological outcomes after Gamma Knife radiosurgery for mesial temporal lobe epilepsy: a prospective multicenter study. Epilepsia. 2011;52(5):909–16.

63. Helmstaedter C, Elger CE, Hufnagel A, Zentner J, Schramm J. Different effects of left anterior temporal lobectomy, selective amygdalohippocampectomy, and temporal cortical lesionectomy on verbal learning, memory, and recognition. J Epilepsy. 1996;9(1):39–45.

64. Hoppe C, Elger CE, Helmstaedter C. Long-term memory impairment in patients with focal epilepsy. Epilepsia. 2007;48(Suppl 9):26–29.

65. Helmstaedter C, Richter S, Roske S, Oltmanns F, Schramm J, Lehmann T-N. Differential effects of temporal pole resection with amygdalohippocampectomy versus selective amygdalohippocampectomy on material-specific memory in patients with mesial temporal lobe epilepsy. Epilepsia. 2008;49(1):88–97.

66. Wendling AS, Hirsch E, Wisniewski I, et al. Selective amygdalohippocampectomy versus standard temporal lobectomy in patients with mesial temporal lobe epilepsy and unilateral hippocampal sclerosis. Epilepsy Res. 2013;104(1–2):94–104.

67. Bujarski KA, Hirashima F, Roberts DW, et al. Long-term seizure, cognitive, and psychiatric outcome following trans–middle temporal gyrus amygdalohippocampectomy and standard temporal lobectomy. J Neurosurg. 2011;55(20):6197–214.

68. Hori T, Yamane F, Ochiai T, et al. Selective subtemporal amygdalohippocampectomy for refractory temporal lobe epilepsy: operative and neuropsychological outcomes. J Neurosurg. 2007;106(1):134–41.

69. Drane DL, Loring DW, Voets NL, et al. Better object recognition and naming outcome with MRI-guided stereotactic laser amygdalohippocampotomy for temporal lobe epilepsy. Epilepsia. 2015;56(1):101–13.

70. Shaw P, Mellers J, Henderson M, Polkey C, David AS, Toone BK. Schizophrenia-like psychosis arising de novo following a temporal lobectomy: timing and risk factors. J Neurol Neurosurg Psychiatry. 2004;75(7):1003–1008.

71. Glosser G, Zwil AS, Glosser DS, O'Connor MJ, Sperling MR. Psychiatric aspects of temporal lobe epilepsy before and after anterior temporal lobectomy. J Neurol Neurosurg Psychiatry. 2000;68(1):53–58.

72. Macrodimitris S, Sherman EMS, Forde S, et al. Psychiatric outcomes of epilepsy surgery: a systematic review. Epilepsia. 2011;52(5):880–90.

73. Devinsky O, Barr WB, Vickrey BG, et al. Changes in depression and anxiety after resective surgery for epilepsy. Neurology. 2005;65(11):1744–49.

74. Shamir RR, Joskowicz L, Tamir I, et al. Reduced risk trajectory planning in image-guided keyhole neurosurgery. Med Phys. 2012;39(5):2885–95.

75. Pope RA, Thompson PJ, Rantell K, Stretton J, Wright M-A, Foong J. Frontal lobe dysfunction as a predictor of depression and anxiety following temporal lobe epilepsy surgery. Epilepsy Res. 2019;152:59–66.

76. Bell GS, Gaitatzis A, Bell CL, Johnson AL, Sander JW. Suicide in people with epilepsy: how great is the risk? Epilepsia. 2009;50(8):1933–42.

77. Casadei CH, Carson KW, Mendiratta A, et al. All-cause mortality and SUDEP in a surgical epilepsy population. Epilepsy Behav. 2020;108:107093.

78. Guarnieri R, Walz R, Hallak JEC, et al. Do psychiatric comorbidities predict postoperative seizure outcome in temporal lobe epilepsy surgery? Epilepsy Behav. 2009;14(3):529–34.

79. Andrade-Machado R, Benjumea-Cuartas V. Temporal plus epilepsy: anatomo-electroclinical subtypes. Iran J Neurol. 2016;15(3):153–63.

80. Lemaitre A-L, Lafargue G, Duffau H, Herbet G. Damage to the left uncinate fasciculus is associated with heightened schizotypal traits: a multimodal lesion-mapping study. Schizophr Res. 2018;197:240–48.

81. Hosking PG. Surgery for frontal lobe epilepsy. Seizure. 2003;12(3):160–66.

82. Englot DJ, Wang DD, Rolston JD, Shih TT, Chang EF. Rates and predictors of long-term seizure freedom after frontal lobe epilepsy surgery: a systematic review and meta-analysis. J Neurosurg. 2012;116(5):1042–48.

83. Bonini F, McGonigal A, Scavarda D, et al. Predictive factors of surgical outcome in frontal lobe epilepsy explored with stereoelectroencephalography. Neurosurgery. 2018;83(2):217–25.

84. McGonigal A, Bartolomei F, Régis J, et al. Stereoelectroencephalography in presurgical assessment of MRI-negative epilepsy. Brain. 2007;130(Pt 12):3169–83.

85. Sarubbo S, De Benedictis A, Merler S, et al. Towards a functional atlas of human white matter. Hum Brain Mapp. 2015;36(8):3117–36.

86. Duffau H. The 'frontal syndrome' revisited: lessons from electrostimulation mapping studies. Cortex. 2012;48(1):120–31.

87. Vilasboas T, Herbet G, Duffau H. Challenging the myth of right nondominant hemisphere: lessons from corticosubcortical stimulation mapping in awake surgery and surgical implications. World Neurosurg. 2017;103:449–56.

88. Zentner J, Hufnagel A, Pechstein U, Wolf HK, Schramm J. Functional results after resective procedures involving the supplementary motor area. J Neurosurg. 1996;85(4):542–49.

89. Busch RM, Floden DP, Ferguson L, et al. Neuropsychological outcome following frontal lobectomy for pharmacoresistant epilepsy in adults. Neurology. 2017;88(7):692–700.

90. Foldvary-Schaefer N, Unnwongse K. Localizing and lateralizing features of auras and seizures. Epilepsy Behav. 2011;20(2):160–66.

91. Laoprasert P, Ojemann JG, Handler MH. Insular epilepsy surgery. Epilepsia. 2017;58:35–45.

92. Malak R, Bouthillier A, Carmant L, et al. Microsurgery of epileptic foci in the insular region. J Neurosurg. 2009;110(6):1153–63.

93. Boucher O, Rouleau I, Escudier F, et al. Neuropsychological performance before and after partial or complete insulectomy in patients with epilepsy. Epilepsy Behav. 2015;43:53–60.

94. Asadollahi M, Sperling MR, Rabiei AH, Asadi-Pooya AA. Drug-resistant parietal lobe epilepsy: clinical manifestations and surgery outcome. Epileptic Disord. 2017;19(1):35–39.

95. Balestrini S, Francione S, Mai R, et al. Multimodal responses induced by cortical stimulation of the parietal lobe: a stereo-electroencephalography study. Brain. 2015;138(9):2596–607.

96. Yagmurlu K, Middlebrooks EH, Tanriover N, Rhotor AL Jr. Fiber tracts of the dorsal language stream in the human brain. 2016;124(5):1396–405.

97. Luerding R, Boesebeck F, Ebner A. Cognitive changes after epilepsy surgery in the posterior cortex. J Neurol Neurosurg Psychiatry. 2004;75(4):583–87.

98. Taylor I, Scheffer IE, Berkovic SF. Occipital epilepsies: identification of specific and newly recognized syndromes. Brain. 2003;126(4):753–69.

99. Harward SC, Chen WC, Rolston JD, Haglund MM, Englot DJ. Seizure outcomes in occipital lobe and posterior quadrant epilepsy surgery: a systematic review and meta-analysis. Clin Neurosurg. 2018;82(3):350–58.

100. Vakharia VN, Sparks RE, Vos SB, et al. Computer-assisted planning for minimally invasive anterior two-thirds laser corpus callosotomy: a feasibility study with probabilistic tractography validation: automated laser callosotomy trajectory planning. NeuroImage Clin. 2020;25:102174.

101. Englot DJ, Birk H, Chang EF. Seizure outcomes in nonresective epilepsy surgery: an update. Neurosurg Rev. 2017;40(2):181–94.

102. Asadi-Pooya AA, Sharan AD, Nei M, Sperling MR. Corpus callosotomy. Epilepsy Behav. 2008;13(1):271–78.

103. Smyth MD, Vellimana AK, Asano E. Corpus callosotomy—open and endoscopic surgical techniques. Epilepsia. 2017;58(Suppl 1):73–79.

104. Bahuleyan B, Robinson S, Nair AR, Sivanandapanicker JL, Cohen AR. Anatomic hemispherectomy: historical perspective. World Neurosurg. 2013;80(3–4):396–98.

105. Schramm J, Kral T, Clusmann H. Transsylvian keyhole functional hemispherectomy. Neurosurgery. 2001;49(4):891–900.

106. Kwan A, Ng WH, Otsubo H, et al. Hemispherectomy for the control of intractable epilepsy in childhood: comparison of 2 surgical techniques in a single institution. Neurosurgery. 2010;67(2 Suppl Operative):429–36.

107. Olin B, Jayewardene AK, Bunker M, Moreno F. Mortality and suicide risk in treatment-resistant depression: an observational study of the long-term impact of intervention. PLoS One. 2012;7(10):e48002.

108. Desbeaumes Jodoin V, Richer F, Miron J-P, Fournier-Gosselin M-P, Lespérance P. Long-term sustained cognitive benefits of vagus nerve stimulation in refractory depression. J ECT. 2018;34(4):283–90.

109. Lancman G, Virk M, Shao H, et al. Vagus nerve stimulation vs. corpus callosotomy in the treatment of Lennox–Gastaut syndrome: a meta-analysis. Seizure. 2013;22(1):3–8.

110. Cukiert A, Cukiert CM, Burattini JA, Mariani PP, Bezerra DF. Seizure outcome after hippocampal deep brain stimulation in patients with refractory temporal lobe epilepsy: a prospective, controlled, randomized, double-blind study. Epilepsia. 2017;58(10):1728–33.

111. Salanova V, Witt T, Worth R, et al. Long-term efficacy and safety of thalamic stimulation for drug-resistant partial epilepsy. Neurology. 2015;84(10):1017–25.

112. Tröster AI, Meador KJ, Irwin CP, Fisher RS. Memory and mood outcomes after anterior thalamic stimulation for refractory partial epilepsy. Seizure. 2017;45:133–41.

113. Alcala-Zermeno JL, Gregg NM, Wirrell EC, et al. Centromedian thalamic nucleus with or without anterior thalamic nucleus deep brain stimulation for epilepsy in children and adults: a retrospective case series. Seizure. 2021;84:101–107.

114. Li MCH, Cook MJ. Deep brain stimulation for drug-resistant epilepsy. Epilepsia. 2018;59(2):273–90.

115. Matias CM, Sharan A, Wu C. Responsive neurostimulation for the treatment of epilepsy. Neurosurg Clin N Am. 2019;30(2):231–42.

116. **Engel J, Wiebe S, French J,** et al. Practice parameter: temporal lobe and localized neocortical resections for epilepsy: report of the Quality Standards Subcommittee of the American Academy of Neurology, in association with the American Epilepsy Society and the American Association of Neurological surgeons. Neurology. 2003;**60**(4):538–47.

117. **Vakharia VN, Vos SB, Winston GP,** et al. Intraoperative overlay of optic radiation tractography during anteromesial temporal resection: a prospective validation study. J Neurosurg. 2021;**136**(2):543–52.

118. **Vakharia VN, Diehl B, Tisdall M.** Visual field defects in temporal lobe epilepsy surgery. Curr Opin Neurol. 2021;**34**(2):188–96.

Section 3

Cognitive, psychological, and systemic comorbidity

Chapter 5

Epilepsy and cognition

John Baker and Chris Butler

Introduction

Cognitive impairment is common among people with epilepsy.[1,2] Almost 50% of people with epilepsy describe difficulties with memory, concentration, or thinking.[3] For many, these symptoms are more problematic than the seizures themselves, and are associated with marked disability and socioeconomic cost.[4-6] For some, cognitive problems persist after adequate seizure control has been established with antiseizure medications (ASMs).[7,8] In some cases, these medications themselves cause additional cognitive side effects.[9,10] The relationship between epilepsy and cognition is bidirectional: many conditions causing cognitive impairment also increase the risk of epilepsy and epilepsy can lead to cognitive impairment itself,[11] a fact which is especially pertinent in conditions where cognitive impairment predates epilepsy onset[12-14] and where seizures can lead to further decline. Despite this intimate relationship between epilepsy and cognition, the neuropsychological assessment of individuals diagnosed with epilepsy is still not standard practice, particularly in adult populations.[15]

In this chapter, we describe the main cognitive deficits associated with different epilepsy syndromes, mechanisms which underlie these deficits, and potential therapeutic approaches (see also Chapter 12).

Cognitive impairment: ictal, postictal, and interictal

The most striking disruption of cognitive function in epilepsy typically occurs during seizures themselves and can range from complete loss of consciousness to subtle disruption in a single cognitive domain such as memory. The nature of the ictal cognitive deficit depends upon the brain networks involved in the seizure. Generalized seizures typically lead to loss of awareness and responsiveness, including disruption of memory, such that unwitnessed seizures may go unrecognized. This is of particular relevance in children and adolescents with frequent absence seizures. These can be readily missed or misinterpreted by family and teachers as momentary lapses in concentration, or children struggling to keep up with schooling as they are thought to be 'daydreaming'. On the other hand, more selective disruption of cognition can occur in the context of focal seizures, such as in the case of transient epileptic amnesia[16,17] or ictal aphasia,[18] which we discuss below.

Cognitive impairment may outlast the seizure itself. The postictal period can be associated with profound disorientation, confusion, and agitation. Marked amplitude attenuation, absence of normal physiological rhythms, and bursting are seen on electroencephalographic (EEG) recordings during the postictal period.[19] The duration of this period depends on the nature and duration of the seizure which has preceded it. Generally, more prolonged seizures lead to a more extensive postictal period.[20–22] Studies of the postictal brain have uncovered several different neurophysiological, metabolic, and vascular abnormalities which underlie this dysfunction, including cerebral hypoperfusion/hypoxia, permeability of the blood–brain barrier,[23,24] and inflammation.[25,26]

Beyond these transient disruptions, cognitive impairment is often a persistent, interictal feature affecting the day-to-day lives of people with epilepsy. This impairment is often present at the time of diagnosis.[27–29] In a study of 247 untreated adults with new-onset epilepsy, Witt and Helmstaedter identified impairments in attention and executive function in 49.4%, and memory deficits in 47.8%, with unimpaired performance in both domains seen in 27.9%.[29] This echoes earlier findings from Taylor and colleagues, in which 155 newly diagnosed, untreated adults with epilepsy underwent comprehensive neuropsychological testing. In this group, 53.5% demonstrated at least one abnormal score (>2 standard deviations below the control mean) in the tested domains.[28]

The severity of cognitive impairment may fluctuate, resolve, or worsen over time as a result of seizures, medications, structural alterations, remodelling, and neuronal loss. It is clear that a baseline neuropsychological assessment in those newly diagnosed with epilepsy is an important tool both in terms of identifying people experiencing, or at risk of, cognitive impairment as a result of their epilepsy, but also as a means of monitoring the efficacy and tolerability of medical and surgical interventions in a manner which looks beyond seizure control.

However, while epilepsy is common, neuropsychologists are a limited resource. Moreover, a thorough neuropsychological assessment is a time-consuming process. Therefore, brief testing which can either be performed in the clinic or in the form of a questionnaire may be a useful means of prioritizing resources to those with the most significant cognitive difficulties. In a study looking at the use of the AD8, a screening questionnaire for cognitive impairment, Aji and Larner identified cognitive impairment in 48% based on self-completed sections and 54% based on the informant-completed components of this questionnaire.[30] Approaches such as this may help to reduce the number of people for whom a full neuropsychological assessment is needed. However, such questionnaires still need to be validated in order to determine their sensitivity and specificity, particularly as subjective and objective cognitive performance in epilepsy are not always aligned.[31]

Cognitive function by domain

Cognitive function can be divided into a number of distinct domains, which include memory, attention, executive function, language, and perception. While advances in our understanding of neuroanatomy and neuropsychology have moved us away from a model in which particular cognitive functions map directly to particular anatomical areas towards a more network-oriented approach, the nature of cognitive symptoms reported by people with epilepsy can still provide useful information regarding the brain areas affected, especially if their seizures have a focal onset.[32–34]

General intelligence

The effects of epilepsy on general intelligence cover a broad spectrum: from subtle impairments to profound intellectual disability.[35,36] These effects are influenced by several factors including age of onset of seizures,[37] duration of epilepsy,[38] frequency of seizures, and episodes of status epilepticus.[39] These effects can increase over time and are also related to the nature of treatment (medical vs surgical, monotherapy vs polytherapy) and its effectiveness in leading to a reduction in seizure frequency.[40,41] Extensive research has also shown that prenatal exposure to antiseizure medications, and sodium valproate in particular, can impact the general cognitive abilities of children born to mothers with epilepsy.[42,43] This includes an increased risk of autism spectrum disorders[44] and attention deficit hyperactivity disorder.[45]

The prevalence of epilepsy is increased in people with a preceding history of intellectual disability.[46] In these cases, seizures are often frequent and difficult to treat; socioeconomic outcomes are poorer and refractory epilepsy may lead to institutionalization.[47] Moreover, the risk of epilepsy-related mortality, including sudden unexpected death in epilepsy (SUDEP) is increased in those with intellectual disability (Chapters 7,9).[48,49]

Several childhood epilepsy syndromes, such as Lennox–Gastaux syndrome, are associated with progressive cognitive impairments and developmental regression. In many cases the onset of seizures may herald the start of this decline. In Dravet syndrome, children experience a range of seizure types with concomitant developmental delays becoming evident from the second year of life. Language skills start to develop at a normal age, but progress very slowly, and often those affected do not develop sufficiently to enable elementary sentence construction. Motor skills are similarly affected, with impairment of walking development and fine motor skills/hand–eye coordination.[50]

Memory

Human memory can be divided into a number of psychologically and neurally distinct memory systems (Figure 5.1). Firstly, short-term or working memory is the ability to keep information 'online' while cognitive operations are being carried out with it, whereas long-term memory refers to memory contents that persist 'offline' and can be retrieved when subsequently needed. Long-term memory can be subdivided into *declarative memory* (knowledge of facts or concepts (semantic memory) and events (episodic memory)) versus *non-declarative memory* (skills, habits, and conditioned responses). Memory can also be thought of as comprising partially distinct processes, which contribute

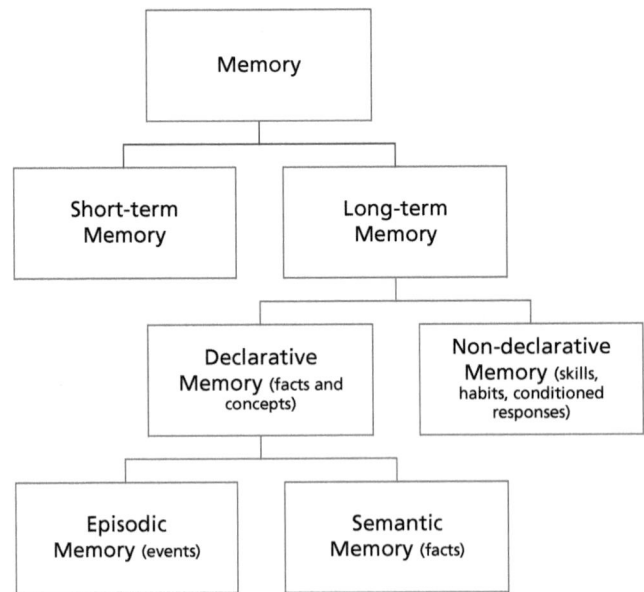

Figure 5.1 Hierarchical framework of memory classification.

to function across the different memory systems: encoding, consolidation, storage, and retrieval. Memory difficulties can result from impairment in any of these systems and/or processes.

The temporal lobes are the brain region most closely associated with the encoding, consolidation, and retrieval of declarative memories.[51,52] Damage to mesial temporal structures, and the hippocampus in particular, leads to amnesia, as well as changes in emotional responses (fear, laughter, crying) due to wider connections between the medial temporal lobes and the rest of the limbic system.[53]

A range of memory problems are associated with temporal lobe epilepsy.[54–59] Where seizures involve the dominant temporal lobe, deficits in verbal memory are particularly common. Mameniskiene et al. have shown that the extent of this impairment is related to the frequency of seizures[60] and, in a follow-up study 13 years later, confirmed that cognitive function remained stable when seizure control had been good.[55] In this population, people with frequent seizures (classified as four or more seizures per month) involving the temporal lobes demonstrated worse memory performance for several types of information tested through a range of neuropsychological tests (Rey Auditory Verbal Learning Test (RAVLT), Verbal Logical Story (VLS), and Rey–Osterrieth Complex Figure Test (ROCFT)) both after a delayed recall interval (30 minutes) and a longer interval (4 weeks).[60] However, more subtle neuropsychological deficits are also evident in those with mild temporal lobe epilepsy. In their study comparing people with mild temporal lobe epilepsy (defined by at least 24 seizure-free months with or without medication) versus healthy controls, Vaccaro and colleagues, again identified impairment in verbal memory (using RAVLT: delayed recall) in those with temporal lobe epilepsy. Moreover, verbal memory performance was found to correlate with subjective memory concerns, independently from its association with mood dysfunction (anxiety and depression).[59]

A particular pattern of memory impairment is seen in individuals with transient epileptic amnesia (TEA).[61] People with TEA present with recurrent episodes of transient amnesia, typically lasting around 15–60 minutes, which often occur on waking.[16,62,63] While some demonstrate other ictal features which help to confirm the diagnosis of epilepsy (orofacial automatisms, periods of unresponsiveness, olfactory hallucinations), for others, the transient amnesia is the sole manifestation of the seizure. Studies of TEA have frequently identified seizures involving the temporal lobes, with subtle hippocampal volume loss described in volumetric studies.[17,64] In addition to the seizures themselves, people with TEA also demonstrate a range of interictal memory difficulties including autobiographical amnesia (typically for salient personal events of the remote past), accelerated long-term forgetting (ALF), and topographical amnesia.

ALF is the excessively rapid loss of access, over extended intervals, of information that appears to have been acquired and initially stored normally, suggesting an isolated deficit in memory consolidation. ALF goes undetected by standard neuropsychological tests of memory, which typically probe memory retention over periods of up to about 30 minutes. It can, however, have a major impact on day-to-day living. ALF has also been described in other forms of temporal lobe epilepsy,[60,65] in paediatric epilepsy populations,[66,67] in antibody-mediated limbic encephalitis,[68-70] and in cases of mild cognitive impairment and mild Alzheimer's disease (AD).[71] Its causes have not yet been fully elucidated, although some work has found a relationship between ALF and the occurrence of seizures or interictal epileptiform discharges on EEG.[72,73]

Attention and executive function

The term executive function encompasses the cognitive processes required for attentional control, planning, reasoning, and problem-solving (Figure 5.2). A broad range of sometimes subtle executive function impairments, which also

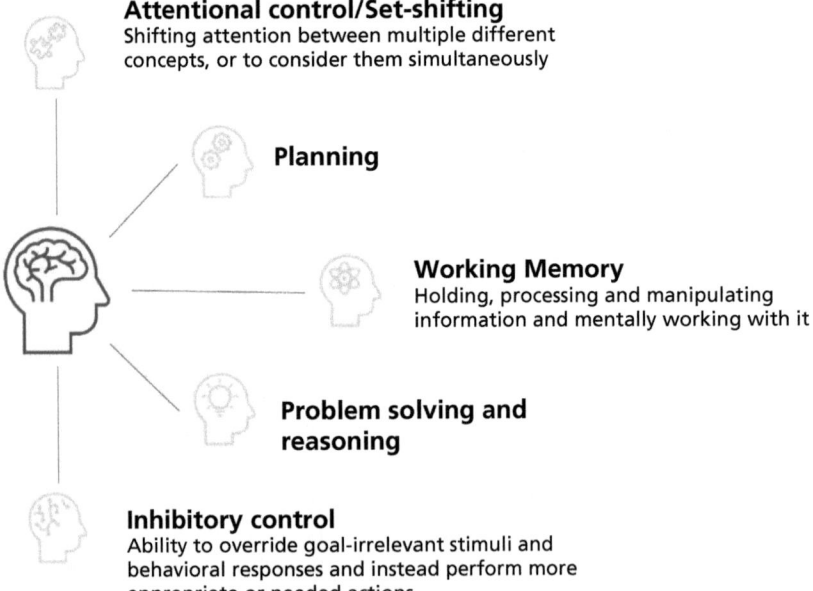

Attentional control/Set-shifting
Shifting attention between multiple different concepts, or to consider them simultaneously

Planning

Working Memory
Holding, processing and manipulating information and mentally working with it

Problem solving and reasoning

Inhibitory control
Ability to override goal-irrelevant stimuli and behavioral responses and instead perform more appropriate or needed actions.

Figure 5.2 Glossary of roles defined by executive function. Processes defined by executive function often overlap and commonly used tests for executive function (including Trail Making Test Part B, verbal fluency testing, Wisconsin card sorting test, and Stroop test) often utilize multiple functions as well as drawing on other cognitive domains (such as visuospatial and language skills).

includes difficulties with working memory and inhibitory control, can be seen in those with frontal lobe epilepsy. These deficits are reflected in poor performance on tasks which involve switching,[33] inhibition,[74] and on classical tests of executive function such as trail-making tasks.[75] Unlike in temporal lobe epilepsy, where the lateralization of the lesion has significant implications for the nature of the cognitive impairment, deficits in frontal lobe epilepsy do not appear to relate as strongly to whether the lesion involves the right or left hemisphere.[76]

The prevalence of attention deficit hyperactivity disorder in children with epilepsy varies widely but has been estimated at between 30% and 40% in focused studies.[77-79] The relationship appears to be bidirectional, and this combination is associated with significantly higher rates of deficits in executive function, increased requirements for school-based remedial services, and poorer long-term educational attainment.[77]

Disorders of attention and executive function have frequently been described in people with juvenile myoclonic epilepsy[80,81] Those with juvenile myoclonic epilepsy can be prone to impulsivity and risk-taking behaviour to a greater extent than in other types of epilepsy.[82] Neuroimaging studies in people with juvenile myoclonic epilepsy have identified functional and structural abnormalities within the frontal cortex and thalamus.[83] Increased functional connectivity between the motor system and frontoparietal cognitive networks, as well as impaired deactivation of the default mode network during cognitive tasks, have been described.[84] These impairments of executive function can have profound impacts on daily life and lead to psychosocial complications and reduced quality of life.[85]

Social cognition

Social cognition refers to the mental processes involved in social interactions including empathy, emotional processing, and theory of mind. People with frontal lobe epilepsy have also been found to demonstrate impairments in this domain.[34,86-88] In addition, impaired emotion recognition is a recognized feature of mesial temporal lobe epilepsy.[89] Studies which have examined facial emotion recognition in people with temporal lobe epilepsy have described a reduction in performance of between 5% and 20% in this measure when compared to healthy controls.[90-92]

Impairments in theory of mind have not been studied extensively. However, in their study looking at characterization and prediction of theory of mind disorders in temporal lobe epilepsy, Hennion and co-workers reported that 84% of participants misunderstood verbal faux pas and around 50% misunderstood sarcasm.[93] Duration of epilepsy and age of onset were risk factors for these impairments, which have been shown to arise from brain areas involved in theory of mind networks, including mesial temporal lobe structures and dorsal medial prefrontal cortex.[89,94]

Language

The generation and understanding of language involves well-known 'language areas' such as Wernicke's area (left posterior superior temporal gyrus) and Broca's area (left insular cortex), as well as more widely distributed networks within the left hemisphere encompassing the perisylvian language network. Language function also requires integration of other regions of the brain including prefrontal cortex for more complex/metaphorical language meaning, as well as premotor, motor, and supplementary motor cortices for the production of language.

Ictal aphasia, a transient impairment of language function resulting from a seizure, can be a manifestation of temporal lobe epilepsy.[18] EEG studies of people with ictal aphasia have identified seizures arising from the temporopolar and the anterior temporobasal cortex.[95] Speech and language disorders are commonly experienced by people with epilepsy, particularly where seizures have started in infancy or childhood. In these individuals, epilepsy in early life appears to impair development of language-related brain regions, with reduced structural connectivity and synchronization.[96] Such disorders in language have been reported in 50% of adolescents with epilepsy.[97] These impairments cover a broad range in terms of severity and prognosis, from relatively mild to more extreme cases leading to language regression. Where aphasia is an ictal phenomenon, effective treatment can lead to stabilization and potentially improvement over time.

In the general population, the 'dominant' brain hemisphere (i.e. that on which language function depends) is usually the left hemisphere in right-handed individuals (92.7% in left hemisphere, 7.5% in right hemisphere) and a mixture of right (27%), left, or both in left-handed individuals.[98,99] However, epilepsy can lead to a reorganization of language networks in the brain. For this reason, functional magnetic resonance imaging (fMRI) scans are commonly performed during evaluation for epilepsy surgery to identify the brain regions upon which language function depends and ensure that these lie outside the areas to be resected. Epilepsy surgery itself can lead to further reorganization of language function to the right hemisphere.[100,101]

Landau–Kleffner syndrome is a rare childhood syndrome of epileptic aphasia, with onset of seizures usually between 3 and 7 years old.[102] Clinically, regression of speech and language functioning, and auditory processing difficulties occur.[103] Neuropsychological evaluation typically demonstrates global impairment, with auditory and linguistic functions significantly below visual/

non-verbal abilities. EEG recordings demonstrate diffuse spike wave abnormalities, sometimes seen only during sleep, and involving the temporal regions, either bilaterally at onset, or unilaterally and spreading to become bilateral.[104] The cause remains unknown, although several candidate genes (including glutamate ionotropic receptor NMDA type subunit 2A (*GRIN2A*), reelin (*RELN*), and bassoon presynaptic cytomatrix protein (*BSN*)) have been reported.[105,106]

Interictal language deficits are also common in adult epilepsy. This can include impairments in object naming, on which people with left temporal lobe epilepsy have been shown to perform less well than those with right-sided epilepsy.[107,108] In these people, this deficit appears to be related to hippocampal pathology,[109] and in particular hippocampal sclerosis.[110] Other language impairments can include disorders of auditory comprehension,[111] spontaneous speech,[112,113] and written language.[114] Language disorders have also been found in those with frontal lobe epilepsy.[115] In an fMRI study of 52 adults with cryptogenic localization-related epilepsy, people with epilepsy had significantly lower functional connectivity than controls in the prefrontal network at rest and functional connectivity in the frontotemporal network correlated with performance on word fluency and text reading tasks.[116]

Perception: visual and auditory hallucinations

Ictal and interictal impairments of visual perception, including hallucinations, are most likely to be a result of seizures involving the occipital lobes. However, seizures involving these regions are far less common than those involving the temporal lobe. Idiopathic childhood occipital epilepsy of Gastaut is a benign syndrome in which sufferers experience visual seizures. Manifestations include elementary and complex visual hallucinations, visual illusions, blindness, or partial visual loss.[117] Investigations show occipital spikes or spike waves on EEG, with normal neuroimaging. Affected individuals commonly experience concomitant migraine, and half will remit within 2–4 years of onset without long-term cognitive sequelae.[117,118] Cases of visual phenomena related to occipital lobe epilepsy have often been reported as single cases.[119–121] In these cases, visual hallucinations are often complex, presenting in a similar manner to Charles Bonnet syndrome,[122] a condition in which visual hallucinations occur on the background of visual loss. Visual field defects also occur in relation to occipital lobe seizures,[123] or more rarely with seizures of the temporal or parietal lobes.[124,125]

Auditory and musical hallucinations are an uncommon feature of epilepsy.[126] In a functional neuroimaging study of 23 people with musical hallucinations, Bernardini and colleagues described a wide range of brain regions involved in auditory seizures. As might be expected, this included primary and secondary auditory cortex, as well as basal ganglia, precuneus, and orbitofrontal areas.[127] Epilepsy with auditory features is often seen in familial cases involving mutations of leucine-rich, glioma-inactivated 1 gene (*LGI1*).[128,129] In these cases, seizures typically involve lateral temporal lobes and auditory manifestations include 'ringing', 'singing', 'humming', and 'whistling' of variable volume which interferes with a sufferer's ability to perceive real-world sounds.[130]

Mechanisms

In this section we review mechanisms through which cognitive impairment may occur in epilepsy. These include seizures themselves, interictal epileptiform activity, focal lesions, wider network dysfunction, medication-related effects, genetics, and psychological factors. In many cases, the cause of cognitive impairment will be multifactorial, resulting from a combination of these factors in different measures.

Seizures and interictal spikes

Transitory cognitive impairment has been described in around 50% of those with subclinical interictal discharges.[131] In this phenomenon, focal interictal discharges have been identified in relation to subtle cognitive impairments, often only noted when a person is tested to the limits of their capability. Transitory cognitive impairment appears to be most easily identified during tests of working memory and language, where discharges occurring during stimulus presentation or within the preceding 2 seconds appear to be most sensitive.[132,133] However, while often momentary and subtle, transitory cognitive impairment can have important day-to-day implications. In a study assessing the impact of subclinical epileptiform EEG changes on driving behaviour, Kasteleijn-Nolst Trenité et al. identified impaired driving performance where subclinical discharges occurred.[134] In a more recent study, Nirkko and colleagues describe an association between interictal epileptiform activity, prolonged reaction times, and virtual accidents, when participants used a car driving computer test.[135]

In a study looking at a paediatric population, there were statistically significant lower scores on several tests (full-scale IQ, block design, auditory reaction time, the Computerized Visual Searching Task (CVST), reading, and Corsi's block tapping) in those with interictal EEG discharges greater than 1% of the time, when compared against a second group with interictal EEG discharges less than 1% of the time.[136] Similar findings have also been identified in adults, where an increase in interictal epileptiform discharges has been shown to be associated with impaired performance on the Wechsler Adult Intelligence Scale (WAIS) and the Wechsler Memory Scale (WMS).[137] Interictal epileptiform abnormalities are particularly common during sleep, where these events are thought to interfere with the normal process of memory consolidation, leading to impairments in memory and learning.[138,139] Such overnight interictal abnormalities may also play a role in ALF by disrupting memory consolidation.[72]

Focal lesions

As we have seen through our domain-based approach, cognitive function in epilepsy is often related to focal structural lesions. A wide range of focal abnormalities (tumour, haemorrhage, infection, traumatic injury) can give rise to epileptic seizures. The probability of identifying a focal lesion in people with epilepsy is increasing with advances in neuroimaging. In a study of 37 people with focal epilepsy with non-lesional 1.5-Tesla (T) or 3 T MRI scans, Feldman et al. identified abnormal findings of 'epileptogenic potential' in 25 (68%) when 7 T scans were performed.[140] Most commonly these abnormalities involved the temporal lobes, including hippocampal asymmetry and hippocampal sclerosis (Figure 5.3). Given the important role played by the hippocampus in multiple memory tasks, it is not surprising that people with hippocampal sclerosis experience cognitive deficits, including impairments of verbal and visual memory, language, and executive function.[112,141]

Focal cortical dysplasia is the most common cause of intractable epilepsy in children. These focal lesions have a high epileptogenic potential and there

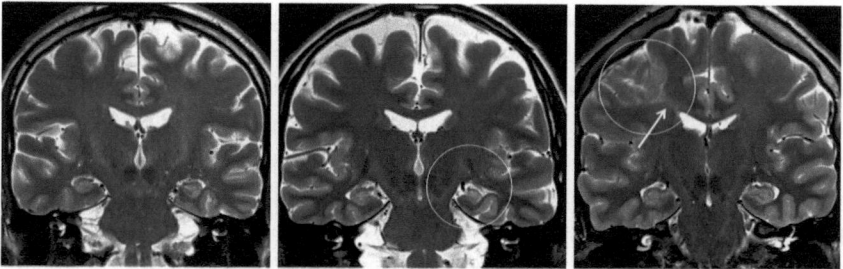

Figure 5.3 Coronal T2-weighted sequences at the level of the hippocampi demonstrating normal appearances (a); the small shrunken appearance of unilateral hippocampal sclerosis (b); and focal cortical dysplasia (c). The arrow highlights the 'transmantle sign' typically associated with focal cortical dysplasia type IIb.
(a) Normal appearance, (b) hippocampal sclerosis, (c) focal cortical dysplasia.

is a high probability of seizure cessation in cases where a complete resection is possible.[142] Focal cortical dysplasia is a term that encompasses several neuropathologically different disorders of neuronal migration and/or lamination occurring both with and without primary structural lesions; as a result, a range of seizure and neurocognitive phenotypes are seen.[143,144] In these instances, cognitive symptoms can relate to the underlying structural abnormality, a high frequency of seizures, or the use of multiple medications. A younger age of seizure onset, high frequency of seizures, and status epilepticus are associated with lower IQ and greater cognitive impairment.[145]

In people who have undergone surgery, cognitive symptoms may change as a result of the resection (Chapter 4). Of 37 children who had undergone surgery for focal cortical dysplasia in childhood and in whom a relevant IQ change could be determined, 24% showed an improvement of at least 10 points, 5% deteriorated by at least 10 points, and 70% had postsurgical scores within 10 IQ points of their presurgical score.[146] In their larger study of memory function following anterior temporal lobe (ATL) resection, Baxendale and colleagues report that 22% of those undergoing right ATL resection (n = 105) and 9% of those with left ATL resection (n = 132) demonstrated improvement in verbal learning postoperatively. For visual learning 9% of right ATL and 16% of left ATL were found to improve postoperatively.[147]

Network dysfunction

While models which emphasize focal lesions and their cognitive impact in epilepsy are useful to a degree, advances in functional neuroimaging have shown that cognitive processes are widely distributed and involve interconnected networks and their interactions.[148] Likewise, even with the most advanced imaging techniques, around 30% of those with epilepsy do not have any evidence of a causative structural lesion on MRI. In a study comparing people with temporal lobe epilepsy (with IQ >70 and no history of epilepsy surgery), divided into three groups (those with normal MRI scans, those with hippocampal sclerosis, and those with MRI abnormalities other than hippocampal sclerosis), with a control group, Rayner et al. reported consistent neuropsychological deficits across all temporal lobe epilepsy groups including autobiographical memory, auditory-verbal learning and recall, and visuospatial recall.[149] It appears that neuronal networks involved in cognition are particularly liable to conduct epileptic activity, partly as a by-product of their interconnectedness 'much as water will be channelled along the existing contours of a landscape' during heavy rain.[150]

While network abnormalities have been shown to be a causative factor in epileptic seizures and in cognitive impairments, it has also been shown that further seizures worsen these network changes, leading to structural reorganization that further impairs cognitive function.[150] Status epilepticus in particular leads to a cascade of injury including neuronal cell death as well as synaptic reorganization in the form of aberrant growth of axons which in turn can lead to hyperexcitability and an increased tendency to synchrony, which can lead to an increased risk of seizures and enduring cognitive impairments.[151] These changes lead to reduced network flexibility, impairing performance in both learning and recall tasks which require dynamic reweighting of network connections.[152]

Several studies have shown that chronic epilepsy leads to structural changes within multiple brain regions, and that these changes progress over time.[153–155] Extensive volume loss in myriad brain regions (including hippocampus, caudate, thalamus, cerebral white and grey matter, pallidum, and brainstem) is seen in people with temporal lobe epilepsy.[154,156] Significant loss of cerebral white matter implicates reductions in connectivity between these regions as a result of chronic epilepsy, a finding further supported by diffusion tensor imaging in similar situations.[157] Although the degree to which these changes correlate with cognitive impairments is less clear, it is probable that such changes will lead to deficits. Dabbs et al. have shown that a longer duration of epilepsy is associated with more extensive volume loss and that concomitant increases in cognitive impairment occur.[32]

Neurodegeneration

Neurodegenerative processes can also lead to a combination of epilepsy and cognitive impairment (see Chapter 10). The prevalence of epilepsy is increased in people with dementia.[158,159] While this has been known about for over a century (it was described by Alois Alzheimer himself in a 1911 case report[160]), the degree to which this risk is increased and whether this increase is seen across all forms of dementia is less clear.

In dementia, the highest risk of developing epilepsy occurs in those with autosomal dominant early-onset forms of AD, involving mutations in one of three genes: presenilin-1 (*PSEN1*), presenilin-2 (*PSEN2*), or amyloid precursor protein (*APP*). An increased risk is also seen in those who have a duplication of *APP*. In these conditions, the prevalence of epilepsy has been shown to be 47.7%.[161] These conditions, as well as in the far larger group with sporadic older-onset AD, the main pathological changes which are described include the formation of amyloid beta (Aβ) plaques and neurofibrillary tangles of hyperphosphorylated tau (p-tau). These changes have been shown to lead to neuronal hyperexcitability and consequent seizures. Studies which have investigated the impact of seizures in those with AD have shown that epilepsy is associated with an accelerated rate of cognitive decline.[162,163]

People with chronic epilepsy have also been shown to have an increase in the deposition of Aβ and p-tau, suggesting that there is a bidirectional relationship between these two conditions (the pathological changes seen in AD lead to epilepsy, recurrent seizures lead to the deposition of AD pathological proteins)[164–166] (Figure 5.4). Recent studies have shown that those who

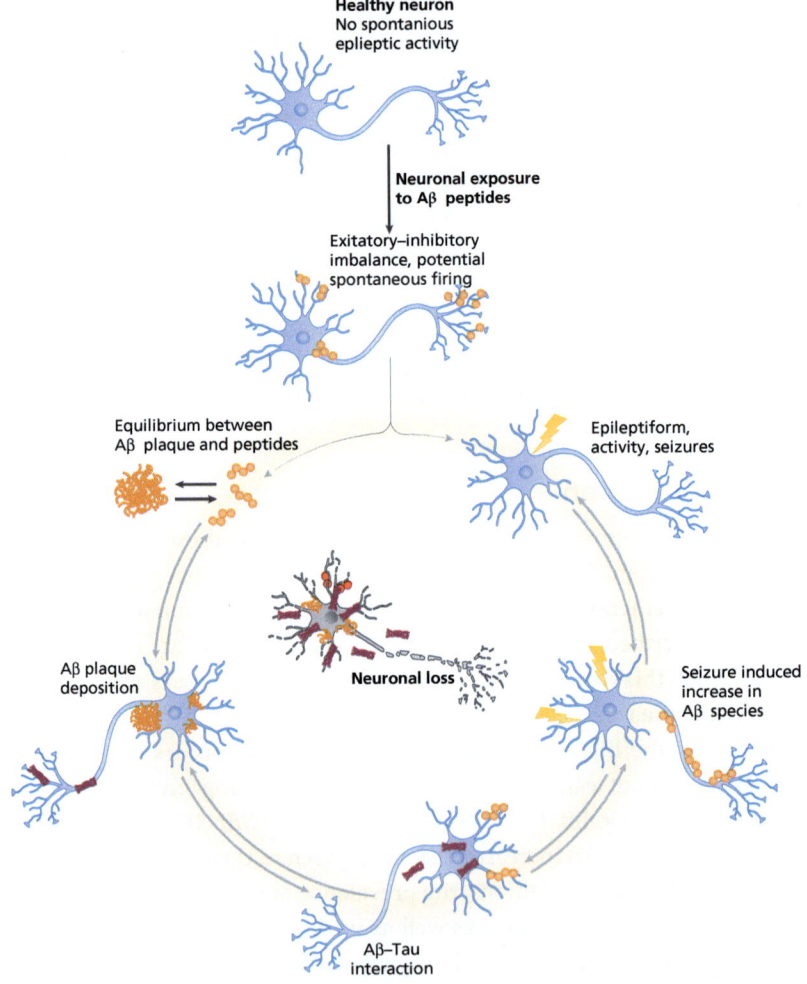

Figure 5.4 Clinical and preclinical studies have described a bidirectional relationship between the deposition of Aβ oligomers and epileptiform activity (Aβ can lead to neuronal hyperexcitability and subsequent epileptic seizures; while seizures can lead to increases in amyloid deposition and neuronal loss).

Reproduced with permission from Romoli M, Sen A, Parnetti L, Calabresi P, Costa C. Amyloid-β: a potential link between epilepsy and cognitive decline. Nat Rev Neurol. 2021;17(8):469–85.

develop epilepsy in later life have an increased risk of subsequently developing dementia.[167]

Medication-related changes in cognition

The initiation of ASMs follows a diagnosis of epilepsy in most people. We know that a majority of these will experience a reduction in seizure frequency, if not complete cessation of seizures, following the initiation of medication. However, for many this does not lead to a concomitant cessation in the cognitive symptoms that they have been experiencing. Some will experience new cognitive impairments once treatments start, including both domain-specific and more general effects. This is attributed to drug-related suppression of neural activity, including dysfunctional network activation in the inferior frontal gyrus and reduced medial temporal lobe activation.[168]

Cognitive symptoms are most common with older ASMs such as phenobarbitone, phenytoin, and carbamazepine,[9,169,170] but are also reported in newer medications such as levetiracetam, lamotrigine, topiramate, and perampanel.[10,171-173] These data suggest that cognitive dysfunction related to new medications is less common and often more subtle than with older treatments,[8,174-176] and that polytherapy increases the risk of cognitive impairment.[177] However, in light of the shorter length of use of these medications and the lack of baseline pretreatment neuropsychological data for most people with epilepsy, these data are limited. In a randomized, double-blind, two-period crossover study which employed 11 neuropsychological tests, Meador and colleagues identified significantly worse effects (p <0.001) in those treated with carbamazepine compared to levetiracetam.[176] In a further study comparing levetiracetam, lamotrigine, and phenobarbital in people with seizures and AD, Cumbo and Ligori demonstrated comparable seizure control in all three groups but an improved cognitive performance in those treated with levetiracetam, particularly on attention and oral fluency items.[178] Studies in this area have led to further investigation into the potential neuroprotective effects of levetiracetam, particularly in dementia.[179-181]

Genetics

Historically, the majority of cases of epilepsy have been described as 'idiopathic', or 'cryptogenic'. However, increasing use of genetic testing has revolutionized understanding of how genetic factors influence the risk of developing epilepsy and a growing number of specific genes are now implicated in seizures.[182] The genetics of epilepsy syndromes influence both the nature of seizures themselves and the cognitive phenotypes with which they are associated.[183]

In several conditions involving both childhood-onset epilepsy and neurocognitive/neurodevelopmental deficits—for example, Dravet syndrome, tuberous sclerosis, and Rett syndrome[182]—the relationship between genetics, epilepsy, and cognition is well defined. For example, most cases of Dravet syndrome are related to mutations in the sodium channel gene *SCN1A*. However, several other genes have been discovered which are associated with similar phenotypes, combining both epilepsy and cognitive impairments including *SCN2A*, *SCN8A*, *SCN9A*, *SCN1B*, *PCDH19*, *GABRA1*, *GABRG2*, *STXBP1*, *HCN1*, *CHD2*, and *KCNA2*.[184] In later-onset forms of epilepsy this relationship is less clear, and studying the relationships between seizures, cognitive function, and genes that confer an increased risk of epilepsy must be a crucial focus for research in the coming years.[185,186] As we have seen, genes involved in familial AD are also associated with an increased risk of epilepsy. Apolipoprotein E4 (*APOE4*) has been identified as one of the most important genetic risk factors for sporadic, late-onset AD and has also been implicated as a cause of later-onset epileptic seizures.[187]

Psychological/social

It has been shown that psychological and social stressors (depression, anxiety, isolation) are associated with an increased frequency of epileptic seizures[188] (see also Chapter 6). It has also been shown that these factors can have a major impact on cognitive function.[189] It can therefore be difficult to disentangle the relationship between psychological factors, epilepsy, and cognition.[190] Although the majority of people with epilepsy experience a reduction in seizure frequency following the initiation of medication, some will continue to experience epileptic seizures despite multiple different treatments being tried, both individually and in combination. Given that people with refractory epilepsy experience ongoing seizures and are typically prescribed multiple different ASMs, cognitive impairment, psychological dysfunction, and reduced quality of life are particularly common in this group.[7,191,192]

Prevention and treatment of cognitive dysfunction in epilepsy

Epilepsy surgery

For people with treatment-resistant epilepsy, for whom a focal epileptogenic zone is identified, epilepsy surgery can provide a potential avenue to seizure freedom. Several studies have shown that, for people with treatment-resistant temporal lobe epilepsy, surgical resection offers the best chance for seizure remission. A person's suitability for epilepsy surgery is determined through a series of investigations and depends upon whether a focus of epileptic activity can be identified and whether the removal of this focus is possible or will cause unacceptable functional damage.

Given that the removal of an epileptogenic focus can lead to a reduction in seizure frequency, it is not surprising that surgery can be associated with the improvement of cognitive impairments in some individuals[193,194] (see Chapter 4). More commonly, though, epilepsy surgery will have negative cognitive sequelae. The nature and extent of these consequences depends on both the site and the size of the resection. In a study of those who had undergone temporal lobe resections, deficits of verbal memory were more common in those who had left temporal surgery.[195] Conversely, those who had undergone right temporal surgery were more likely to have stable or improved cognitive function.[194] Tanriverdi and colleagues have shown that selective surgery can minimize the ensuing cognitive impairment when compared to larger surgical areas, suggesting that the size of the operation is important in minimizing postoperative cognitive impairments and emphasizing the importance of thorough preoperative investigations to characterize the site of seizure generation. It is, however, recognized that more limited resection may be less likely to result in seizure control.[196]

Laser interstitial thermal therapy and stereotactic laser ablation have evolved out of this desire for ultra-selective minimally invasive surgery. In these approaches, MRI-guided lasers are focused onto the regions of the brain which have previously been identified as being responsible for seizure generation. The heat generated by the lasers ablates the epileptogenic tissue. These procedures reduce the volume of brain affected by surgery, reduce anaesthetic requirements, remove the need for craniotomy, and through a combination of these factors, reduce the length of hospital admission. Research is ongoing into the efficacy of this procedure in the epilepsy population.[197,198]

Cognitive rehabilitation in epilepsy

The role of rehabilitation to limit cognitive impairment has been investigated in people who have undergone epilepsy surgery as well as those who have been managed medically.[199] Reaching a conclusion on the role and efficacy of rehabilitation in these populations is complicated by heterogeneity in the studies which have evaluated this issue—both in terms of the populations studied and the interventions which have been employed.[200,201] Beneficial effects of cognitive rehabilitation have been shown for verbal learning in those who have undergone surgery for left temporal lobe epilepsy[202,203] as well as improvements in mood.[204] Also, cognitive rehabilitation programmes can lead to increased levels of employment postoperatively.[205] Cognitive rehabilitation takes a holistic view of the individual, looking to improve quality of life through a number of strategies, measured across several different outcomes. In a study of 77 adults with temporal lobe epilepsy, Thompson and colleagues investigated a mixture of traditional and online cognitive rehabilitation approaches, both alone and in combination.[206] They report improved verbal recall (p <0.001) and improved subjective memory ratings (p <0.007) after training, when compared to those who did not receive a cognitive training programme.

Conclusion

Cognitive impairment is common among people with epilepsy. There are multiple potential causes and the nature of the impairment depends on many factors including premorbid cognitive function, age of onset, site of seizure onset, frequency and duration of seizures, psychological comorbidities, and treatments used. Neuropsychological deficits can often be detected at the time of epilepsy diagnosis and recurrent seizures may lead to permanent and progressive changes within the brain networks underpinning cognition. Cognitive impairment may have profound educational, employment, and psychosocial impacts for people with epilepsy, and its prompt recognition and monitoring by clinicians is a crucial and often underemphasized part of epilepsy management.

References

1. **Motamedi G, Meador K.** Epilepsy and cognition. Epilepsy Behav. 2003;4(Suppl 2):S25–38.
2. **Vingerhoets G.** Cognitive effects of seizures. Seizure. 2006;15(4):221–26.
3. **Fisher RS, Vickrey BG, Gibson P,** et al. The impact of epilepsy from the patient's perspective I. Descriptions and subjective perceptions. Epilepsy Res. 2000;41(1):39–51.
4. **Allers K, Essue BM, Hackett ML,** et al. The economic impact of epilepsy: a systematic review. BMC Neurol. 2015;15:245.
5. **Pickrell WO, Lacey AS, Bodger OG,** et al. Epilepsy and deprivation, a data linkage study. Epilepsia. 2015;56(4):585–91.
6. **Steer S, Pickrell WO, Kerr MP, Thomas RH.** Epilepsy prevalence and socioeconomic deprivation in England. Epilepsia. 2014;55(10):1634–41.
7. **Laxer KD, Trinka E, Hirsch LJ,** et al. The consequences of refractory epilepsy and its treatment. Epilepsy Behav. 2014;37:59–70.
8. **Barr WB.** Understanding the cognitive side effects of antiepileptic drugs: can functional imaging be helpful? Epilepsy Curr. 2019;19(1):22–23.
9. **Ortinski P, Meador KJ.** Cognitive side effects of antiepileptic drugs. Epilepsy Behav. 2004;5(Suppl 1):S60–65.
10. **Meador KJ.** Cognitive and memory effects of the new antiepileptic drugs. Epilepsy Res. 2006;68(1):63–67.
11. **Helmstaedter C, Witt JA.** Epilepsy and cognition—a bidirectional relationship? Seizure. 2017;49:83–89.

12. **Mullen SA, Berkovic SF.** Genetic generalized epilepsies. Epilepsia. 2018;**59**(6):1148–53.

13. **Nickels KC, Zaccariello MJ, Hamiwka LD, Wirrell EC.** Cognitive and neurodevelopmental comorbidities in paediatric epilepsy. Nat Rev Neurol. 2016;**12**(8):465–76.

14. **Prince E, Ring H.** Causes of learning disability and epilepsy: a review. Curr Opin Neurol. 2011;**24**(2):154–58.

15. **Vogt VL, Aikia M, Del Barrio A, et al.** Current standards of neuropsychological assessment in epilepsy surgery centers across Europe. Epilepsia. 2017;**58**(3):343–55.

16. **Butler CR, Graham KS, Hodges JR, Kapur N, Wardlaw JM, Zeman AZ.** The syndrome of transient epileptic amnesia. Ann Neurol. 2007;**61**(6):587–98.

17. **Butler CR, Zeman A.** The causes and consequences of transient epileptic amnesia. Behav Neurol. 2011;**24**(4):299–305.

18. **Benatar M.** Ictal aphasia. Epilepsy Behav. 2002;**3**(5):413–19.

19. **Bateman LM, Mendiratta A, Liou JY, et al.** Postictal clinical and electroencephalographic activity following intracranially recorded bilateral tonic-clonic seizures. Epilepsia. 2019;**60**(1):74–84.

20. **Fisher RS, Engel JJ Jr.** Definition of the postictal state: when does it start and end? Epilepsy Behav. 2010;**19**(2):100–104.

21. **Helmstaedter C, Elger CE, Lendt M.** Postictal courses of cognitive deficits in focal epilepsies. Epilepsia. 1994;**35**(5):1073–78.

22. **Remi J, Noachtar S.** Clinical features of the postictal state: correlation with seizure variables. Epilepsy Behav. 2010;**19**(2):114–17.

23. **Farrell JS, Colangeli R, Wolff MD, et al.** Postictal hypoperfusion/hypoxia provides the foundation for a unified theory of seizure-induced brain abnormalities and behavioral dysfunction. Epilepsia. 2017;**58**(9):1493–501.

24. **van Vliet EA, da Costa Araujo S, Redeker S, van Schaik R, Aronica E, Gorter JA.** Blood-brain barrier leakage may lead to progression of temporal lobe epilepsy. Brain. 2007;**130**(Pt 2):521–34.

25. **Vezzani A, French J, Bartfai T, Baram TZ.** The role of inflammation in epilepsy. Nat Rev Neurol. 2011;**7**(1):31–40.

26. **Khurgel M, Switzer RC 3rd, Teskey GC, Spiller AE, Racine RJ, Ivy GO.** Activation of astrocytes during epileptogenesis in the absence of neuronal degeneration. Neurobiol Dis. 1995;**2**(1):23–35.

27. **Pulliainen V, Kuikka P, Jokelainen M.** Motor and cognitive functions in newly diagnosed adult seizure patients before antiepileptic medication. Acta Neurol Scand. 2000;**101**(2):73–78.

28. **Taylor J, Kolamunnage-Dona R, Marson AG, Smith PE, Aldenkamp AP, Baker GA.** Patients with epilepsy: cognitively compromised before the start of antiepileptic drug treatment? Epilepsia. 2010;**51**(1):48–56.

29. **Witt JA, Helmstaedter C.** Should cognition be screened in new-onset epilepsies? A study in 247 untreated patients. J Neurol. 2012;**259**(8):1727–31.

30. **Aji BM, Larner AJ.** Cognitive assessment in an epilepsy clinic using the AD8 questionnaire. Epilepsy Behav. 2018;**85**:234–36.

31. **Galioto R, Blum AS, Tremont G.** Subjective cognitive complaints versus objective neuropsychological performance in older adults with epilepsy. Epilepsy Behav. 2015;**51**:48–52.

32. Dabbs K, Jones J, Seidenberg M, Hermann B. Neuroanatomical correlates of cognitive phenotypes in temporal lobe epilepsy. Epilepsy Behav. 2009;15(4):445–51.

33. McDonald CR, Delis DC, Norman MA, Tecoma ES, Iragui VJ. Discriminating patients with frontal-lobe epilepsy and temporal-lobe epilepsy: utility of a multilevel design fluency test. Neuropsychology. 2005;19(6):806–13.

34. Helmstaedter C, Witt JA. Multifactorial etiology of interictal behavior in frontal and temporal lobe epilepsy. Epilepsia. 2012;53(10):1765–73.

35. Wo SW, Ong LC, Low WY, Lai PSM. The impact of epilepsy on academic achievement in children with normal intelligence and without major comorbidities: a systematic review. Epilepsy Res. 2017;136:35–45.

36. Reilly C, Atkinson P, Das KB, et al. Cognition in school-aged children with 'active' epilepsy: a population-based study. J Clin Exp Neuropsychol. 2015;37(4):429–38.

37. Hermann BP, Seidenberg M, Bell B. The neurodevelopmental impact of childhood onset temporal lobe epilepsy on brain structure and function and the risk of progressive cognitive effects. Prog Brain Res. 2002;135:429–38.

38. Jokeit H, Ebner A. Long term effects of refractory temporal lobe epilepsy on cognitive abilities: a cross sectional study. J Neurol Neurosurg Psychiatry. 1999;67(1):44–50.

39. Pujar SS, Martinos MM, Cortina-Borja M, et al. Long-term prognosis after childhood convulsive status epilepticus: a prospective cohort study. Lancet Child Adolesc Health. 2018;2(2):103–11.

40. Puka K, Khattab M, Kerr EN, Smith ML. Academic achievement one year after resective epilepsy surgery in children. Epilepsy Behav. 2015;47:1–5.

41. Nadebaum C, Anderson V, Vajda F, Reutens D, Barton S, Wood A. The Australian brain and cognition and antiepileptic drugs study: IQ in school-aged children exposed to sodium valproate and polytherapy. J Int Neuropsychol Soc. 2011;17(1):133–42.

42. Andrade C. Valproate in pregnancy: recent research and regulatory responses. J Clin Psychiatry. 2018;79(3):18f12351.

43. Barton S, Nadebaum C, Anderson VA, Vajda F, Reutens DC, Wood AG. Memory dysfunction in school-aged children exposed prenatally to antiepileptic drugs. Neuropsychology. 2018;32(7):784–96.

44. Christensen J, Grønborg TK, Sørensen MJ, et al. Prenatal valproate exposure and risk of autism spectrum disorders and childhood autism. JAMA. 2013;309(16):1696–703.

45. Christensen J, Pedersen L, Sun Y, Dreier JW, Brikell I, Dalsgaard S. Association of prenatal exposure to valproate and other antiepileptic drugs with risk for attention-deficit/hyperactivity disorder in offspring. JAMA Netw Open. 2019;2(1):e186606.

46. Robertson J, Hatton C, Emerson E, Baines S. Prevalence of epilepsy among people with intellectual disabilities: a systematic review. Seizure. 2015;29:46–62.

47. van Blarikom W, Tan IY, Aldenkamp AP, van Gennep AT. Epilepsy, intellectual disability, and living environment: a critical review. Epilepsy Behav. 2006;9(1):14–18.

48. Robertson J, Hatton C, Emerson E, Baines S. Mortality in people with intellectual disabilities and epilepsy: a systematic review. Seizure. 2015;29:123–33.

49. Young C, Shankar R, Palmer J, et al. Does intellectual disability increase sudden unexpected death in epilepsy (SUDEP) risk? Seizure. 2015;25:112–16.

50. Dravet C. The core Dravet syndrome phenotype. Epilepsia. 2011;52(Suppl 2):3–9.

51. **Squire LR, Stark CE, Clark RE.** The medial temporal lobe. Annu Rev Neurosci. 2004;**27**:279–306.

52. **Lech RK, Suchan B.** The medial temporal lobe: memory and beyond. Behav Brain Res. 2013;**254**:45–49.

53. **Blair RD.** Temporal lobe epilepsy semiology. Epilepsy Res Treat. 2012;**2012**:751510.

54. **Lah S, Castles A, Smith ML.** Reading in children with temporal lobe epilepsy: a systematic review. Epilepsy Behav. 2017;**68**:84–94.

55. **Mameniskiene R, Rimsiene J, Puronaite R.** Cognitive changes in people with temporal lobe epilepsy over a 13-year period. Epilepsy Behav. 2016;**63**:89–97.

56. **Riley JD, Fling BW, Cramer SC, Lin JJ.** Altered organization of face-processing networks in temporal lobe epilepsy. Epilepsia. 2015;**56**(5):762–71.

57. **Tramoni-Negre E, Lambert I, Bartolomei F, Felician O.** Long-term memory deficits in temporal lobe epilepsy. Rev Neurol (Paris). 2017;**173**(7–8):490–97.

58. **Trebuchon A, Lambert I, Guisiano B, et al.** The different patterns of seizure-induced aphasia in temporal lobe epilepsies. Epilepsy Behav. 2018;**78**:256–64.

59. **Vaccaro MG, Trimboli M, Scarpazza C, et al.** Neuropsychological profile of mild temporal lobe epilepsy. Epilepsy Behav. 2018;**85**:222–26.

60. **Mameniskiene R, Jatuzis D, Kaubrys G, Budrys V.** The decay of memory between delayed and long-term recall in patients with temporal lobe epilepsy. Epilepsy Behav. 2006;**8**(1):278–88.

61. **Zeman A, Butler C, Muhlert N, Milton F.** Novel forms of forgetting in temporal lobe epilepsy. Epilepsy Behav. 2013;**26**(3):335–42.

62. **Zeman AZ, Boniface SJ, Hodges JR.** Transient epileptic amnesia: a description of the clinical and neuropsychological features in 10 cases and a review of the literature. J Neurol Neurosurg Psychiatry. 1998;**64**(4):435–43.

63. **Mosbah A, Tramoni E, Guedj E, et al.** Clinical, neuropsychological, and metabolic characteristics of transient epileptic amnesia syndrome. Epilepsia. 2014;**55**(5):699–706.

64. **Butler C, van Erp W, Bhaduri A, Hammers A, Heckemann R, Zeman A.** Magnetic resonance volumetry reveals focal brain atrophy in transient epileptic amnesia. Epilepsy Behav. 2013;**28**(3):363–69.

65. **Lah S, Mohamed A, Thayer Z, Miller L, Diamond K.** Accelerated long-term forgetting of verbal information in unilateral temporal lobe epilepsy: is it related to structural hippocampal abnormalities and/or incomplete learning? J Clin Exp Neuropsychol. 2014;**36**(2):158–69.

66. **Cronel-Ohayon S, Zesiger P, Davidoff V, Boni A, Roulet E, Deonna T.** Deficit in memory consolidation (abnormal forgetting rate) in childhood temporal lobe epilepsy. Pre and postoperative long-term observation. Neuropediatrics. 2006;**37**(6):317–24.

67. **Gascoigne MB, Barton B, Webster R, Gill D, Antony J, Lah SS.** Accelerated long-term forgetting in children with idiopathic generalized epilepsy. Epilepsia. 2012;**53**(12):2135–40.

68. **Witt JA, Vogt VL, Widman G, Langen KJ, Elger CE, Helmstaedter C.** Loss of autonoetic awareness of recent autobiographical episodes and accelerated long-term forgetting in a patient with previously unrecognized glutamic acid decarboxylase antibody related limbic encephalitis. Front Neurol. 2015;**6**:130.

69. Savage SA, Irani SR, Leite MI, Zeman AZ. NMDA receptor antibody encephalitis presenting as transient epileptic amnesia. J Neuroimmunol. 2019;327:41–43.

70. Loane C, Argyropoulos GPD, Roca-Fernandez A, et al. Hippocampal network abnormalities explain amnesia after VGKCC-Ab related autoimmune limbic encephalitis. J Neurol Neurosurg Psychiatry. 2019;90(9):965–74.

71. Walsh CM, Wilkins S, Bettcher BM, Butler CR, Miller BL, Kramer JH. Memory consolidation in aging and MCI after 1 week. Neuropsychology. 2014;28(2):273–80.

72. Lambert I, Tramoni-Negre E, Lagarde S, et al. Hippocampal interictal spikes during sleep impact long-term memory consolidation. Ann Neurol. 2020;87(6):976–87.

73. Burkholder DB, Jones AL, Jones DT, et al. Frequent sleep-related bitemporal focal seizures in transient epileptic amnesia syndrome: evidence from ictal video-EEG. Epilepsia Open. 2017;2(2):255–59.

74. McDonald CR, Delis DC, Norman MA, Wetter SR, Tecoma ES, Iragui VJ. Response inhibition and set shifting in patients with frontal lobe epilepsy or temporal lobe epilepsy. Epilepsy Behav. 2005;7(3):438–46.

75. Upton D, Thompson PJ. General neuropsychological characteristics of frontal lobe epilepsy. Epilepsy Res. 1996;23(2):169–77.

76. O'Muircheartaigh J, Richardson MP. Epilepsy and the frontal lobes. Cortex. 2012;48(2):144–55.

77. Auvin S, Wirrell E, Donald KA, et al. Systematic review of the screening, diagnosis, and management of ADHD in children with epilepsy. Consensus paper of the Task Force on Comorbidities of the ILAE Pediatric Commission. Epilepsia. 2018;59(10):1867–80.

78. Dunn DW, Austin JK, Harezlak J, Ambrosius WT. ADHD and epilepsy in childhood. Dev Med Child Neurol. 2003;45(1):50–54.

79. Cohen R, Senecky Y, Shuper A, et al. Prevalence of epilepsy and attention-deficit hyperactivity (ADHD) disorder: a population-based study. J Child Neurol. 2013;28(1):120–23.

80. Syvertsen M, Selmer K, Enger U, et al. Psychosocial complications in juvenile myoclonic epilepsy. Epilepsy Behav. 2019;90:122–28.

81. Schmitz B, Yacubian EM, Feucht M, Hermann B, Trimble M. Neuropsychology and behavior in juvenile myoclonic epilepsy. Epilepsy Behav. 2013;28(Suppl 1):S72–73.

82. Moschetta S, Valente KD. Impulsivity and seizure frequency, but not cognitive deficits, impact social adjustment in patients with juvenile myoclonic epilepsy. Epilepsia. 2013;54(5):866–70.

83. Wandschneider B, Thompson PJ, Vollmar C, Koepp MJ. Frontal lobe function and structure in juvenile myoclonic epilepsy: a comprehensive review of neuropsychological and imaging data. Epilepsia. 2012;53(12):2091–98.

84. Vollmar C, O'Muircheartaigh J, Barker GJ, et al. Motor system hyperconnectivity in juvenile myoclonic epilepsy: a cognitive functional magnetic resonance imaging study. Brain. 2011;134(Pt 6):1710–19.

85. Holtkamp M, Senf P, Kirschbaum A, Janz D. Psychosocial long-term outcome in juvenile myoclonic epilepsy. Epilepsia. 2014;55(11):1732–38.

86. Farrant A, Morris RG, Russell T, et al. Social cognition in frontal lobe epilepsy. Epilepsy Behav. 2005;7(3):506–16.

87. **Cahn-Weiner DA, Wittenberg D, McDonald C.** Everyday cognition in temporal lobe and frontal lobe epilepsy. Epileptic Disord. 2009;**11**(3):222–27.

88. **Patrikelis P, Angelakis E, Gatzonis S.** Neurocognitive and behavioral functioning in frontal lobe epilepsy: a review. Epilepsy Behav. 2009;**14**(1):19–26.

89. **Ives-Deliperi VL, Jokeit H.** Impaired social cognition in epilepsy: a review of what we have learnt from neuroimaging studies. Front Neurol. 2019;**10**:940.

90. **Monti G, Meletti S.** Emotion recognition in temporal lobe epilepsy: a systematic review. Neurosci Biobehav Rev. 2015;**55**:280–93.

91. **Young AW, Hellawell DJ, Van De Wal C, Johnson M.** Facial expression processing after amygdalotomy. Neuropsychologia. 1996;**34**(1):31–39.

92. **Meletti S, Cantalupo G, Santoro F,** et al. Temporal lobe epilepsy and emotion recognition without amygdala: a case study of Urbach–Wiethe disease and review of the literature. Epileptic Disord. 2014;**16**(4):518–27.

93. **Hennion S, Delbeuck X, Duhamel A,** et al. Characterization and prediction of theory of mind disorders in temporal lobe epilepsy. Neuropsychology. 2015;**29**(3):485–92.

94. **Hennion S, Delbeuck X, Koelkebeck K,** et al. A functional magnetic resonance imaging investigation of theory of mind impairments in patients with temporal lobe epilepsy. Neuropsychologia. 2016;**93**(Pt A):271–79.

95. **Toledano R, Jiménez-Huete A, García-Morales I,** et al. Aphasic seizures in patients with temporopolar and anterior temporobasal lesions: a video-EEG study. Epilepsy Behav. 2013;**29**(1):172–77.

96. **Pal DK.** Epilepsy and neurodevelopmental disorders of language. Curr Opin Neurol. 2011;**24**(2):126–31.

97. **Baumer FM, Cardon AL, Porter BE.** Language dysfunction in pediatric epilepsy. J Pediatr. 2018;**194**:13–21.

98. **Knecht S, Deppe M, Dräger B,** et al. Language lateralization in healthy right-handers. Brain. 2000;**123** (Pt 1):74–81.

99. **Knecht S, Dräger B, Deppe M,** et al. Handedness and hemispheric language dominance in healthy humans. Brain. 2000;**123**(Pt 12):2512–18.

100. **de Bode S, Smets L, Mathern GW, Dubinsky S.** Complex syntax in the isolated right hemisphere: receptive grammatical abilities after cerebral hemispherectomy. Epilepsy Behav. 2015;**51**:33–39.

101. **Gröppel G, Dorfer C, Mühlebner-Fahrngruber A,** et al. Improvement of language development after successful hemispherotomy. Seizure. 2015;**30**:70–75.

102. **Landau WM, Kleffner FR.** Syndrome of acquired aphasia with convulsive disorder in children. Neurology. 1957;**7**(8):523–30.

103. **Riccio CA, Vidrine SM, Cohen MJ, Acosta-Cotte D, Park Y.** Neurocognitive and behavioral profiles of children with Landau–Kleffner syndrome. Appl Neuropsychol Child. 2017;**6**(4):345–54.

104. **Hughes JR.** A review of the relationships between Landau–Kleffner syndrome, electrical status epilepticus during sleep, and continuous spike-waves during sleep. Epilepsy Behav. 2011;**20**(2):247–53.

105. **Yang X, Qian P, Xu X,** et al. GRIN2A mutations in epilepsy-aphasia spectrum disorders. Brain Dev. 2018;**40**(3):205–10.

106. Conroy J, McGettigan PA, McCreary D, et al. Towards the identification of a genetic basis for Landau–Kleffner syndrome. Epilepsia. 2014;55(6):858–65.

107. Schefft BK, Testa SM, Dulay MF, Privitera MD, Yeh HS. Preoperative assessment of confrontation naming ability and interictal paraphasia production in unilateral temporal lobe epilepsy. Epilepsy Behav. 2003;4(2):161–68.

108. Hamberger MJ, Tamny TR. Auditory naming and temporal lobe epilepsy. Epilepsy Res. 1999;35(3):229–43.

109. Davies KG, Bell BD, Bush AJ, Hermann BP, Dohan FC Jr, Jaap AS. Naming decline after left anterior temporal lobectomy correlates with pathological status of resected hippocampus. Epilepsia. 1998;39(4):407–19.

110. Hermann BP, Seidenberg M, Schoenfeld J, Davies K. Neuropsychological characteristics of the syndrome of mesial temporal lobe epilepsy. Arch Neurol. 1997;54(4):369–76.

111. Wang WH, Liou HH, Chen CC, et al. Neuropsychological performance and seizure-related risk factors in patients with temporal lobe epilepsy: a retrospective cross-sectional study. Epilepsy Behav. 2011;22(4):728–34.

112. Oddo S, Solís P, Consalvo D, et al. Mesial temporal lobe epilepsy and hippocampal sclerosis: cognitive function assessment in Hispanic patients. Epilepsy Behav. 2003;4(6):717–22.

113. Bartha L, Trinka E, Ortler M, et al. Linguistic deficits following left selective amygdalohippocampectomy: a prospective study. Epilepsy Behav. 2004;5(3):348–57.

114. Bartha L, Benke T, Bauer G, Trinka E. Interictal language functions in temporal lobe epilepsy. J Neurol Neurosurg Psychiatry. 2005;76(6):808–14.

115. Ramirez MJ, Schefft BK, Howe SR, Hovanitz C, Yeh HS, Privitera MD. The effects of perceived emotional distress on language performance in intractable epilepsy. Epilepsy Behav. 2010;18(1–2):64–73.

116. Vlooswijk MC, Jansen JF, Majoie HJ, et al. Functional connectivity and language impairment in cryptogenic localization-related epilepsy. Neurology. 2010;75(5):395–402.

117. Caraballo RH, Cersósimo RO, Fejerman N. Childhood occipital epilepsy of Gastaut: a study of 33 patients. Epilepsia. 2008;49(2):288–97.

118. Panayiotopoulos CP, Michael M, Sanders S, Valeta T, Koutroumanidis M. Benign childhood focal epilepsies: assessment of established and newly recognized syndromes. Brain. 2008;131(Pt 9):2264–86.

119. Brown-Vargas D, Cienki JJ. Occipital lobe epilepsy presenting as Charles Bonnet syndrome. Am J Emerg Med. 2012;30(9):2102.e5–6.

120. Doud A, Julius A, Ransom CB. Visual phenomena in occipital lobe epilepsy: 'it's beautiful!'. JAMA Neurol. 2018;75(9):1146–47.

121. Sakamoto Y, Suzuki R, Ohara T, et al. Complex visual hallucinations as the sole manifestation of symptomatic temporo-occipital lobe epilepsy due to old intracerebral hemorrhage. Seizure. 2014;23(3):244–46.

122. Adcock JE, Panayiotopoulos CP. Occipital lobe seizures and epilepsies. J Clin Neurophysiol. 2012;29(5):397–407.

123. Spatt J, Mamoli B. Ictal visual hallucinations and post-ictal hemianopia with anosognosia. Seizure. 2000;9(7):502–504.

124. **Shaw S, Kim P, Millett D.** Status epilepticus amauroticus revisited: ictal and peri-ictal homonymous hemianopsia. Arch Neurol. 2012;**69**(11):1504–507.

125. **Kurşun O, Karataş H, Dericioğlu N, Saygi S.** Refractory lesional parietal lobe epilepsy: clinical, electroencephalographic and neurodiagnostic findings. Noro Psikiyatr Ars. 2016;**53**(3):213–21.

126. **Coebergh JAF, Lauw RF, Sommer IEC, Blom JD.** Musical hallucinations and their relation with epilepsy. J Neurol. 2019;**266**(6):1501–15.

127. **Bernardini F, Attademo L, Blackmon K, Devinsky O.** Musical hallucinations: a brief review of functional neuroimaging findings. CNS Spectr. 2017;**22**(5):397–403.

128. **Kalachikov S, Evgrafov O, Ross B, et al.** Mutations in LGI1 cause autosomal-dominant partial epilepsy with auditory features. Nat Genet. 2002;**30**(3):335–41.

129. **Bisulli F, Menghi V, Vignatelli L, et al.** Epilepsy with auditory features: long-term outcome and predictors of terminal remission. Epilepsia. 2018;**59**(4):834–43.

130. **Winawer MR, Ottman R, Hauser WA, Pedley TA.** Autosomal dominant partial epilepsy with auditory features: defining the phenotype. Neurology. 2000;**54**(11):2173–76.

131. **Binnie CD.** Cognitive impairment during epileptiform discharges: is it ever justifiable to treat the EEG? Lancet Neurol. 2003;**2**(12):725–30.

132. **Binnie CD, Kasteleijn-Nolst Trenité DG, Smit AM, Wilkins AJ.** Interactions of epileptiform EEG discharges and cognition. Epilepsy Res. 1987;**1**(4):239–45.

133. **Landi S, Petrucco L, Sicca F, Ratto GM.** Transient cognitive impairment in epilepsy. Front Mol Neurosci. 2018;**11**:458.

134. **Kasteleijn-Nolst Trenité DG, Riemersma JB, Binnie CD, Smit AM, Meinardi H.** The influence of subclinical epileptiform EEG discharges on driving behaviour. Electroencephalogr Clin Neurophysiol. 1987;**67**(2):167–70.

135. **Nirkko AC, Bernasconi C, von Allmen A, Liechti C, Mathis J, Krestel H.** Virtual car accidents of epilepsy patients, interictal epileptic activity, and medication. Epilepsia. 2016;**57**(5):832–40.

136. **Nicolai J, Ebus S, Biemans DP, et al.** The cognitive effects of interictal epileptiform EEG discharges and short nonconvulsive epileptic seizures. Epilepsia. 2012;**53**(6):1051–59.

137. **Lv Y, Wang Z, Cui L, Ma D, Meng H.** Cognitive correlates of interictal epileptiform discharges in adult patients with epilepsy in China. Epilepsy Behav. 2013;**29**(1):205–10.

138. **Holmes GL, Lenck-Santini PP.** Role of interictal epileptiform abnormalities in cognitive impairment. Epilepsy Behav. 2006;**8**(3):504–15.

139. **Rasch B, Born J.** About sleep's role in memory. Physiol Rev. 2013;**93**(2):681–766.

140. **Feldman RE, Delman BN, Pawha PS, et al.** 7T MRI in epilepsy patients with previously normal clinical MRI exams compared against healthy controls. PLoS One. 2019;**14**(3):e0213642.

141. **Zalonis I, Christidi F, Artemiadis A, et al.** Verbal and figural fluency in temporal lobe epilepsy: does hippocampal sclerosis affect performance? Cogn Behav Neurol. 2017;**30**(2):48–56.

142. **Choi SA, Kim KJ.** The surgical and cognitive outcomes of focal cortical dysplasia. J Korean Neurosurg Soc. 2019;**62**(3):321–27.

143. **Spreafico R, Blümcke I.** Focal cortical dysplasias: clinical implication of neuropathological classification systems. Acta Neuropathol. 2010;**120**(3):359–67.

144. **Blümcke I, Thom M, Aronica E, et al.** The clinicopathologic spectrum of focal cortical dysplasias: a consensus classification proposed by an ad hoc Task Force of the ILAE Diagnostic Methods Commission. Epilepsia. 2011;**52**(1):158–74.

145. **Kimura N, Takahashi Y, Shigematsu H, et al.** Risk factors of cognitive impairment in pediatric epilepsy patients with focal cortical dysplasia. Brain Dev. 2019;**41**(1):77–84.

146. **Veersema TJ, van Schooneveld MMJ, Ferrier CH, et al.** Cognitive functioning after epilepsy surgery in children with mild malformation of cortical development and focal cortical dysplasia. Epilepsy Behav. 2019;**94**:209–15.

147. **Baxendale S, Thompson PJ, Duncan JS.** Improvements in memory function following anterior temporal lobe resection for epilepsy. Neurology. 2008;**71**(17):1319–25.

148. **Park HJ, Friston K.** Structural and functional brain networks: from connections to cognition. Science. 2013;**342**(6158):1238411.

149. **Rayner G, Tailby C, Jackson G, Wilson S.** Looking beyond lesions for causes of neuropsychological impairment in epilepsy. Neurology. 2019;**92**(7):e680–89.

150. **Rayner G, Tailby C.** Current concepts of memory disorder in epilepsy: edging towards a network account. Curr Neurol Neurosci Rep. 2017;**17**(8):55.

151. **Holmes GL.** Cognitive impairment in epilepsy: the role of network abnormalities. Epileptic Disord. 2015;**17**(2):101–16.

152. **Tailby C, Kowalczyk MA, Jackson GD.** Cognitive impairment in epilepsy: the role of reduced network flexibility. Ann Clin Transl Neurol. 2018;**5**(1):29–40.

153. **Dabbs K, Becker T, Jones J, Rutecki P, Seidenberg M, Hermann B.** Brain structure and aging in chronic temporal lobe epilepsy. Epilepsia. 2012;**53**(6):1033–43.

154. **McMillan AB, Hermann BP, Johnson SC, Hansen RR, Seidenberg M, Meyerand ME.** Voxel-based morphometry of unilateral temporal lobe epilepsy reveals abnormalities in cerebral white matter. Neuroimage. 2004;**23**(1):167–74.

155. **Seidenberg M, Kelly KG, Parrish J, et al.** Ipsilateral and contralateral MRI volumetric abnormalities in chronic unilateral temporal lobe epilepsy and their clinical correlates. Epilepsia. 2005;**46**(3):420–30.

156. **Bernasconi N, Duchesne S, Janke A, Lerch J, Collins DL, Bernasconi A.** Whole-brain voxel-based statistical analysis of gray matter and white matter in temporal lobe epilepsy. Neuroimage. 2004;**23**(2):717–23.

157. **Gross DW.** Diffusion tensor imaging in temporal lobe epilepsy. Epilepsia. 2011;**52**(Suppl 4):32–34.

158. **Romoli M, Sen A, Parnetti L, Calabresi P, Costa C.** Amyloid-β: a potential link between epilepsy and cognitive decline. Nat Rev Neurol. 2021;**17**(8):469–85.

159. **Baker J, Libretto T, Henley W, Zeman A.** The prevalence and clinical features of epileptic seizures in a memory clinic population. Seizure. 2019;**71**:83–92.

160. **Alzheimer A.** Über eigenartige Krankheitsfälle des späteren Alters. Neurologie und Psychiatrie. 1911;**4**(1):356.

161. **Zarea A, Charbonnier C, Rovelet-Lecrux A, et al.** Seizures in dominantly inherited Alzheimer disease. Neurology. 2016;**87**(9):912–19.

162. **Baker J, Libretto T, Henley W, Zeman A.** The prevalence and clinical features of epileptic seizures in a memory clinic population. Seizure. 2019;**71**:83–92.

163. **Vossel KA, Ranasinghe KG, Beagle AJ**, et al. Incidence and impact of subclinical epileptiform activity in Alzheimer's disease. Ann Neurol. 2016;**80**(6):858–70.

164. **Yan XX, Cai Y, Shelton J**, et al. Chronic temporal lobe epilepsy is associated with enhanced Alzheimer-like neuropathology in 3×Tg-AD mice. PLoS One. 2012;**7**(11):e48782.

165. **Li BY, Chen SD.** Potential similarities in temporal lobe epilepsy and Alzheimer's disease: from clinic to pathology. Am J Alzheimers Dis Other Demen. 2015;**30**(8):723–28.

166. **Sen A, Capelli V, Husain M.** Cognition and dementia in older patients with epilepsy. Brain. 2018;**141**(6):1592–608.

167. **Johnson EL, Krauss GL, Kucharska-Newton A**, et al. Dementia in late-onset epilepsy: the Atherosclerosis Risk in Communities Study. Neurology. 2020;**95**(24):e3248–56.

168. **Xiao F, Caciagli L, Wandschneider B**, et al. Effects of carbamazepine and lamotrigine on functional magnetic resonance imaging cognitive networks. Epilepsia. 2018;**59**(7):1362–71.

169. **Meador KJ, Loring DW, Huh K, Gallagher BB, King DW.** Comparative cognitive effects of anticonvulsants. Neurology. 1990;**40**(3 Pt 1):391–94.

170. **Meador KJ, Loring DW, Moore EE**, et al. Comparative cognitive effects of phenobarbital, phenytoin, and valproate in healthy adults. Neurology. 1995;**45**(8):1494–99.

171. **Meador KJ, Loring DW, Boyd A**, et al. Randomized double-blind comparison of cognitive and EEG effects of lacosamide and carbamazepine. Epilepsy Behav. 2016;**62**:267–75.

172. **Pina-Garza JE, Lagae L, Villanueva V**, et al. Long-term effects of adjunctive perampanel on cognition in adolescents with partial seizures. Epilepsy Behav. 2018;**83**:50–58.

173. **Schoenberg MR, Rum RS, Osborn KE, Werz MA.** A randomized, double-blind, placebo-controlled crossover study of the effects of levetiracetam on cognition, mood, and balance in healthy older adults. Epilepsia. 2017;**58**(9):1566–74.

174. **Meador KJ, Loring DW, Ray PG**, et al. Differential cognitive and behavioral effects of carbamazepine and lamotrigine. Neurology. 2001;**56**(9):1177–82.

175. **Akter N, Rahman MM, Akhter S, Fatema K.** A randomized controlled trial of phenobarbital and levetiracetam in childhood epilepsy. Mymensingh Med J. 2018;**27**(4):776–84.

176. **Meador KJ, Gevins A, Loring DW**, et al. Neuropsychological and neurophysiologic effects of carbamazepine and levetiracetam. Neurology. 2007;**69**(22):2076–84.

177. **Park SP, Kwon SH.** Cognitive effects of antiepileptic drugs. J Clin Neurol. 2008;**4**(3):99–106.

178. **Cumbo E, Ligori LD.** Levetiracetam, lamotrigine, and phenobarbital in patients with epileptic seizures and Alzheimer's disease. Epilepsy Behav. 2010;**17**(4):461–66.

179. **Musaeus CS, Shafi MM, Santarnecchi E, Herman ST, Press DZ.** Levetiracetam alters oscillatory connectivity in Alzheimer's disease. J Alzheimers Dis. 2017;**58**(4):1065–76.

180. **Devi L, Ohno M.** Effects of levetiracetam, an antiepileptic drug, on memory impairments associated with aging and Alzheimer's disease in mice. Neurobiol Learn Mem. 2013;**102**:7–11.

181. Inaba T, Miyamoto N, Hira K, et al. Protective role of levetiracetam against cognitive impairment and brain white matter damage in mouse prolonged cerebral hypoperfusion. Neuroscience. 2019;**414**:255–64.

182. Myers KA, Johnstone DL, Dyment DA. Epilepsy genetics: current knowledge, applications, and future directions. Clin Genet. 2019;**95**(1):95–111.

183. Thomas RH, Berkovic SF. The hidden genetics of epilepsy—a clinically important new paradigm. Nat Rev Neurol. 2014;**10**(5):283–92.

184. Steel D, Symonds JD, Zuberi SM, Brunklaus A. Dravet syndrome and its mimics: beyond SCN1A. Epilepsia. 2017;**58**(11):1807–16.

185. Baxendale S, Thompson P. Reprint of: The new approach to epilepsy classification: cognition and behavior in adult epilepsy syndromes. Epilepsy Behav. 2016;**64**(Pt B):318–21.

186. Johnson MR, Shkura K, Langley SR, et al. Systems genetics identifies a convergent gene network for cognition and neurodevelopmental disease. Nat Neurosci. 2016;**19**(2):223–32.

187. Di Battista AM, Heinsinger NM, Rebeck GW. Alzheimer's disease genetic risk factor APOE-ε4 also affects normal brain function. Curr Alzheimer Res. 2016;**13**(11):1200–207.

188. Kanner AM. Management of psychiatric and neurological comorbidities in epilepsy. Nat Rev Neurol. 2016;**12**(2):106–16.

189. Disner SG, Beevers CG, Haigh EA, Beck AT. Neural mechanisms of the cognitive model of depression. Nat Rev Neurosci. 2011;**12**(8):467–77.

190. Feldman L, Lapin B, Busch RM, Bautista JF. Evaluating subjective cognitive impairment in the adult epilepsy clinic: effects of depression, number of antiepileptic medications, and seizure frequency. Epilepsy Behav. 2018;**81**:18–24.

191. Gaitatzis A, Johnson AL, Chadwick DW, Shorvon SD, Sander JW. Life expectancy in people with newly diagnosed epilepsy. Brain. 2004;**127**(Pt 11):2427–32.

192. Sperling MR. The consequences of uncontrolled epilepsy. CNS Spectr. 2004;**9**(2):98–101, 106–109.

193. Bell BD, Giovagnoli AR. Memory after temporal lobe epilepsy surgery: risk and reward. Neurology. 2008;**71**(17):1302–303.

194. Helmstaedter C. Cognitive outcomes of different surgical approaches in temporal lobe epilepsy. Epileptic Disord. 2013;**15**(3):221–39.

195. Clusmann H, Schramm J, Kral T, et al. Prognostic factors and outcome after different types of resection for temporal lobe epilepsy. J Neurosurg. 2002;**97**(5):1131–41.

196. Tanriverdi T, Dudley RW, Hasan A, et al. Memory outcome after temporal lobe epilepsy surgery: corticoamygdalohippocampectomy versus selective amygdalohippocampectomy. J Neurosurg. 2010;**113**(6):1164–75.

197. Kim AH, Tatter S, Rao G, et al. Laser Ablation of Abnormal Neurological Tissue Using Robotic NeuroBlate System (LAANTERN): 12-month outcomes and quality of life after brain tumor ablation. Neurosurgery. 2020;**87**(3):E338–46.

198. Sperling MR, Gross RE, Alvarez GE, McKhann GM, Salanova V, Gilmore J. Stereotactic laser ablation for mesial temporal lobe epilepsy: a prospective, multicenter, single-arm study. Epilepsia. 2020;**61**(6):1183–89.

199. Farina E, Raglio A, Giovagnoli AR. Cognitive rehabilitation in epilepsy: an evidence-based review. Epilepsy Res. 2015;**109**:210–18.

200. Joplin S, Stewart E, Gascoigne M, Lah S. Memory rehabilitation in patients with epilepsy: a systematic review. Neuropsychol Rev. 2018;28(1):88–110.

201. Mazur-Mosiewicz A, Carlson HL, Hartwick C, et al. Effectiveness of cognitive rehabilitation following epilepsy surgery: current state of knowledge. Epilepsia. 2015;56(5):735–44.

202. Helmstaedter C, Loer B, Wohlfahrt R, et al. The effects of cognitive rehabilitation on memory outcome after temporal lobe epilepsy surgery. Epilepsy Behav. 2008;12(3):402–409.

203. Mosca C, Zoubrinetzy R, Baciu M, et al. Rehabilitation of verbal memory by means of preserved nonverbal memory abilities after epilepsy surgery. Epilepsy Behav Case Rep. 2014;2:167–73.

204. Koorenhof L, Baxendale S, Smith N, Thompson P. Memory rehabilitation and brain training for surgical temporal lobe epilepsy patients: a preliminary report. Seizure. 2012;21(3):178–82.

205. Thorbecke R, May TW, Koch-Stoecker S, Ebner A, Bien CG, Specht U. Effects of an inpatient rehabilitation program after temporal lobe epilepsy surgery and other factors on employment 2 years after epilepsy surgery. Epilepsia. 2014;55(5):725–33.

206. Thompson PJ, Conn H, Baxendale SA, et al. Optimizing memory function in temporal lobe epilepsy. Seizure. 2016;38:68–74.

Chapter 6

Epilepsy and psychopathological comorbidities

Marco Mula, Dale C. Hesdorffer, and
Michael R. Trimble

Introduction

The modern era of neuropsychiatry may have started with Hughlings Jackson (1835–1911) whose work with epilepsy not only covered such observations as 'auras' and 'dreamy states', but also involved states of 'insanity' and speculations about the development of 'positive' and 'negative' symptoms in cerebral diseases. In 1962, Guerrant and collaborators summarized the history of the relationship between epilepsy and psychiatry over the previous 100 years.[1] They outlined four periods as shown in Table 6.1. Period 1 refers to 'the era of degeneration', an idea that dominated the clinical neurosciences for much of the 19th century. Defined by Bénédict Morel (1809–1873) as 'a morbid deviation from the human type', this circumscribed such conditions as epilepsy, running through families, and in the individual leading to dementia, states that were not only incurable but could be contagious.[2] This seemingly pessimistic outlook then was countered by the second period, which was a part of the psychoanalytic era, when the personality of the patient was integral to the onset of epilepsy and was linked to its development. A 'psychic factor', as part of 'a predisposition to seizures and associated with inheritance was an expression of the same nervous constitution which gives rise to the convulsion'.[3] These theories considered epilepsy a constitutional disorder, the latter implying even more direct psychoanalytic views, such that the seizure itself was simply a psychological regression, protecting an overstressed ego. Thus, seizures were viewed as arising out of the personality and this gave rise to the 'epileptic character', lined up with various other 'psychosomatic' disorders, such as the diabetic or the cancer personality.

These ideas were firmly rejected by, among others, the epileptologist William Lennox (1884–1960), whose book *Epilepsy and Related Disorders* was, for a long time, the revered text. While *people* with epilepsy could have psychological

Table 6.1 A summary of the relationship between epilepsy and personality disorders

Period	Years
1. Of epileptic deterioration	−1900
2. Of the epileptic character	1900–1930
3. Of normality	1930–present time?
4. Of psychomotor peculiarity	1950–present time

After Guerrant et al. (1962).[1]

disorders, these were secondary to factors such as head injury, effects of sedative medications, and social stigma, but were not directly due to the seizures. The personality of *people* with epilepsy was considered quite ordinary, hence the 'normality' referred to in the table; there could be no link with psychiatry, or for that matter with intellectual disability. This view was embraced by many neurologists and lay societies, and is still widely held, especially by social psychologists, reinforcing the cataract between neurology and psychiatry that was a feature of clinical practice through much of the 20th century.

The term 'period of psychomotor peculiarity' (period 4) altered everything. The discovery of, and then the clinical application of, the electroencephalogram (EEG) heralded a 're-volution' (re-turning) within clinical neuroscience. The French epileptologist Henri Gastaut (1915–1995) emphasized the underlying neuropathology of 'psychomotor' seizures (Ammon's horn sclerosis as it was then), and the personality differences between people with psychomotor epilepsy and those with generalized epilepsy. He pointed out the high frequency of people with epilepsy in mental hospitals. He noted that many of those with temporal lobe epilepsy presented 'bizarre' behaviours interictally, and concluded 'psychical troubles in epileptics result, not from the repetition of the epileptic fits, but from the lesion which causes them'.[4] With regard to temporal lobe epilepsy he noted that the 'lesions are known to be in the rhinencephalon, a region long ago shown by Herrick and by Papez to be concerned with affect'.[4]

The resulting debates, which are still to some extent unresolved, related to whether recurrent seizures or the organic lesions were the causes of psychological and psychiatric comorbidities, and what was the importance of the underlying site of the pathology (the useful designation temporal lobe epilepsy being cast aside, even by those interested in neuroanatomy).

The introduction of the EEG and an expanding interest in epilepsy and its management was central to the development of modern neuropsychiatry, aided by a clearer understanding of limbic system neuroanatomy.

It was within this palimpsest of observations and ideas that psychological and psychiatric comorbidities of epilepsy became a focus of attention, recognized by lay organizations, accepted by a newer generation of neurologists, and, once again, central to neuropsychiatry.[5]

Epidemiology

While cross-sectional studies of epilepsy and psychiatric disorders provide useful public health information and inform epileptologists, they have significant limitations. The greatest limitation is the inability of cross-sectional studies to test hypotheses that might explain the co-occurrence of psychiatric disorders and epilepsy. An 11-item US cross-sectional survey included validated questions for epilepsy history and neuropsychiatric comorbidities including anxiety, depression, bipolar disorder, and attention deficit hyperactivity disorder (ADHD).[6] Pain disorders included migraine, chronic pain, fibromyalgia, and neuropathic pain. Additional comorbidities were asthma, diabetes, and high blood pressure. Survey questions were mailed to 190,000 households generally representative of the non-institutionalized US population aged 18 years and older. There were 172,959 respondent self-reports. Two per cent of 172,959 respondents reported having epilepsy. Those with self-reported epilepsy were more likely to self-report (than those without epilepsy) (p <0.001) for neuropsychiatric disorders, pain disorders, and asthma.[6]

While evidence from cross-sectional studies of neuropsychiatric disorders and epilepsy overlap, they do not consider time order. Instead, studies of incident cohorts with epilepsy or incident psychiatric disorders are better able to address the sequence of unidirectional and bidirectional associations, answers to which are crucial to our understanding.

Unidirectional and bidirectional relationships

To prove causation, there must be a unidirectional temporal relationship where the exposure occurs before the disease develops. The bidirectional relationship arises from two chronological sequences, that is, incident psychiatric disorder and incident epilepsy need reciprocal temporal relationships to demonstrate causation.[7] There is also a need for consistency of the findings across studies to make a persuasive argument for causality.

Unidirectional relationships

Several studies in children and adults have found that a history of depression prior to incident epilepsy was associated with continued seizures in the first

12 months,[8] felt stigma at diagnosis of incident epilepsy,[9] and poor quality of life,[10] which is more strongly associated with depression in epilepsy than with seizure frequency.

ADHD and risk for incident seizures in children

In a population-based, case–control study of newly diagnosed unprovoked seizures in Iceland, children were matched to the next two same-sex births.[11] The Diagnostic Interview Schedule for Children (DISC) was used to diagnose ADHD in cases and controls aged 3–16 years. A history of ADHD was 2.5-fold higher in those with newly diagnosed seizures when compared to controls (95% confidence interval (CI) 1.1–5.5). The odds ratio (OR) for ADHD, predominately inattentive type, was 3.7 (95% CI 1.1–12.8). Neither ADHD impulsive type nor the ADHD combined type was statistically significant nor was seizure type, sex, aetiology, and seizure frequency at diagnosis.

Major depression and risk for seizures in adults

In a case–control study of newly diagnosed idiopathic/cryptogenic seizure in older adults, the *Diagnostic and Statistical Manual of Mental Disorders*, third edition, revised (DSM-III-R) criteria were used to diagnose depression as a risk factor for a first unprovoked seizure.[12] If a person had more than one episode of depression, only the most severe episode was used. Features of DSM-II-R criteria were included. Crude odds ratios were 6.0 (95% CI 1.56–22.0) for major depression, 2.2 (95% CI 1.1–4.5) for tricyclic antidepressants, 1.6 (95% CI 1.0–2.5) for phenothiazines, 4.7 (95% CI 1.2–18) for electroconvulsive therapy, and 4.4 (95% CI 1.5–13.0) for at least five depressive symptoms for less than 2 weeks.

Bidirectional relationship between psychiatric disorders and seizures

Two studies address the bidirectional associations between incident epilepsy, suicidality, and psychiatric disorders: one using the UK General Practice Research Database[13] and another one using the Stockholm Epilepsy Register[14] (Table 6.2).

Bidirectional relationship between psychosis/ schizophrenia and epilepsy

Studies examining the time order of the relationship between psychosis/schizophrenia and epilepsy have been conducted in large population-based registries. Hesdorffer has shown that the cumulative data suggest a bidirectional relationship between incident epilepsy and incident psychosis.[13] Psychosis was

Table 6.2 Bidirectional relationship between psychiatric disorders and incident epilepsy

A. United Kingdom

Disorder	Time before and after epilepsy onset					
	−3 to −2 years	−2 to <−1 years	−1 to 0 years	>0 to 1 years	<1 to 2 years	>2 to 3 years
	IRR (95% CI)	IRR (95% CI)	IRR (95% CI)	IRR (95% CI)	IRR (95% CI)	IRR (95% CI)
Depression	1.9 (1.5–2.4)	1.5 (1.2–2.0)	2.5 (2.0–3.2)	2.3 (1.8–3.0)	2.5 (1.9–3.4)	2.2 (1.5–3.2)
Bipolar disorder	2.5 (0.4–14.8)	2.5 (0.4–14.8)	12.4 (3.4–45.0)	5.1 (1.1–22.7)	0.9 (0.1–8.2)	14.2 (1.6–127.1)
Anxiety	1.8 (1.4–2.3)	1.8 (1.4–2.3)	2.1 (1.7–2.5)	2.2 (1.8–2.8)	1.8 (1.4–2.3)	1.4 (1.0–1.9)
Psychosis	15.7 (5.3–46.8)	8.5 (3.5–20.6)	7.7 (3.8–15.9)	10.9 (4.9–24.4)	4.8 (2.1–10.9)	4.0 (1.5–10.3)
Suicide attempt[a]	3.8 (2.1–7.2)	2.7 (1.4–5.1)	4.0 (2.3–7.0)	5.1 (2.9–8.8)	2.1 (1.1–3.9)	1.7 (0.8–3.6)
Psychiatric disorders[b]	1.9 (1.5–2.4)	1.9 (1.5–2.3)	2.3 (1.9–2.7)	2.2 (1.8–2.8)	2.1 (1.6–2.7)	1.7 (1.2–2.3)

CI, confidence interval; IRR, incidence rate ratio.

[a] Suicide attempt before epilepsy onset and suicide attempt or completion after onset; [b] depression, anxiety or psychosis.

B. Sweden

Time before/ after seizure diagnosis	Psychiatric disorders combined		Depression		Psychosis		Suicide attempt	
	OR	CI	OR	CI	OR	CI	OR	CI
>5 years before	2.6	1.8–3.7	2.2	1.3–3.7	2.1	1.3–3.4	2.2	1.3–3.8
2–5 years before	2.7	1.4–5.2	1.6	0.6–4.2	2.5	0.7–8.9	3.8	1.6–9.4
<2 years before	3.9	1.9–7.9	6.3	2.8–14.6	5.6	1.2–25.8	4.7	1.2–18.8
0–2 years after	4.5	2.7–7.6	4.1	2.2–7.7	6.4	1.9–21.3	4.4	1.8–11.0
>2 years after	1.9	1.3–3.0	1.7	1.0–2.8	2.5	1.0–6.3	2.2	1.1–4.4

CI, confidence interval; OR, odds ratio.

associated with a statistically significant increased risk for developing epilepsy in each of the 3 years before epilepsy onset (incident rate ratio (IRR) =15.7, 8.5, and 7.7 in the third to first year before epilepsy onset, respectively) and incident epilepsy was associated with a statistically significant increased risk for developing a first-ever psychosis in each of the 3 years after epilepsy onset (IRR = 10.9, 4.8, and 4.0, respectively). Similar results were observed when epilepsy of unknown aetiology was examined. In a Swedish study,[14] hospitalized psychosis was associated with an increased risk for developing epilepsy (OR = 2.7; 95% CI 1.6–4.8).

An early Danish record-linkage study assessed the risk for non-organic non-affective psychosis, non-affective psychosis, and schizophrenia in people with epilepsy compared to controls, excluding all people with a learning disability and/or substance misuse as these are, of themselves, associated with epilepsy.[15] The standardized incidence ratio was significantly increased 2.15-fold for schizophrenia (p < 0.001) for men and women, 2.74-fold for non-affective psychosis (p < 0.0001), and 2.75-fold for non-organic non-affective psychoses (p < 0.001). Psychomotor epilepsy was associated with a 5.07-fold increased risk for non-organic non-affective psychosis (95% CI 3.42–7.24) in males, greater than other epilepsy types. Data for females and for both females and males did not differ. In general, the risk for schizophrenia was increased most for psychomotor epilepsy (standardized incidence ratio = 2.35; 95% CI 1.17–4.21). In terms of sex differences, this was seen in males (standardized incidence ratio = 2.56; 95% CI 1.03–5.27) but it was not statistically significant in females. There was overlap across epilepsy types for non-affective psychosis.

A second Danish registry study[16] examined the association between epilepsy and risk for schizophrenia and schizophrenia-like psychosis in the presence and absence of a personal history of epilepsy, and a family history of psychoses, adjusting for age, sex, calendar year of diagnosis, place of birth, paternal and maternal age at birth, and birth order. Among those with no family history of psychosis, a personal history of epilepsy was associated with an increased risk for schizophrenia (adjusted relative risk (RR) = 2.61; 95% CI 2.29–2.99) and with an increased risk for schizophrenia-like psychosis (adjusted RR = 3.12; 95% CI 2.83–3.42). However, a family history of epilepsy was associated with a minor risk for schizophrenia (adjusted RR = 1.17; 95% CI 1.05–1.31) and for schizophrenia-like psychosis (adjusted RR = 1.26; 95% CI 1.15–1.37). A personal history of epilepsy was associated with a greater risk for schizophrenia and schizophrenia-like psychosis compared to a family history of epilepsy, family history of schizophrenia, family history of schizophrenia-like psychosis, and family history of affective psychosis.

There were no sex differences, but increasing age was associated with a statistically significant increased risk for developing schizophrenia in people with epilepsy.[17]

Premature mortality

Fazel and colleagues[18] studied the risk and causes of premature mortality between 1954 and 2009 for inpatients and outpatients, comparing individuals with epilepsy to age- and sex-matched general population controls and to unaffected siblings. The adjusted odds of premature mortality was 11.1 (95% CI 10.6–11.6) compared to the general population and 11.4 (95% CI 10.4–12.5) compared with unaffected siblings. Death owing to external causes was associated with non-vehicle accidents (adjusted OR = 5.5 (95% CI 4.7–6.5)) and suicide (adjusted OR = 3.7 (95% CI 3.3–4.2)). Among those dying from external causes, comorbid psychiatric disorders were strongly associated with depression and substance misuse.

Clinical aspects

The phenomenology of psychiatric disorders of epilepsy has been a matter of debate for many years. Although people with epilepsy can obviously develop psychiatric disorders identical to those of people without epilepsy, several authors have pointed out that many people with epilepsy present with atypical symptoms that are poorly reflected by conventional classificatory systems such as the DSM or the International Classification of Diseases (ICD).[19,20] In general terms, the psychopathological spectrum in epilepsy is likely to be large and it is entirely reasonable that the underlying brain pathology shapes the final psychopathological phenotype of a specific psychiatric condition, masking, or minimizing, some aspects and emphasizing others.

Table 6.3 Classification of psychiatric symptoms in relationship to seizure activity

Relationship with seizures		Description
Peri-ictal	Pre-ictal	Preceding seizures from hours to days
	Ictal	Seizures with psychic symptoms (e.g. ictal fear) or non-convulsive status epilepticus
	Postictal	Mostly after tonic–clonic seizures (isolated or in cluster), rarely after focal seizures
Para-ictal		Forced normalization phenomenon (i.e. alternative psychoses)
Interictal		Unrelated to seizures. Mostly chronic disorders

This point has relevant clinical implications and does not represent just an academic exercise. In fact, the existence of epilepsy-specific psychiatric conditions implies the need for specific clinical instruments for the diagnosis, adopting specific guidelines of treatment and ultimately a different prognosis as compared to psychiatric disorders outside epilepsy. Research in this area is still at an early stage with limited evidence-based guidelines. From a clinical perspective, variables to consider in the assessment of a subject with epilepsy and a psychiatric condition are (1) the temporal relationship between psychiatric symptoms and seizures; (2) the high rates of multiple psychiatric comorbidities (e.g. mood and anxiety disorders); (3) the presence of cognitive problems due to the underlying neurological condition; and (4) the psychotropic effect of antiepileptic drugs.

The practicality of classifying psychiatric symptoms according to their temporal relationship to seizure occurrence (peri-ictal/para-ictal symptoms vs interictal symptoms) is well established (Table 6.3). Peri-ictal symptoms have been well described by Gowers and Jackson but also by Kraepelin and Bleuler and the differentiation between peri-ictal and interictal psychiatric symptoms has relevant clinical implications.[21,22]

Peri-ictal psychopathology

Premonitory symptoms or behavioural changes preceding seizures seem to be reported by at least one-third of patients and usually precede tonic–clonic rather than focal seizures. These symptoms are described as mood changes, for example, dysphoria, insomnia, or irritability lasting hours up to days, while hallucinations or perceptual abnormalities tend to be less frequent.[23,24]

The so-called ictal psychiatric symptoms are prolonged focal seizures or episodes of non-convulsive status epilepticus, mostly of temporal lobe origin and more rarely extratemporal. The presence of automatisms or other epileptic phenomena can point towards an epileptic origin along with EEG confirming epileptic abnormalities. Fear or panic as an ictal phenomenon has a strong localizing value as it is associated with the right mesial temporal lobe structures, usually the amygdala, and seems to have a poor prognostic value for seizure control after surgery.[21]

Psychopathological manifestations following seizures have been the main interest of several clinicians and researchers. There is a large literature on postictal psychoses whose phenomenology and clinical implications have been described in detail by many authors. Postictal psychoses represent one-quarter of all psychotic episodes in epilepsy. They seem to occur in people with focal epilepsies, mainly of temporal lobe origin though extratemporal structural lesions are frequently reported in these subjects. The majority of these individuals present with what is defined as the 'nuclear type' of postictal psychosis.[25] This type is characterized by a lucid interval after a seizure (i.e. a period of normal mental state preceding the onset of the psychotic episode), lasting from 1 to 6 days, usually 48 hours.[26] The phenomenology of the delusion is characterized by abnormal moods (either depressed or manic) and a paranoid/mystic delusion. Some people are confused throughout the episode but others present with fluctuating consciousness and disorientation. Psychotic symptoms usually remit spontaneously within days or weeks, with no real need for long-term antipsychotic drug treatment, which is mainly prescribed in the acute phase to reduce mortality and morbidity due to severe aggressive behaviour and high self-harm or suicidal risk. Outside epilepsy, benzodiazepines alone do not represent usual pharmacological options in patients with psychotic disorders. However, the use of benzodiazepines, especially clobazam, is quite a popular treatment for postictal psychoses among clinicians[27] although this is not based on any evidence.

In one out of four cases, postictal psychoses may progress into a chronic interictal psychosis.[28]

Although less well described than postictal psychoses, postictal mood changes, either mania or depressed mood, are frequently reported by people with epilepsy. A case series from a video-telemetry unit suggests that up to 25% of those with drug-resistant focal epilepsy present with postictal mood changes while postictal anxiety can occur in up to 45%.[29] These symptoms are relatively short, usually lasting hours rather than days. It is now recognized that individuals with chronic unremitted interictal psychiatric disorders can present with postictal deterioration of the underlying psychiatric disorder. The same case series from a video-telemetry unit showed that 58% of patients with interictal depression present a postictal deterioration, 33% postictal anxiety, and up to 77% postictal suicidal ideation.[29]

Among seizure-related psychopathological manifestations, it is important to mention the so-called forced normalization phenomenon. This concept refers to the publications of Heinrich Landolt who described a group of patients who had florid psychotic episodes with 'forced' or 'paradoxical' normalization of the EEG. Subsequently, Tellenbach introduced the term 'alternative psychosis' for the clinical phenomenon of the reciprocal relationship between abnormal mental states and seizures, which did not, as Landolt's term did, rely on EEG findings.[30] Since the early observations of Landolt, a number of patients with alternative psychoses have been documented to put the existence of this phenomenon beyond doubt and an association with the prescription of all antiseizure medications was noted, suggesting that this is not a drug-specific phenomenon but it is rather linked to the neurobiological mechanisms underlying seizure control. Initially, drug-refractory temporal lobe epilepsy was claimed to be the prototype but subsequent literature on alternative psychoses favoured generalized epilepsies. Nowadays, there is agreement that the forced normalization phenomenon occurs with both generalized and focal epilepsies.[31]

Interictal psychopathology

As already discussed, many different factors can contribute to the atypical phenomenology of interictal psychiatric disorders in epilepsy. The atypical features of depression in epilepsy are not only due to the presence of peri-ictal mood changes but also to the high comorbidity rates with anxiety disorders and the effect of antiseizure medications. In recent times, many authors have discussed a specific condition named interictal dysphoric disorder of epilepsy.[19] This is a somatoform-depressive syndrome characterized by mood instability and somatic complaints. Although now established that this is not specific to epilepsy per se, some people do develop this condition that seems to benefit mainly from mood stabilizers rather than antidepressant drug treatment.[32]

Interictal psychoses are linked to temporal lobe epilepsy and this has been demonstrated by clinical and imaging studies.[33,34] A number of authors have pointed out the phenomenological peculiarities of interictal psychoses as compared to schizophrenia such as the preserved affect, the presence of religious/mystical delusions, and the lack of negative symptoms.[34] This is in keeping with prospective studies showing that the long-term prognosis of interictal psychoses of epilepsy is better than that of schizophrenia, with less reported long-term institutionalization.[35]

Functional seizures

Functional seizures (also known as psychogenic non-epileptic attacks or dissociative seizures) are paroxysmal, time-limited, alterations in motor, sensory, autonomic, and/or cognitive signs, and symptoms. Superficially, they resemble epileptic seizures, but they are not caused by ictal epileptiform activity.[36] They are typically reported as being beyond voluntary control, and most fulfil the diagnostic criteria of dissociative (conversion) disorder (ICD-10), or conversion (functional neurological symptom) disorder (DSM-5). The incidence of functional seizures is between 1.4 and 4.9 per 1000,000 per year, and its prevalence between 2 and 33 per 100,000 with an onset between the second and fourth decades of life.[37] Data on the occurrence of functional seizures in people with epilepsy are limited. A meta-analysis showed a pooled prevalence for functional seizures in people with epilepsy of 12% (95% CI 10–14%) while the prevalence of epilepsy in people with functional seizures is around 22% (95% CI 20–25%).

Treatment issues

In general terms, evidence-based data on the management of psychiatric disorders in epilepsy are limited. However, it seems reasonable to follow internationally accepted guidelines of treatment outside epilepsy, applying individually tailored adjustments according to the epilepsy type and the concomitant use of antiseizure medications. Based on this, the International League Against Epilepsy published a number of recommendations to guide clinicians in treating major psychiatric conditions in epilepsy.[38]

Psychological treatments

In the general population, psychological treatments are first line for all anxiety disorders[39] and for mild to moderate depression.[40] It seems, therefore, reasonable to apply this guidance also to people with epilepsy but the evidence is still limited and mainly based on quality of life data.[41] An International League Against Epilepsy report confirmed that psychological interventions are recommended in people with epilepsy and mild to moderate depression, although again the evidence level is still low.[42]

Psychoeducation and psychological treatments still represent first-line treatments in people with functional seizures.[43] However, data are still controversial. Data from a US multicentre, pilot, randomized clinical trial of cognitive behavioural therapy–informed therapy with or without sertraline in people with functional seizures showed a significant seizure reduction as compared to people treated with sertraline only.[44] However, a UK pragmatic, parallel-arm, multicentre, randomized controlled trial failed to show any benefit of cognitive behavioural therapy in addition to standard medical care for the reduction of monthly seizures.[45] Further studies are needed to identify which patient group may benefit from specific interventions.[46] There are no studies on the treatment of functional seizures in people with epilepsy.

Pharmacological treatment of mood and anxiety disorders

Firstly, it is important to explore a few basic concepts in the treatment of depression that, for example, neurologists may not always be familiar with. The acute treatment of depression is aimed at remission and recovery, meaning full control of all symptoms (*remission*) for a period of 6–12 months (*recovery*). The long-term treatment of depression is aimed at preventing relapse and recurrence. A clinical deterioration before remission is reached or a new depressive episode before remission has turned into a recovery is called *relapse* while a new depressive episode after complete recovery is called *recurrence*.

Epidemiological studies of depression outside epilepsy show that up to 90% of patients go into remission with one treatment or a combination of therapeutic interventions and among these subjects about 50% go into recovery within 6 months and up to 75% in 2 years.[47] It is still unknown whether people with epilepsy and depression have similar remission and recovery rates.

Another important point is that drug treatment is not always recommended. In fact, antidepressants should not be routinely prescribed to treat persistent sub-threshold symptoms or mild depression because the risk:benefit ratio is poor. Antidepressants should be considered for patients with a past history of moderate to severe depression and sub-threshold depressive symptoms that have been present for at least 2 years or have persisted despite psychological interventions. For people with sub-threshold depressive symptoms or mild depression, low-intensity psychosocial interventions (i.e. individual guided self-help groups, computerized cognitive behavioural therapy, or structured group physical activity programmes or group cognitive behavioural therapy) should be recommended first.

In case of drug treatment, there are enough data to suggest that selective serotonin reuptake inhibitors (SSRIs), especially citalopram and sertraline, are safe and well tolerated in epilepsy although the evidence is still low and based mainly on open studies. Clinicians need to consider the potential risk of pharmacokinetic interactions with enzyme inducers (i.e. carbamazepine, phenytoin, and barbiturates; see Chapter 3) leading to at least a 25% reduction in blood levels of SSRIs. For this reason, doses should be adjusted according to response. Prescribers need also to be aware of the spectrum of side effects of antidepressants and the potential for pharmacodynamic interactions with antiepileptic drugs. Sexual dysfunction, hyponatraemia, and extrapyramidal side effects are well-known side effects of SSRIs, while weight gain and sedation are typical of tricyclics or other antidepressants like mirtazapine. For these reasons, special attention should be paid when antidepressants are prescribed alongside antiseizure medications with a similar spectrum of side effects.[48]

Pharmacological treatment of psychoses

As already discussed for antidepressants, it is important that prescribers become familiar at least with the potential risk for interactions and the spectrum of side effects of individual drugs. Enzyme inducers (i.e. carbamazepine, phenytoin, and barbiturates) can reduce the blood levels of almost all antipsychotics and this is particularly evident for quetiapine. The introduction of carbamaze-pine to a stable regimen with quetiapine can lead to undetectable levels of the antipsychotic up to a dose of 700 mg per day.[48] This should also be considered in case of discontinuation of any inducer to avoid quetiapine toxicity. In terms of side effects, apart from sedation, weight gain is the major problem with the majority of antipsychotics. This is particularly evident with olanzapine and for this reason patients should be informed about the risk of severe weight gain when olanzapine is combined with valproate, carbamazepine, gabapentin, or pregabalin. Clozapine can be potentially associated with neutropenia and for this reason the combined treatment with carbamazepine should be avoided.

Seizure risk during psychotropic drug treatment

That psychotropic drugs may be associated with an increased risk of seizures has been a matter of debate for a long time. While this seems to be established for some antipsychotic drugs, namely clozapine, evidence about antidepres-sants is still controversial. In fact, historically, the supposed proconvulsant effect of psychotropic drugs was based on a priori assumptions rather than on clinical evidence.

For antidepressants, the supposed increased risk of seizures was based on case reports and, subsequently, EEG studies showing epileptic abnormalities with tricyclics (i.e. amitriptyline and imipramine).[48] These data, despite not being systematic and based just on a few specific agents, led to the general im-pression that all antidepressants were proconvulsants. In reality, an increased risk of seizures has been demonstrated only for a minority of compounds such as maprotiline, high doses of clomipramine and amitriptyline (>200 mg), and high doses of bupropion immediate-release formulation (>450 mg). The issue of drug-related seizures is quite complex and multiple factors have to be taken into account. In fact, studies in animal models suggest that serotonin potenti-ation is actually anticonvulsant[49] and if one takes into account epidemiological data about the bidirectional relationship between epilepsy and mood disorders, the reported prevalence of epileptic seizures during treatment with antidepres-sants, especially SSRIs, is even lower than expected, suggesting a potential antiseizure effect of SSRIs.[48]

For antipsychotics the occurrence of seizures as a side effect is more estab-lished than for antidepressants, although such risk is mainly evident for clo-zapine while all other antipsychotics, especially second-generation atypical antipsychotics, seem to have a low proconvulsant risk.[48] The risk of seizures during treatment with clozapine seems to be both titration and dose dependent going up to 4.4% for dosages higher than 600 mg. Up to 5% of people treated with clozapine present EEG abnormalities[50] but whether this is a predictive factor for clozapine-induced seizures is still unknown. In general terms, clo-zapine seems to mainly worsen myoclonic jerks but generalized tonic–clonic seizures or even focal seizures have been reported in predisposed subjects.

Conclusion

Psychiatric disorders represent a relatively frequent comorbidity in people with epilepsy involving around one in three patients. Mood and anxiety disorders are the most frequently encountered with a lifetime history in one in four people. Psychoses are relatively rare in epilepsy but represent a serious comorbidity with prevalence rates up to 6% in temporal lobe epilepsy.

Data on treatment are still limited but promising in terms of efficacy and tolerability of existing guidelines of treatments used outside epilepsy. SSRIs have been shown to be effective and well tolerated in people with epilepsy as well as new atypical antipsychotics. Seizure risk and interactions with antiseizure medications need to be considered on an individual basis and are mostly related to antiseizure medications with inducing properties. Seizure worsening has to be considered for clozapine and tricyclics as well as clomipramine at high doses.

Integrated clinical pathways shaped on resources are advisable to offer access to appropriate mental healthcare to people with epilepsy.

References

1. **Guerrant J, Anderson W, Fischer A, Weinstein M, Jaros R.** Personality in epilepsy. Springfield, IL: Thomas; 1962.
2. **Pick D.** Faces of degeneration: a European disorder, c.1848–1918. Cambridge: Cambridge University Press; 1993.
3. **Turner A.** Epilepsy. London: Macmillan; 1907.
4. **Gastaut H.** The epilepsies: electroclinical correlations. Springfield, IL: Thomas; 1954.
5. **Trimble MR.** The intentional brain: motion, emotion, and the development of modern neuropsychiatry. Baltimore, MD: Johns Hopkins University Press; 2016.
6. **Ottman R, Lipton RB, Ettinger AB,** et al. Comorbidities of epilepsy: results from the Epilepsy Comorbidities and Health (EPIC) survey. Epilepsia. 2011;52(2):308–15.
7. **Keezer MR, Sisodiya SM, Sander JW.** Comorbidities of epilepsy: current concepts and future perspectives. Lancet Neurol. 2016;15(1):106–15.
8. **Hitiris N, Mohanraj R, Norrie J, Sills GJ, Brodie MJ.** Predictors of pharmacoresistant epilepsy. Epilepsy Res. 2007;75(2–3):192–96.
9. **Leaffer EB, Jacoby A, Benn E,** et al. Associates of stigma in an incident epilepsy population from northern Manhattan, New York City. Epilepsy Behav. 2011;21(1):60–64.
10. **Gilliam F.** Optimizing health outcomes in active epilepsy. Neurology. 2002;58(8 Suppl 5):S9–20.

11. **Hesdorffer DC, Ludvigsson P, Olafsson E, Gudmundsson G, Kjartansson O, Hauser WA.** ADHD as a risk factor for incident unprovoked seizures and epilepsy in children. Arch Gen Psychiatry. 2004;**61**(7):731–36.

12. **Hesdorffer DC, Hauser WA, Annegers JF, Cascino G.** Major depression is a risk factor for seizures in older adults. Ann Neurol. 2000;**47**(2):246–49.

13. **Hesdorffer DC, Ishihara L, Mynepalli L, Webb DJ, Weil J, Hauser WA.** Epilepsy, suicidality, and psychiatric disorders: a bidirectional association. Ann Neurol. 2012;**72**(2):184–91.

14. **Adelow C, Andersson T, Ahlbom A, Tomson T.** Hospitalization for psychiatric disorders before and after onset of unprovoked seizures/epilepsy. Neurology. 2012;**78**(6):396–401.

15. **Bredkjaer SR, Mortensen PB, Parnas J.** Epilepsy and non-organic non-affective psychosis. National epidemiologic study. Br J Psychiatry. 1998;**172**:235–38.

16. **Qin P, Xu H, Laursen TM, Vestergaard M, Mortensen PB.** Risk for schizophrenia and schizophrenia-like psychosis among patients with epilepsy: population based cohort study. BMJ. 2005;**331**(7507):23.

17. **Thorup A, Waltoft BL, Pedersen CB, Mortensen PB, Nordentoft M.** Young males have a higher risk of developing schizophrenia: a Danish register study. Psychol Med. 2007;**37**(4):479–84.

18. **Fazel S, Wolf A, Långström N, Newton CR, Lichtenstein P.** Premature mortality in epilepsy and the role of psychiatric comorbidity: a total population study. Lancet. 2013;**382**(9905):1646–54.

19. **Mula M.** The interictal dysphoric disorder of epilepsy: a still open debate. Curr Neurol Neurosci Rep. 2013;**13**(6):355.

20. **Kanner AM.** Depression and epilepsy: a new perspective on two closely related disorders. Epilepsy Curr. 2006;**6**(5):141–46.

21. **Mula M.** Epilepsy-induced behavioral changes during the ictal phase. Epilepsy Behav. 2014;**30**:14–16.

22. **Mula M.** Neuropsychiatric symptoms of epilepsy. London: Springer; 2015.

23. **Mula M, Jauch R, Cavanna A, et al.** Interictal dysphoric disorder and periictal dysphoric symptoms in patients with epilepsy. Epilepsia. 2010;**51**(7):1139–45.

24. **Scaramelli A, Braga P, Avellanal A, et al.** Prodromal symptoms in epileptic patients: clinical characterization of the pre-ictal phase. Seizure. 2009;**18**(4):246–50.

25. **Oshima T, Tadokoro Y, Kanemoto K.** A prospective study of postictal psychoses with emphasis on the periictal type. Epilepsia. 2006;**47**(12):2131–34.

26. **Adachi N, Ito M, Kanemoto K, et al.** Duration of postictal psychotic episodes. Epilepsia. 2007;**48**(8):1531–37.

27. **de Toffol B, Trimble M, Hesdorffer DC, et al.** Pharmacotherapy in patients with epilepsy and psychosis. Epilepsy Behav. 2018;**88**:54–60.

28. **Adachi N, Kato M, Sekimoto M, et al.** Recurrent postictal psychosis after remission of interictal psychosis: further evidence of bimodal psychosis. Epilepsia. 2003;**44**(9):1218–22.

29. **Kanner AM, Soto A, Gross-Kanner H.** Prevalence and clinical characteristics of postictal psychiatric symptoms in partial epilepsy. Neurology. 2004;**62**(5):708–13.

30. **Trimble MR, Schmitz B.** Forced normalization and alternative psychoses of epilepsy. Petersfield: Wrightson Biomedical Publishing; 1998.

31. **Mula M.** The Landolt's phenomenon: an update. Epileptologia. 2010;18:39–44.

32. **Blumer D, Montouris G, Davies K.** The interictal dysphoric disorder: recognition, pathogenesis, and treatment of the major psychiatric disorder of epilepsy. Epilepsy Behav. 2004;5:826–40.

33. **Mula M, Cavanna A, Collimedaglia L,** et al. Clinical correlates of schizotypy in patients with epilepsy. J Neuropsychiatry Clin Neurosci. 2008;20(6):441–46.

34. **Trimble MR.** The psychoses of epilepsy. New York: Raven Press; 1991.

35. **Ashidate N.** [Clinical study on epilepsy and psychosis]. Seishin Shinkeigaku Zasshi. 2006;108(4):260–65.

36. **LaFrance WC Jr, Baker GA, Duncan R, Goldstein LH, Reuber M.** Minimum requirements for the diagnosis of psychogenic nonepileptic seizures: a staged approach: a report from the International League Against Epilepsy Nonepileptic Seizures Task Force. Epilepsia. 2013;54(3):2005–18.

37. **Asadi-Pooya AA, Sperling MR,** Epidemiology of psychogenic nonepileptic seizures. Epilepsy Behav. 2015;46:60–65.

38. **Kerr MP, Mensah S, Besag F,** et al. International consensus clinical practice statements for the treatment of neuropsychiatric conditions associated with epilepsy. Epilepsia. 2011;52(11):2133–38.

39. **National Institute for Health and Care Excellence.** Generalised anxiety disorder and panic disorder in adults: management. Clinical guideline [CG113]. London: National Institute for Health and Care Excellence; 2019.

40. **National Institute for Health and Care Excellence.** Depression in adults: recognition and management. Clinical guideline [CG90]. London: National Institute for Health and Care Excellence; 2009.

41. **Michaelis R, Tang V, Nevitt SJ,** et al. Cochrane systematic review and meta-analysis of the impact of psychological treatments for people with epilepsy on health-related quality of life. Epilepsia. 2018;59(2):315–32.

42. **Michaelis R, Tang V, Goldstein LH,** et al. Psychological treatments for adults and children with epilepsy: evidence-based recommendations by the International League Against Epilepsy Psychology Task Force. Epilepsia. 2018;59(7):1282–302.

43. **Gasparini S, Beghi E, Ferlazzo E,** et al. Management of psychogenic non-epileptic seizures: a multidisciplinary approach. Eur J Neurol. 2019;26(2):205.e15.

44. **LaFrance WC Jr, Baird GL, Barry JJ,** et al. Multicenter pilot treatment trial for psychogenic nonepileptic seizures: a randomized clinical trial. JAMA Psychiatry. 2014;71(9):997–1005.

45. **Goldstein LH, Robinson EJ, Mellers JDC,** et al. Cognitive behavioural therapy for adults with dissociative seizures (CODES): a pragmatic, multicentre, randomised controlled trial. Lancet Psychiatry. 2020;7(6):491–505.

46. **Agrawal N, Gaynor D, Lomax A, Mula M.** Multimodular psychotherapy intervention for nonepileptic attack disorder: an individualized pragmatic approach. Epilepsy Behav. 2014;41:144–48.

47. **Kanner A.** Depression in neurologic disorders: diagnosis and management. New York: John Wiley & Sons; 2012.

48. **Mula M.** The pharmacological management of psychiatric comorbidities in patients with epilepsy. Pharmacol Res. 2016;**107**:147–53.

49. **Hamid H, Kanner AM.** Should antidepressant drugs of the selective serotonin reuptake inhibitor family be tested as antiepileptic drugs? Epilepsy Behav. 2013;**26**(3):261–65.

50. **Devinsky O, Honigfeld G, Patin J.** Clozapine-related seizures. Neurology. 1991;**41**(3):369–71.

Chapter 7

Epilepsy and intellectual disabilities

Tim Andrews and Rohit Shankar

Introduction

Intellectual disability (ID) is characterized by significant impairments of intellectual and adaptive functioning with onset before adulthood. Epilepsy is significantly more common in people with ID, with prevalence estimates ranging from 20% to 30% in the UK for people with ID who are known to clinical services.[1] Up to half of people with severe/profound ID may have a seizure disorder.[2] Table 7.1 provides a brief overview of the differing severity of ID and key characteristics.

Treatment-resistant epilepsy and adverse reactions to antiseizure medications (ASMs) are more frequent in people with ID, which makes balancing quality of life issues with seizure control particularly challenging. Two-thirds of people with ID and epilepsy show a poor response to AMSs.[3] People with ID and epilepsy often have more physical disabilities than those with ID without epilepsy.[4] Also, an earlier age of seizure onset and severity of epilepsy are both correlated with more severe learning disabilities.[2]

Psychiatric disorders are a common comorbid finding in people with epilepsy (see Chapter 6), and this association is even more evident in people with both epilepsy and ID.[5,6] Findings from epidemiological studies have shown increased prevalence of mood disorders, anxiety disorders, and attention deficit disorders compared to the general population.[1,2,6,7] There may be genetic and environmental factors that cause the brain to display both structural and functional abnormalities, which may increase the occurrence of ID, epilepsy, and psychiatric disorders.[1,2,6,7] Behavioural disorders may coexist with psychiatric disorders or autistic spectrum disorders (ASD).[1,2,6,7] Behavioural disorders are more likely to be associated with poorly controlled epilepsy, and polypharmacy.[1,2,6,7] The link between epilepsy and other neurodevelopmental disorders is easily missed.[8]

Table 7.1 Classifications of intellectual disability severity and other relevant characteristics

Severity category	Approximate per cent distribution of cases by severity	DSM-IV criteria (severity levels were based only on IQ categories)	DSM-5 criteria (severity classified on the basis of daily skills)	Epilepsy prevalence
Mild	85%	Approximate IQ range 50–69	Can live independently with minimum levels of support	8–10%
Moderate	10%	Approximate IQ range 36–49	Independent living may be achieved with moderate levels of support, such as those available in group homes	30%
Severe	3.5%	Approximate IQ range 20–35	Requires daily assistance with self-care activities and safety supervision	30–50%
Profound	1.5%	IQ <20	Requires 24-hour care	30–50%

DSM, *Diagnostic and Statistical Manual of Mental Disorders*.

Modified from Mental Disorders and Disabilities Among Low-Income Children. Committee to Evaluate the Supplemental Security Income Disability Program for Children with Mental Disorders; Board on the Health of Select Populations; Board on Children, Youth, and Families; Institute of Medicine; Division of Behavioral and Social Sciences and Education; The National Academies of Sciences, Engineering, and Medicine; Boat TF, Wu JT, editors. Washington (DC): National Academies Press (US); 2015 Oct 28.

Increasingly, more genetic associations between epilepsy and ID have been identified with the widespread use of gene panels and whole genome sequencing.

Two prominent dimensions exists. There are paediatric encephalopathies such as West syndrome, Landu–Kleffner syndrome, Lennox–Gastaut syndrome, Rett syndrome, Dravet syndrome, and so forth which are significantly associated with a ID. This is due to early developmental processes being interfered with by the destructive epilepsy patterns. The other dimension is ID syndromes which are likely to have a higher prevalence of epilepsy. Examples include Angelman syndrome and Down syndrome. A third category where a syndrome has high rates of epilepsy but is not always associated with ID, such as Sturge–Weber syndrome and tuberous sclerosis, also exists. The different aetiologies are outlined in Table 7.2.

Table 7.2 Aetiology of epilepsy in people with intellectual disabilities

Structural with underlying genetic component	Tuberous sclerosis
	Neurofibromatosis
	Sturge–Weber syndrome
	Acquired
	Perinatal brain injury: birth trauma/hypoxia
	Vascular: arteriovenous malformations, stroke
	Neurodegenerative
	Dementia
	Rett syndrome
	Lafora body disease
	Batten's disease
Genetic	*Chromosomal*
	Down syndrome
	Aicardi syndrome
	Sex aneuploidies (Klinefelter syndrome, Turner syndrome, etc.)
	Miller–Dieker syndrome
	Ring chromosome 14 and 20 syndromes
	Trisomy 12p
	Single gene/microdeletion
	Tuberous sclerosis: *TSC1, TSC2*
	Neurofibromatosis: *NF1, NF2*
	Angelman syndrome: *UBE3A*
	Fragile X: *FMR1*
	Rett syndrome: *MECP2*
	Landau–Kleffner syndrome: *GRIN2A* in 20%
	Wolf Hirshorn syndrome: microdeletion

(*continued*)

Table 7.2 Continued

Infections	Tuberculosis
	HIV
	Congenital
	Cytomegalovirus/Zika
	Meningitis/encephalitis
	Toxoplasmosis
	Parasitic causes
	Neurocysticercosis
	Falciparum malaria
	Toxocara canis
	Onchocerca volvulus
Metabolic	Hypoglycaemia
	Uraemia
	Aminoacidopathies
	Pyridoxine-dependent seizures
Autoimmune (examples)	NMDA receptor encephalitis
	Anti-LGI1 encephalitis
Drug related (examples)	Cholinesterase inhibitors
	Withdrawal seizures

Modified from Woodbury-Smith M, ed. *Clinical Topics in Disorders of Intellectual Development* (2015) RCPsych Publications.

Neurodevelopmental, psychiatric, and neurocognitive comorbidities and epilepsy

Epilepsy is associated with increased rates of psychosis, mood disorders, anxiety disorders, attention deficit hyperactivity disorder (ADHD), dementia, and autism in the general population in both adults and children (see Chapters 5 and 6).[9] There may be genetic and environmental factors that cause the brain to display both structural and functional abnormalities, which may increase the occurrence of ID, epilepsy, psychiatric disorders, and, in later life, cognitive deficits.[2] Specific challenges in the field of ID can make the diagnosis of comorbid psychiatric and neurodevelopmental disorders difficult.[10] People with ID can experience communication difficulties that vary from problems expressing psychological experiences to being unable to produce speech.[1] As may be expected, this results in an under-reporting of psychiatric symptoms. Clinicians must be aware of this and place greater emphasis on observing the individual and on obtaining collateral history from family and care staff. There can be a tendency to attribute any behavioural or psychological disturbance to a person's ID (known as diagnostic overshadowing). It is thus important to have a good understanding of specific and relevant comorbidities.

Neurodevelopment and epilepsy

Autism

A meta-analysis of people with epilepsy showed an epilepsy prevalence of 22% in people with ASD and ID compared to 8% in people with ASD without ID.[11] Certain conditions such as tuberous sclerosis (particularly when associated with the *TSC2* gene), Dravet syndrome, and Rett syndrome are strongly associated with autistic-like conditions.[12]

Epilepsy is reported to occur in 10–20% of individuals with fragile X syndrome. Fragile X syndrome is strongly associated with ASD. A frequent seizure and electroencephalogram pattern in fragile X syndrome appears to resemble that of self-limited epilepsy with centrotemporal spikes (previously known as benign Rolandic epilepsy of childhood).[13]

Early life seizures may induce a variety of changes in the hippocampus, including short-term enhancement of excitation and long-term enhancement of inhibitory neurotransmission and reductions in excitatory neurotransmission. This may, in part, explain enhanced risk of ASD in people with early-onset seizures. Imbalances of excitatory and inhibitory neurotransmission, resulting either from genetic mutations or effects of early-onset seizures, may provide a common mechanism for both ASD and epilepsy and provide a basis for understanding the frequent co-occurrence of these disorders.[14]

Some epileptic encephalopathies are closely associated with autism. In 2018, a study in China found autism to be much more prevalent in people with Dravet syndrome compared to a similar group of people with Lennox–Gastaut syndrome with a similar level of ID.[14]

Some syndromes such as Landau–Kleffner syndrome are also associated with autism-like features.[15] However, there are certain differences. Onset tends to be later than in typical ASD, and regression tends to mainly affect language with these children retaining their social awareness, use of gestures, and measured non-verbal cognitive abilities.[16]

Attention deficit hyperactivity disorder

ADHD has been associated with epilepsy in childhood epidemiological studies. Compared with children never diagnosed with epilepsy, children with ADHD were found to be nearly four times more likely to have epilepsy (23% vs 6%).[17] There is no evidence ADHD rates are higher in other people with seizures who also have ID than in those without epilepsy. The use of methylphenidate, the most commonly used drug in ADHD, appears relatively safe from an epilepsy perspective.[18]

Major psychiatric disorders and epilepsy

A recent study compared a population of people with ID in the Netherlands and the UK.[7] The populations had broadly similar rates of psychosis (1.6–2.4%), mood disorders (12–12.7%), and anxiety disorders (4.2%). The study emphasized that epilepsy in people with ID is not a standalone condition but part of a broader neurodevelopmental syndrome where ASMs are only partly effective and their usage needs to be balanced against side effects and overall quality of life.

Psychosis

People with ID have up to three times higher rates of schizophrenia than the general population, for a number of reasons. Firstly, early-onset schizophrenia may represent a more severe form of the disorder. Secondly, cognitive impairment may enhance susceptibility to psychosis. Thirdly, there may be some final common pathway that gives rise to both conditions.[19] Epilepsy does not increase the risk of psychosis further, but the same factors causing psychosis in the general population are likely to apply.

Historically, temporal lobe epilepsy (TLE) has been most closely linked to psychosis and affective disorders.[20] While an early study noted an association between psychosis and left-sided temporal lobe lesions, subsequent work has confirmed a laterality effect, but with inconsistency concerning the affected side. Temporal lobe lesions that develop *in utero* or during the perinatal period seem to be most associated with psychosis in later life.

Rates of psychosis are higher in people with epilepsy (see Chapter 6).[21] This relationship is complex and psychotic symptoms may be transient and closely associated with seizures either ictally, or postictally, or not associated at all. Postictal psychosis is seen in 7% of people with TLE.[22] Postictal psychosis in this context has been conceptualized as a phenomenon akin to Todd's paralysis, indicating the postictal inactivation of cortical regions involved in the ictal event, which usually include bilateral medial temporal structures. Seizures cause a release of a number of other neurotransmitters which include acetylcholine, glutamate, catecholamines, serotonin, opiates, adenosine, and nitric oxide. Endogenous opiates appear to play a special role in the postictal state. It is possible that the repeated release of neurotransmitters during seizure activity leads to postsynaptic receptor changes and this may be relevant to postictal psychosis.

A 2016 study found one in seven people with epilepsy who developed psychosis had an ASM-induced psychotic disorder.[23] Around half the study population had ID, but there was no statistical difference in rates of psychosis in people with ID and those without. In these individuals, female sex, temporal lobe involvement, and current use of levetiracetam were significantly associated with ASM-induced psychotic disorder compared to other types of psychosis. Carbamazepine had a negative association. Disorganized behaviours and thinking were predominant in ASM-induced psychotic disorder. People with ASM-induced psychotic disorder differed from non-ASM-induced psychotic disorders in having better outcomes.

Mood disorders

In people without ID, rates of depression are higher in those with seizures, and depression tends to be associated with more severe seizures.[24] ID is also associated with higher rates of depression, but this is not further increased by the presence of seizures. Risk factors for developing depression are complex and involve biological factors (neurotransmitter abnormalities and temporal lobe abnormalities), psychological factors (coping with chronic Illness), and social factors (stigmatization and impact on independence and family relationships).[25,26] Hippocampal atrophy has been correlated with depression in TLE.[27] Amygdala hypertrophy has also been linked to depression in children exposed to early life stress and also in TLE.[28]

Anxiety disorders

The overall pooled prevalence of anxiety disorders in people with epilepsy has been estimated at 20.2% in the general non-ID population.[24] These data included people with obsessive–compulsive disorder and post-traumatic stress disorder. One 2019 study in people with ID and epilepsy from a tertiary referral centre did show higher rates of anxiety (12.7%).[29] A 2003 study found a rate of 28.6% for neurotic disorders as detected by the Psychiatric Assessment Schedule for Adults with Developmental Disabilities (PAS-ADD) checklist in a Scottish community sample of people with ID and epilepsy, but this sample would have also included mood disorders.[30]

Functional seizures (psychogenic non-epileptic seizures)

Previous studies have reported moderate rates of association with panic in psychogenic non-epileptic seizures (PNES/functional seizures (FS)), though the proportions vary considerably across the literature. Some theories suggest panic and/or hyperventilation have aetiological roles in PNES/FS, though these remain unproven.[31] They concluded that there was an important, although not essential, role for panic and hyperventilation in the pathogenesis of PNES events. Hyperventilation is an effective inducer of PNES events in a minority of patients.

A 2008 study compared people with PNES with and without ID, although most people included had mild ID.[32] Rates of non-epileptic status were statistically higher in the ID group (44% vs 16%). It was concluded that a diagnosis of epilepsy, the use of ASMs, episodes of psychogenic non-epileptic status, and situational or emotional triggers were more common among those with ID. It was suggested that PNES in people with ID is less likely to present as an emotional conflict, but more as a reinforced behavioural pattern, which can be considered a subcategory of PNES. By displaying this reinforced behavioural pattern, a secondary gain may be sought such as receiving attention and avoidance of demands or unpleasant situations.

Other relevant comorbidities

Sleep disorders

Sleep disorders occur in 30–60% of adults with ID and are frequently missed. Poor sleep hygiene can be associated with an adverse impact on seizure profile. Severity of ID, epilepsy, and cerebral palsy are all associated with an increased risk of sleep disorders. Contributing factors may include pain, muscle spasms, sleep apnoea, reflux and aspiration, and inability to change body position at night.[33] ASMs with sedative properties may help people with epilepsy who have insomnia, whereas stimulating ASMs may benefit those with epilepsy and daytime somnolence. ASMs affect sleep architecture in highly variable ways, and benzodiazepines in particular may not necessarily improve the quality of sleep, even though they may prolong it.[34]

Challenging behaviour/behaviours that challenge

One of the most widely used definitions of challenging behaviour comes from the Royal College of Psychiatrists, British Psychological Society, and Royal College of Speech and Language Therapists 2007 joint statement[35]:

> Behaviour can be described as challenging when it is of such an intensity, frequency, or duration as to threaten the quality of life and/or the physical safety of the individual or others and it is likely to lead to responses that are restrictive, aversive or result in exclusion.

High rates of challenging behaviour have been reported in people with ID and epilepsy.[10] Various factors have been to be associated with behavioural disorders and epilepsy in ID.[10] Factors include high seizure frequency, presence of tonic–clonic seizures, and polypharmacy.[36] Certain drugs such as levetiracetam, perampanel, topiramate, vigabatrin, and zonisamide have been linked to behavioural disturbance and psychiatric disorders.[37]

There is no clear evidence that behavioural disorders are significantly different in people with ID with or without seizures. A recent review of the literature found no clear and consistent relationship between epilepsy and overall rates of challenging behaviour but highlighted major methodological flaws in the studies included.[38] Furthermore, certain conditions such as tuberous sclerosis, Conelia de Lange syndrome, and fragile X syndrome may be associated with phenotypes that may increase association with behavioural issues irrespective of whether they have seizures or not.

Dementia

Old retrospective reports describing 'epileptic dementia' have been discredited, although the intersection between epilepsy and dementia is complex and an area of active study (see Chapter 5). It is probably better to consider how the interrelated nature of epilepsy and underlying brain pathology determines potential cognitive decline.[39]

People with Down syndrome have much higher rates of dementia than the age-matched general population owing to trisomy 21 and overexpression of the *APOE4* gene. However, people with ID who do not have Down syndrome have four times the rate of dementia compared to the general population.[40]

Dementia is one of the factors that leads to increased rates of epilepsy in Down syndrome and a triphasic presentation has been suggested.[41] The three phases are seizures occurring in infancy, typically infantile spasms; then in the third decade of life usually focal seizures or focal to bilateral tonic–clonic seizures; and finally generalized tonic–clonic and myoclonus seizures associated with dementia.[41,42]

Stigma

Those with ID and epilepsy are vulnerable to double stigma.[43] From a psychological perspective, the stigmatization associated with epilepsy is compounded by social exclusion, often experienced by people with ID. Stigma may be subdivided into different categories. Internalized stigma (or self-stigma) reflects the feelings of a person with epilepsy (and/or ID) about being different. Interpersonal stigma is the negative actions or reactions of significant others towards the person with epilepsy. Institutionalized stigma refers to the position taken by society towards people with epilepsy. Reflected stigma can affect people in close personal proximity to someone with epilepsy. This can include family members and even professionals involved in their care (see Chapter 15).

Fear of reflected stigma is likely to contribute to the social isolation of people with epilepsy and ID and may adversely impact healthcare service provision. Internalized stigma affects self-esteem and may cause people to 'give up' on trying to be more independent and compound any comorbid mood disorder.[43,44]

Sudden unexpected death in epilepsy and direct seizure-related mortality

People with ID and epilepsy are more likely to die prematurely than both the general population and those with ID but no epilepsy, for a whole variety of reasons.[45,46] They are also at higher risk of sudden unexpected death in epilepsy (SUDEP; see Chapter 9) than the general population with ID.[47] A significant number of deaths in people with epilepsy may be potentially preventable through better seizure control, regular monitoring, and raising awareness among patients and carers.[45-49] SUDEP was the second most common cause of death in adults with ID and epilepsy after respiratory diseases.[50] In a UK-based retrospective study of 904 adults, over 90% had an epilepsy review but only 25% had an epilepsy care plan and only 61% had a documented discussion about SUDEP.[6] There was also a high level of polypharmacy identified. In those with nocturnal seizures about 75% had some form of nocturnal monitoring. The authors concluded that, particularly in people with moderate to severe ID who are at greater risk of SUDEP, there should be more integrated and holistic care for this vulnerable group.

The complex risks to people with epilepsy in general and particularly those with ID are well identified.[51-53] Focus needs to be on improved and optimized seizure control as well as identification and mitigation of impacting biopsychosocial factors.[54,55] Equally, there need to be regular, suitable, and dynamic risk assessments to enable capture of any change in risk status to enable people to receive more proactive care, for example, those in primary care being easily referred back to specialist care when needs arise.[56] Where possible, using evidence-based tools, such as the SUDEP and Seizure Safety Checklist, can help identify modifiable risk and action proactive interventions, for example, avoiding bathing in isolation and installing nocturnal monitoring.[57,58]

Assessment and treatment

Assessment

The diagnosis of epilepsy still depends largely on a detailed history and informant reports including witness descriptions of seizures. This increasingly may include use of technology such as recorded video on mobile phones. Where individuals are supported by multiple paid carers, it may be quite difficult to obtain a consistent history and accurate witness accounts of seizures, due to variability in accounts.[1] Confusion may arise between stereotypies or other behaviours and seizure activity.[1] Neuropsychological testing can be helpful where the seizures are thought to be focal and localize where the epileptic focus might be. Neuroimaging may also be helpful in this regard as may video-telemetry and possibly magnetoencephalography, although this is not widely used in the UK. For many of these investigations, patient cooperation is needed and best efforts should be made to enable this.

Treatment

Treatment of people with ID and epilepsy is a complex area because of the co-existence of multiple pathologies and the potential for certain ASMs to have an adverse impact on behaviour.[2,8,37] (see Chapter 3). Box 7.1 sets out basic

---

Box 7.1 Minimum care standards for adults with intellectual and developmental disabilities and epilepsy

Health care providers should be educated about the medical, cognitive, and behavioral comorbidities.

Health care providers should be instructed to be patient-centered in communication: for example, to make eye contact, to speak to the person even if he or she is nonverbal, and to show the same respect as for any other patient.

In every patient, the diagnosis should be carefully assessed, no matter what the age of the patient, with regard to underlying cause, epilepsy syndrome, and comorbid disorders.

Consider genetic disorders that could impact therapy (e.g. Dravet syndrome).

Consider atypical presentations of epilepsy syndromes (e.g. Lennox–Gastaut syndrome without slow spike and wave or daytime tonic seizures).

Autism spectrum and other psychiatric disorders are often comorbid; their identification may improve care access and help tailor therapy.

As children reach adolescence, they and their caregivers should be educated about their care and transition to adult care should be planned in advance; adult epilepsy specialist care is usually required.

Families should be educated on the nature of adult epilepsy care and an adult care provider identified.

(continued)

Box 7.1 (*Continued*)

A brief personal and medical summary should be prepared and updated annually, and be available for all individuals involved in the care of the patient with IDD-E; this should include past and current diagnoses, medications and beneficial adverse effects, allergies, and personal preferences (e.g. ways to calm the patient in a stressful setting).

Assess the ASM regimen efficacy and safety during every clinical visit; consider misattribution of ASM side effects to the IDD (diagnostic overshadowing).

For patients with treatment-resistant epilepsy, consider dietary or surgical therapies.

Consider preventive strategies to reduce chances of injury or premature death, including risk from injury, drowning, and SUDEP; assess living accommodations and consider social work involvement if needed.

Consider the needs of family members and the potential burden they are experiencing and refer for support as needed.

An individualized seizure emergency management plan should be part of the medical summary.

Integration of care among all health providers, with one provider identified as the coordinator; care should always include careful listening to the patient with IDD-E and inclusion of his or her input with respect to care decisions.

Mental health should be reviewed at every visit; referral to mental health support should be considered when concerns arise.

Ongoing awareness is needed to assess for changes in neurologic and medical health; be aware of red flags such as weight loss, behavior change, and loss of appetite for unrecognized physical comorbidity.

Abbreviations. AED = antiepileptic drug; IDD = intellectual and developmental disabilities; IDD-E = intellectual and developmental disabilities and epilepsy; SUDEP = sudden unexpected death in epilepsy.

Reproduced from Devinsky O, Asato M, Camfield P, Geller E, Kanner AM, Keller S, et al. Delivery of epilepsy care to adults with intellectual and developmental disabilities. Neurology. 2015;85(17):1512–21.

minimum care standards for people with epilepsy and ID. This has been further expanded in the Step Together guidance, an England-wide effort to systemize care delivery for epilepsy in people with ID across all clinical and commissioning stakeholders.[46] These highlight the importance of monitoring mental health and being vigilant about side effects. It is also important to ensure good case coordination and transitional arrangements between child and adult services in addition to suitable resourcing and relevant monitoring.

Antiseizure medications

People with ID are more susceptible to the side effects from ASMs, and also less able to communicate the difficulties when they experience side effects. It has been recommended that in people with ID initial doses should be as low as possible and titration should be slower than the general population.[37] This should aid monitoring of efficacy and also in particular side effects that manifest as behavioural change.

There is only weak evidence in the use of ASMs and their effects in randomized controlled trials specifically in people with ID.[59] Most studies are either underpowered and/or have other methodological issues. Current evidence is most supportive of lamotrigine and sodium valproate.[37,60] There is some positive evidence for the use of topiramate, levetiracetam, rufinamide, perampanel, lacosamide, and eslicarbazepine.[60–66] The current evidence does not support use of phenobarbitone, phenytoin, or vigabatrin in adults.[1,2,37,60] It is recommended that the management of epilepsy in people with ID needs to be person-centred and based on a good understanding of the combination of factors related to ID and those related to epilepsy.[1,2,60]

An underexplored area is the management of epilepsy in older adults with ID.[67] While there are no obvious red flags identified to date, few studies have considered the older ID population especially given their unique risk factors, thus this is an area needing further exploration.[68] Other issues, such as impact on bone health especially given that many people with ID and epilepsy are on long-term ASMs, remain poorly explored.[69,70] (see Chapters 3 and 10).

Genetic investigations and antiseizure medication prescribing

The field of genetics is rapidly changing and it can be difficult to keep up to date with every new discovery of an epilepsy-related gene. Nonetheless, it is perhaps particularly important to genetically investigate people with ID and epilepsy especially those who have no diagnosis to account for their comorbid neurodevelopmental disorders.[8] Whole genome sequencing is now becoming widely available in economically developed countries although it is also important to perform aligned orthogonal tests such as array comparative hybridization and karyotyping.

The findings from genetic investigations may influence epilepsy treatment, including the choice of ASM medication. Identification of an *SCN1A* gene mutation in a person presenting with a Dravet syndrome phenotype should lead to the avoidance or withdrawal of lamotrigine, phenytoin, carbamazepine, or any other sodium channel-blocking ASM, which can aggravate seizures in this population.[71] Instead, ASMs such as sodium valproate, clonazepam, stiripentol, and cannabidiol are indicated.

A mutation of the *SLC2A1* gene in the presence of abnormal movements and/or a family history of seizures helps in the diagnosis of glucose transporter type 1 (GLUT1) deficiency, which responds very well to a ketogenic diet.[72] Some mitochondrial disorders and cerebral creatine deficiency syndromes are also associated with ID and epilepsy, and may respond to specific treatments.[73]

Genetic testing can also help avoid serious medication side effects. The recessive polymerase gamma (POLG)-related disorders form part of the group of mitochondrial disorders and are commonly associated with seizures and may have a complex and variable presentation.[74,75] Sodium valproate can cause irreversible liver failure in people with a POLG mutation, and consideration should be given to testing for POLG mutations when presenting with seizures and liver dysfunction.[76]

Ketogenic diet

The ketogenic diet is regarded as the treatment of choice for certain metabolic disorders such as the glucose transporter type 1 and pyruvate dehydrogenase complex deficiencies.[72,77] There is some evidence it may be helpful in Dravet syndrome and tuberous sclerosis.[78] The ketogenic diet is not without side effects and dropout rates tend to be high.[79] The ketogenic diet is quite restrictive. There are challenges regarding people with ID making informed choices and balancing their quality of life. It may specifically pose concerns where a person with moderate to severe ID will be further restricted in an area of their life where they have the enjoyment of some choice in the food they eat. More research in this direction is needed.

Epilepsy surgery for people with intellectual disabilities

ID is not a contraindication for epilepsy surgery, and a presurgical evaluation should be offered in refractory cases as for other people with epilepsy.[1,37] The number of individuals with a low IQ who are offered surgery, however, remains fewer than the number of those functioning within the normal intelligence range.[80] Probably the most widely used surgical intervention used in the UK in people with ID and drug-resistant epilepsy is vagus nerve stimulation (VNS; see Chapter 4). A large number of people with ID and epilepsy are treatment resistant and VNS has been shown to be effective in treatment-resistant epilepsy.[81] A 2021 study explored the use of ambulatory outpatient VNS implantation in 26 outpatients with ID and found it to be safe and feasible.[82] A 2017 systematic review exploring evidence of benefit of VNS in children with ID demonstrated less effectiveness in seizure frequency reduction in children with ID compared to those children with normal cognitive abilities.[83] Nevertheless, the absence of side effects and drug interactions highlighted some advantages of VNS, compared to adding an extra ASM. Also, there is suggestive evidence of VNS benefit on quality of life of people with ID and epilepsy although this needs further exploration.[84]

The future direction of travel

Recent research suggests that epilepsy in people with ID is a bellwether for multimorbidity, polypharmacy, siloed care, and premature mortality.[6] There is emergence of key risk factors which are associated with premature mortality in this vulnerable group. Further work has outlined that older populations with ID and epilepsy are at higher risk.[85] A case–control study using multiple variable logistic regression analysis for risk of epilepsy-related death in people with ID compared 190 deaths in people with ID and epilepsy to 910 controls.[86] It has shown age over 50 years, increased antipsychotic medication use, and lack of an epilepsy review within a 12-month. This as was associated with an increased risk of death. It also highlighted that being open to the services supporting people with ID could reduce odds of death by 72% compared to just being open to neurology services. This could possibly be due to the holistic care which ID specialist services offer including assessment and management of communication, dysphagia, diet, bowel and bladder, physiotherapy, and psychiatric issues.

As people with ID and epilepsy have multimorbidity and access a myriad of settings and services, there is a growing awareness of the need for all stakeholders associated with such vulnerable individuals being aware of epilepsy and its risks.[87] This concept of 'capable communities' for people with ID and epilepsy has been furthered with a toolkit to understand and evidence the capabilities of a particular health and social care system to be able to support the diverse needs of individuals with ID and epilepsy in their region.[88]

Conclusion

Epilepsy is more common in people with ID, and the presentation is often more complex. Stereotypic or other behaviours may make clinical diagnosis more difficult.

Psychiatric disorders are not more common in people with ID and epilepsy than those without seizures, but are much more common than in the general population. Understanding of the interrelationship between developmental brain disorders and seizures may be helped in many cases by the rapidly expanding field of genomics. Side effects of medication are easier to miss in people with ID and may be complicated by polypharmacy. Efforts to systemize care delivery for epilepsy in people with ID across all clinical and commissioning stakeholders is recommended, as is good case coordination and transitional arrangements between child and adult services. ASMs should be started at the lowest possible dose and slowly up-titrated. Phenytoin, phenobarbitone, and vigabatrin are best avoided. Surgery, perhaps particularly VNS, should be considered in certain cases. SUDEP is more common in people with ID and some deaths may be potentially preventable through better seizure control, regular monitoring (particularly overnight), environmental risk assessments, avoiding sleeping prone, and raising awareness among people with ID, their families, and their carers as well as healthcare professionals.

References

1. **Royal College of Psychiatrists.** Management of epilepsy in adults with intellectual disability (CR203). 2017. Available at: https://www.rcpsych.ac.uk/improving-care/camp aigning-for-better-mental-health-policy/college-reports/2017-college-reports/man agement-of-epilepsy-in-adults-with-intellectual-disability-cr203-may-2017 [accessed 9 February 2022].
2. **Watkins LV, Linehan C, Brandt C,** et al. Epilepsy in adults with neurodevelopmental disability—what every neurologist should know. Epileptic Disord. 2022;24(1):9–25.
3. **McGrother CW, Bhaumik S, Thorp CF, Hauck A, Branford D, Watson JM.** Epilepsy in adults with intellectual disabilities: prevalence, associations and service implications. Seizure. 2006;15(6):376–86.
4. **Robertson J, Hatton C, Emerson E, Baines S.** Prevalence of epilepsy among people with intellectual disabilities: a systematic review. Seizure. 2015;29:46–62.
5. **Doran Z, Shankar R, Keezer MR,** et al. Managing anti-epileptic drug treatment in adult patients with intellectual disability: a serious conundrum. Eur J Neurol. 2016;23(7):1152–57.
6. **Sun JJ, Perera B, Henley W,** et al. Epilepsy related multimorbidity, polypharmacy and risks in adults with intellectual disabilities: a national study. J Neurol 2022;269(5):2750–60.
7. **Snoeijen-Schouwenaars FM, Young C, Rowe C, van Ool JS, Schelhaas HJ, Shankar R.** People with epilepsy and intellectual disability: more than a sum of two conditions. Epilepsy Behav. 2021;124:108355.

8. **Shankar R, Perera B, Thomas R.** Epilepsy, an orphan disorder within the neurodevelopmental family. J Neurol Neurosurg Psychiatry. 2020;**91**(12):1245–47.

9. **Rai D, Kerr MP, McManus S,** et al. Epilepsy and psychiatric comorbidity: a nationally representative population-based study. Epilepsia. 2012;**53**(6):1095–103.

10. **Kinney MO, Chester V, Alexander RT.** Epilepsy, anti-seizure medication, intellectual disability and challenging behaviour—everyone's business, no one's priority. Seizure. 2020:**81**:111–16.

11. **Amiet C, Gourfinkel-An I, Bouzamondo A,** et al. Epilepsy in autism is associated with intellectual disability and gender: evidence from a meta-analysis. Biol Psychiatry. 2008;**64**(7):577–82.

12. **Berg AT.** Epilepsy, cognition, and behavior: the clinical picture. Epilepsia. 2011;**52**(Suppl 1):7–12.

13. **Hagerman PJ.** The fragile X prevalence paradox. J Med Genet. 2008;**45**(8):498–99.

14. **Brooks-Kayal A.** Epilepsy and autism spectrum disorders: are there common developmental mechanisms? Brain Dev. 2010;**32**(9):731–38.

15. **Pearl PL, Carrazana EJ, Holmes GL.** The Landau–Kleffner syndrome. Epilepsy Curr. 2001;**1**(2):39–45.

16. **Russ SA, Larson K, Halfon N.** A national profile of childhood epilepsy and seizure disorder. Pediatrics. 2012;**129**(2):256–64.

17. **Ravi M, Ickowicz A.** Epilepsy, attention-deficit/hyperactivity disorder and methylphenidate: critical examination of guiding evidence. J Can Acad Child Adolesc Psychiatry. 2015;**25**(1):50–58.

18. **Doody GA, Johnstone EC, Sanderson TL, Owens DG, Muir WJ.** 'Pfropfschizophrenie' revisited. Schizophrenia in people with mild learning disability. Br J Psychiatry. 1998;**173**(2):145–53.

19. **Flor-Henry P.** Psychosis and temporal lobe epilepsy; a controlled investigation. Epilepsia. 1969;**10**(3):363–95.

20. **Toone B.** The psychoses of epilepsy. In: **Alarcón G, Valentín A,** eds. Introduction to epilepsy. Cambridge: Cambridge University Press; 2012:522–23.

21. <TBC>

22. **Cleary RA, Thompson PJ, Thom M, Foong J.** Postictal psychosis in temporal lobe epilepsy: risk factors and postsurgical outcome? Epilepsy Res. 2013;**106**(1–2):264–72.

23. **Chen Z, Lusicic A, O'Brien TJ, Velakoulis D, Adams SJ, Kwan P.** Psychotic disorders induced by antiepileptic drugs in people with epilepsy. Brain. 2016;**139**(10):2668–78.

24. **Scott AJ, Sharpe L, Hunt C, Gandy M.** Anxiety and depressive disorders in people with epilepsy: a meta-analysis. Epilepsia. 2017;**58**(6):973–82.

25. **Fiest KM, Birbeck GL, Jacoby A, Jette N.** Stigma in epilepsy. Curr Neurol Neurosci Rep. 2014;**14**(5):444.

26. **Mula M, Schmitz B.** Depression in epilepsy: mechanisms and therapeutic approach. Ther Adv Neurol Disord. 2009;**2**(5):337–44.

27. **Shamim S, Hasler G, Liew C, Sato S, Theodore WH.** Temporal lobe epilepsy, depression, and hippocampal volume. Epilepsia. 2009;**50**(5):1067–71.

28. **Daley M, Siddarth P, Levitt J,** et al. Amygdala volume and psychopathology in childhood complex partial seizures. Epilepsy Behav. 2008;**13**(1):212–17.

29. Snoeijen-Schouwenaars FM, van Ool JS, Tan IY, Aldenkamp AP, Schelhaas HJ, Hendriksen JGM. Mood, anxiety, and perceived quality of life in adults with epilepsy and intellectual disability. Acta Neurol Scand. 2019;**139**(6):519–25.

30. Espie CA, Watkins J, Curtice L, et al. Psychopathology in people with epilepsy and intellectual disability; an investigation of potential explanatory variables. J Neurol Neurosurg Psychiatry. 2003;**74**(11):1485–92.

31. Indranada AM, Mullen SA, Duncan R, Berlowitz DJ, Kanaan RAA. The association of panic and hyperventilation with psychogenic non-epileptic seizures: a systematic review and meta-analysis. Seizure. 2018;**59**(1):108–15.

32. Duncan R, Oto M. Psychogenic nonepileptic seizures in patients with learning disability: comparison with patients with no learning disability. Epilepsy Behav. 2008;**12**(1):183–86.

33. Kotagal S, Gibbons VP, Stith JA. Sleep abnormalities in patients with severe cerebral palsy. Dev Med Child Neurol. 1994;**36**:304–11.

34. Geurkink EA, Sheth RD, Gidal BE, Hermann BP. Effects of anticonvulsant medication on EEG sleep architecture. Epilepsy Behav. 2000;**1**(6):378–83.

35. Royal College of Psychiatrists, British Psychological Society, Royal College of Speech and Language Therapists. Challenging behaviour—a unified approach. 2007. Available at: https://www.rcpsych.ac.uk/docs/default-source/improving-care/better-mh-policy/college-reports/college-report-cr144.pdf

36. Kerr M, Gil-Nagel A, Glynn M, Mula M, Thompson R, Zuberi SM. Treatment of behavioral problems in intellectually disabled adult patients with epilepsy. Epilepsia. 2013;**54**(Suppl 1):34–40.

37. Royal College of Psychiatrists. Prescribing antiepileptic drugs for people with epilepsy and intellectual disability (CR206). 2017. Available at: https://www.rcpsych.ac.uk/improving-care/campaigning-for-better-mental-health-policy/college-reports/2017-college-reports/prescribing-anti-epileptic-drugs-for-people-with-epilepsy-and-intellectual-disability-cr206-oct-2017

38. Deb S, Akrout Brizard B, Limbu B. Association between epilepsy and challenging behaviour in adults with intellectual disabilities: systematic review and meta-analysis. BJPsych Open. 2020;**6**(5):e114.

39. Helmstaedter C, Witt JA. Epilepsy and cognition—a bidirectional relationship? Seizure. 2017;**49**:83–89.

40. Strydom A, Hassiotis A, King M, Livingston G. The relationship of dementia prevalence in older adults with intellectual disability (ID) to age and severity of ID. Psychol Med. 2009;**39**(1):13–21.

41. Johannsen P, Christensen JEJ, Goldstein H, Kamp Nielsen V, Mai J. Epilepsy in Down syndrome—prevalence in three age groups. Seizure. 1996;**5**(2):121–25.

42. Pueschel SM, Louis S, Mcknight P. Seizure disorders in Down syndrome. Arch Neurol. 1991;**48**(3):318–20.

43. Mula M, Kaufman KR. Double stigma in mental health: epilepsy and mental illness. BJPsych Open. 2020;**6**(4):e72.

44. Fiest KM, Birbeck GL, Jacoby A, Jette N. Stigma in epilepsy. Curr Neurol Neurosci Rep. 2014;**14**(5):444.

45. The Learning Disabilities Mortality Review (LeDeR) Programme. Annual report 2020. 2020. Available at: http://www.bristol.ac.uk/media-library/sites/sps/leder/LeDeR_2020_annual_report_FINAL.pdf [accessed 11 February 2022].

46. Shankar R, Mitchell S. Step together. 2020. Available at: https://www.bild.org.uk/wp-content/uploads/2020/11/Step-Together-17-November-2020-Download-Link-.pdf [accessed 11 February 2022].

47. Young C, Shankar R, Palmer J, et al. Does intellectual disability increase sudden unexpected death in epilepsy (SUDEP) risk? Seizure. 2015;25:112–16.

48. Young C, Shankar R, Henley W, Rose A, Cheatle K, Sander, JW. SUDEP and seizure safety communication: assessing if people hear and act. Epilepsy Behav. 2018;86:200–203.

49. Sun, J, Perera B, Henley W, Ashby S, Shankar R. Seizure and sudden unexpected death in epilepsy (SUDEP) characteristics in an urban UK intellectual disability service. Seizure. 2020;80:18–23.

50. Kiani R, Tyrer F, Jesu A, et al. Mortality from sudden unexpected death in epilepsy (SUDEP) in a cohort of adults with intellectual disability. J Intellect Disabil Res. 2014;58(6):508–20.

51. Shankar R, Donner EJ, McLean B, Nashef L, Tomson T. Sudden unexpected death in epilepsy (SUDEP): what every neurologist should know. Epileptic Disord. 2017;19(1):1–9.

52. Watkins L, Shankar R. Reducing the risk of sudden unexpected death in epilepsy (SUDEP). Curr Treat Options Neurol. 2018;20(10):40.

53. Watkins L, Shankar R, Sander JW. Identifying and mitigating sudden unexpected death in epilepsy (SUDEP) risk factors. Expert Rev Neurother. 2018;18(4):265–74.

54. Shankar R, Henley W, Boland C, et al. Decreasing the risk of sudden unexpected death in epilepsy: structured communication of risk factors for premature mortality in people with epilepsy. Eur J Neurol. 2018;25(9):1121–27.

55. Shankar R, Newman C, Gales A, et al. Has the time come to stratify and score SUDEP risk to inform people with epilepsy of their changes in safety? Front Neurol. 2018;9:281.

56. McCabe J, McLean B, Henley W, et al. Sudden unexpected death in epilepsy (SUDEP) and seizure safety: modifiable and non-modifiable risk factors differences between primary and secondary care. Epilepsy Behav. 2021;115:107637.

57. Shankar R, Walker M, McLean B, et al. Steps to prevent SUDEP: the validity of risk factors in the SUDEP and seizure safety checklist: a case control study. J Neurol. 2016;263(9):1840–46.

58. Shankar R, Ashby S, McLean B, Newman, C. Bridging the gap of risk communication and management using the SUDEP and Seizure Safety Checklist. Epilepsy Behav. 2020;103(Pt B):106419.

59. Doran Z, Shankar R, Keezer MR, et al. Managing anti-epileptic drug treatment in adult patients with intellectual disability: a serious conundrum. Eur J Neurol. 2016;23(7):1152–57.

60. Watkins L, O'Dwyer M, Kerr M, Scheepers M, Courtenay K, Shankar R. Quality improvement in the management of people with epilepsy and intellectual disability: the development of clinical guidance. Expert Opin Pharmacother. 2020;21(2):173–81.

61. Shankar R, Henley W, Wehner T, et al. Perampanel in the general population and in people with intellectual disability: differing responses. Seizure. 2017;**49**:30–35.

62. Wehner T, Mannan S, Turaga S, et al. Retention of perampanel in adults with pharmacoresistant epilepsy at a single tertiary care center. Epilepsy Behav. 2017;**73**:106–10.

63. Allard J, Henley W, Snoeijen-Schouwenaars F, et al. European perspective of perampanel response in people with intellectual disability. Acta Neurol Scand. 2020;**142**(3):255–59.

64. Trinka E, Lattanzi S, Carpenter K, et al. Exploring the evidence for broad-spectrum effectiveness of perampanel: a systematic review of clinical data in generalised seizures. CNS Drugs. 2021;**35**:821–37.

65. Allard J, Henley W, Mclean B, et al. Lacosamide in the general population and in people with intellectual disability: similar responses? Seizure. 2020;**76**:161–66.

66. Allard J, Lawthom C, Henley W, et al. Eslicarbazepine acetate response in intellectual disability population versus general population. Acta Neurol Scand. 2021;**143**(3):256–60.

67. O'Dwyer M, Watkins L, McCallion P, McCarron M, Hennman M, Shankar R Optimising medicines use in older adults with intellectual disability who have epilepsy: challenges and perspectives. Ther Adv Drug Saf. 2021;**12**:20420986211025157.

68. Watkins L, O'Dwyer M, Shankar R. New anti-seizure medication for elderly epileptic patients. Expert Opin Pharmacother. 2019;**20**(13):1601–608.

69. Sawhney I, Zia A, Yazdi B, Shankar R. Awareness of bone health risks in people with epilepsy and intellectual disability. Br J Learn Disabil. 2020;**48**(3):224–31.

70. Winterhalder R, Shankar R. Bone health in adults with epilepsy and intellectual disability Br J Gen Pract. 2022;**72**(716):100–101.

71. Miller IO, Sotero de Menezes MA. SCN1A seizure disorders. In: Adam MP, Ardinger HH, Pagon RA, et al., eds. GeneReviews˚. Seattle, WA: University of Washington, Seattle; 29 November 2007 [updated 18 April 2019]. Available at: https://www.ncbi.nlm.nih.gov/books/NBK1318/

72. Sandu C, Burloiu CM, Barca DG, Magureanu SA, Craiu DC. Ketogenic diet in patients with GLUT1 deficiency syndrome. Maedica (Bucur). 2019;**14**(2):93–97.

73. Mercimek-Andrews S, Salomons GS. Creatine deficiency disorders. In: Adam MP, Ardinger HH, Pagon RA, et al., eds. GeneReviews˚. Seattle, WA: University of Washington, Seattle; 15 January 2009 [updated 10 February 2022]. Available at: https://www.ncbi.nlm.nih.gov/books/NBK3794/

74. Hikmat O, Eichele T, Tzoulis C, Bindoff LA. Understanding the epilepsy in POLG related disease. Int J Mol Sci. 2017;**18**(9):1845.

75. Specchio N, Pietrafusa N, Calabrese C, et al. POLG1-related epilepsy: review of diagnostic and therapeutic findings. Brain Sci. 2020;**10**(11):768.

76. Stewart JD, Horvath R, Baruffini E, et al. Polymerase γ gene POLG determines the risk of sodium valproate-induced liver toxicity. Hepatology. 2010;**52**(5):1791–96.

77. Sofou K, Dahlin M, Hallböök T, Lindefeldt M, Viggedal G, Darin N. Ketogenic diet in pyruvate dehydrogenase complex deficiency: short- and long-term outcomes. J Inherit Metab Dis. 2017;**40**(2):237–45.

78. **Ismayilova N, Leung MA, Kumar R, Smith M, Williams RE.** Ketogenic diet therapy in infants less than two years of age for medically refractory epilepsy. Seizure. 2018;57:5–7.

79. **Schoeler NE, Cross JH, Sander JW, Sisodiya SM.** Can we predict a favourable response to ketogenic diet therapies for drug-resistant epilepsy? Epilepsy Res. 2013;106(1–2):1–16.

80. **Kerr M, Linehan C, Brandt C, et al.** Behavioral disorder in people with an intellectual disability and epilepsy: a report of the intellectual disability task force of the neuropsychiatric commission of ILAE. Epilepsia Open. 2016;1(3–4):102–11.

81. **Batson S, Shankar R, Conry J, et al.** Efficacy and safety of VNS therapy or continued medication management for treatment of adults with drug-resistant epilepsy: systematic review and meta-analysis. J Neurol. 2022;269(6):2874–91.

82. **Mezjan I, Gourfinkel-An I, Degos V, et al.** Outpatient vagus nerve stimulation surgery in patients with drug-resistant epilepsy with severe intellectual disability. Epilepsy Behav. 2021;118:107931.

83. **Sourbron J, Klinkenberg S, Kessels A, Schelhaas HJ, Lagae L, Majoie M.** Vagus nerve stimulation in children: a focus on intellectual disability. Eur J Paediatr Neurol. 2017;21(3):427–40.

84. **Satya-Murti S, Shepard KM, Helmers SL.** Vagus nerve stimulation in the treatment of epilepsy: payment policy perspectives. Neurol Clin Pract. 2013;3(5):431–35.

85. **Watkins LV, Henley W, Sun JJ, et al.** Tackling increased risks in older adults with intellectual disability and epilepsy: data from a national multicentre cohort study. Seizure. 2022;101:15–21.

86. **Sun JJ, Watkins L, Henley W, et al.** Mortality risk in adults with intellectual disabilities and epilepsy: an England and Wales case-control study. J Neurol. 2023;270(7):3527–36.

87. **Shankar R.** Managing epilepsy in people with intellectual disabilities—creating capable communities. BJPsych Adv. 2023;29(5):305–307.

88. **Epilepsy Action.** Step together. n. d. Available at: https://www.epilepsy.org.uk/professio nal/step-together

Chapter 8

Epilepsy and systemic disease

Patricia Dugan

Introduction

Seizures may arise acutely during the course of medical illnesses that do not
principally originate in the central nervous system (CNS). In the acute hospital setting, disturbances of electrolyte and fluid balance predominate, and
seizures may occur in the setting of toxic-metabolic encephalopathies due to
hyponatraemia, hypomagnesaemia, hypocalcaemia, hypophosphataemia,
disorders of glucose metabolism, meningoencephalitis, systemic infections,
hepatic and renal failure, anoxia, and hypoxia. Seizures may also result as
an adverse effect of drugs, or may be precipitated when medications are
abruptly discontinued after chronic use.[1,2] Comorbid health conditions
are common in people with epilepsy; for example, cardiovascular disease,
stroke, low bone mineral density, depression, anxiety, and migraine headache. This is due to complex relationships between epilepsy, its treatment,
and various biological and environmental factors.[3-6] This chapter reviews
the major systemic disorders that are associated with epilepsy due to a
shared underlying genetic predisposition or pathogenesis, direct or indirect
causal associations, or bidirectional relationships, emphasizing clinical
features and pathophysiology that may facilitate targeted diagnostic and
therapeutic strategies (Figure 8.1). These systemic disorders involve multiple organ systems, including the CNS, and seizures may be the presenting
symptom.

Epilepsy may also complicate systemic disorders through a variety of mechanisms, including direct immunological effects on the brain, vascular abnormalities, and cortical structural abnormalities. Recognizing the underlying
relationship between epilepsy and these systemic disorders is paramount, as
comorbid organ dysfunction or neuropsychiatric involvement may have important implications for epilepsy treatment.[3]

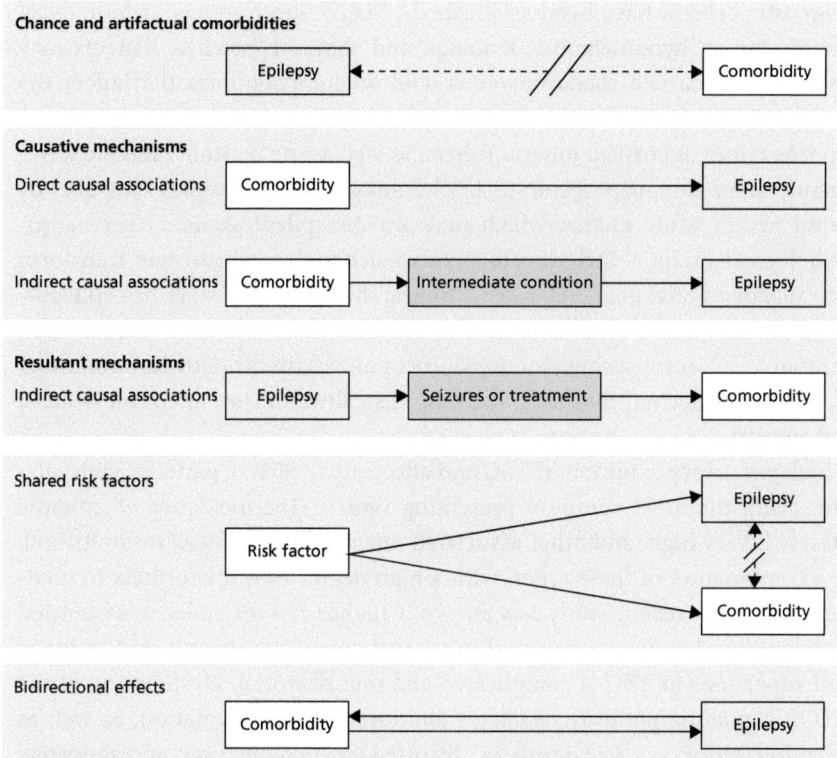

Figure 8.1 Schema illustrating possible ways by which epilepsy can inter-relate with systemic illness.

Neurocutaneous disorders

Neurocutaneous disorders are a heterogeneous group of genetic disorders exemplified by abnormalities of the nervous and cutaneous systems and affecting the skin, brain, and other organs. Epilepsy may be a feature of the three most common neurocutaneous disorders, tuberous sclerosis complex (TSC), neurofibromatosis type 1 (NF1), and Sturge–Weber syndrome (SWS).

Tuberous sclerosis complex

TSC is an autosomal dominant multisystem disorder with variable frequency, penetrance, and severity.[7] While it can affect numerous organs, the most common finding is benign tumours (hamartomas) in the skin, brain, kidneys, lungs, and heart.[8] It is caused by mutations in either of the tumour suppressor genes *TSC1* and *TSC2*, which encode hamartin and tuberin, respectively. Mutations cause dysregulation of the mammalian/mechanistic target of rapamycin (mTOR) signalling pathway, resulting in the development of hamartomas that are responsible for the clinical features of TSC. Clinical diagnostic criteria have been established.[9] Major skin findings include facial angiofibromas, hypomelanotic macules, and shagreen patches. Patients may also develop cardiac rhabdomyomas, and angiomyolipomas that affect the kidneys. In the brain, hamartomas may be found in the cerebral cortex, and are referred to as cortical tubers. Tubers, as well as the perituberal cortex, frequently serve as epileptogenic foci.[10,11] Subcortical heterotopias may also be found within white matter, which may also be epileptogenic. Other neuropathological findings include subependymal nodules, which may transform into subependymal giant cell astrocytomas; these structures are not epileptogenic but may cause obstructive hydrocephalus when located by the foramen of Monro.[7,10] Neuropsychiatric and neurocognitive comorbidities are common, including intellectual disability, learning disability, autism, attention deficits, and anxiety.

Epilepsy is very common in TSC and affects up to 90% of patients, with seizures being the most common presenting sign.[7,10] The incidence of infantile spasms is very high, and other associated seizures may be focal, or multifocal, or a combination of these types, with a high degree of refractoriness to medical therapy. A recent study has shown a higher risk of epilepsy associated with cardiac rhabdomyomas, and other systemic tumours and skin lesions.[8] Epileptogenesis in TSC is complicated and multifactorial. Dysfunction of the mTOR signalling pathway results in abnormal cellular excitation, as well as cell proliferation, cortical dysplasia, distorted vascular anatomy, and abnormal neuronal circuits.[12–14]

The treatment of epilepsy in the setting of TSC typically involves the use of conventional antiseizure medications (ASMs). However, because the percentage of people with tuberous sclerosis who have drug-resistant epilepsy is high (approximately 70%), non-pharmacological therapies are commonly employed, such as the ketogenic diet and vagus nerve stimulation. The role of palliative resective epilepsy surgery in the treatment of TSC has also been established, with multiple surgical strategies available to identify and remove epileptogenic tubers or perituberal cortex.[15,16] Vigabatrin is the first choice for the treatment of infantile spasms associated with TSC. Novel treatment utilizing the mTOR inhibitor everolimus has shown to significantly reduce seizures in a recent phase III randomized, double-blind, placebo-controlled study.[17]

Sturge–Weber syndrome

SWS is a sporadically occurring neurocutaneous disorder and refers to the association of a characteristic facial angioma (port-wine birthmark), leptomeningeal vascular malformations, and ocular angiomas. It is caused by a sporadic somatic mosaic mutation in the *GNAQ* gene. Facial involvement, with a port-wine stain on the forehead or upper eyelid, is associated with an increased risk of brain involvement. The cerebral vascular malformations are usually unilateral; bilateral involvement confers a worse prognosis. These vascular malformations may be associated with cortical malformations, and may result in epilepsy, hemiparesis, intellectual disability, and migraine headaches.[10] Eye involvement includes increased vascularity of the conjunctiva, buphthalmos, or glaucoma.

Epilepsy occurs very frequently in SWS: up to 72% of cases with unilateral cerebral involvement, and over 90% of those with bilateral involvement, with 90% of individuals presenting with seizure onset within the first 2 years of life.[10,18,19]

Seizures in SWS are typically focal or focal to bilateral tonic–clonic, and may occur in clusters or as episodes of status epilepticus. The mechanism of epileptogenesis in SWS is unclear but is likely related to abnormal blood vessel development, abnormal regional perfusion, and accompanying cortical malformations. Conventional ASMs such as oxcarbazepine, levetiracetam, and phenobarbital are often used. Topiramate may be used cautiously because of the possibility of exacerbating glaucoma, primarily in adults with SWS. The ketogenic diet as well as surgical strategies such as hemispherectomy or focal resections may be indicated in refractory cases.

The somatic mosaic mutation in *GNAQ* causes hyperactivation of downstream pathways of Gαq, including the mTOR and extracellular signal-regulated kinase (ERK) pathway. Several case series have been published detailing the use of the mTOR inhibitor, sirolimus, in individuals with SWS and showed that this is well tolerated and has the potential to improve cognitive functioning.[19] Adjunctive treatment with aspirin is often recommended to reduce the risk for stroke.

Neurofibromatosis type 1

NF1 is the most common neurocutaneous disorder with an autosomal dominant mode of inheritance; mutations are *de novo* in approximately half of cases.[10,20] The diagnosis of NF1 is made on the basis of clinical criteria[20]; distinctive findings include café au lait macules, cutaneous or subcutaneous neurofibromas (benign nerve sheath tumours), axillary or groin freckling, optic pathway gliomas, and Lisch nodules (iris hamartomas). Cognitive deficits may be present, as well as sleep disorders, anxiety, and migraine headaches.

Epilepsy is less frequently observed, occurring in 6–10% of affected individuals, and is likely due to cortical dysgenesis. The *NF1* gene encodes the tumour suppressor protein, neurofibromin; the exact role the lack of neurofibromin plays in the predisposition to epilepsy is not yet clear.[10] Seizures are focal or focal to bilateral tonic–clonic, and are typically treated with conventional ASM therapy.

Connective tissue diseases

Connective tissue diseases are a heterogeneous group of multisystem disorders that typically affect joints, skin, and muscles, but may also involve the CNS, lungs, kidneys, gastrointestinal tract, and cardiovascular system. Aetiologies may be autoimmune or inherited (genetic).

Systemic lupus erythematosus

Systemic lupus erythematosus (SLE) is an autoantibody-mediated multiorgan disease with a relapsing and remitting course, typically characterized by arthritis, pericarditis, nephritis, photosensitivity, and malar rash. Neuropsychiatric SLE may involve both the CNS and peripheral nervous system (PNS); the prevalence of CNS involvement is noted in 25–75% of cases, with cognitive dysfunction, cerebrovascular disease, and headaches commonly reported. Seizures are among the most serious symptoms associated with SLE, and are reported in 6–51% of affected individuals.[21-23] Generalized tonic–clonic seizures are more commonly observed than focal seizures, and can occur at the onset of SLE, often in the setting of active disease.

The relationship between epilepsy and SLE is complex and multifactorial. Antiphospholipid antibodies, particularly lupus anticoagulant and anticardiolipin antibodies, are found to be elevated in many people with SLE and epilepsy.[22,24] Antiphospholipid antibodies are also prothrombotic and may secondarily produce seizures through thrombotic occlusion and inflammation. Antithrombotic drugs may be necessary for secondary stroke prevention in people with antiphospholipid syndrome with a history of stroke or transient ischaemic attack. Seizures may also be precipitated by concomitant infection, metabolic derangements, renal failure, or malignant hypertension. ASM therapy is typically initiated after the onset of seizures, but adjunctive therapy with a corticosteroid and possibly an immunosuppressive agent should be considered if seizures occur in the setting of an acute inflammatory event.[21]

Sjögren syndrome

Sjögren syndrome is systemic autoimmune disease characterized by lymphocytic infiltration of the salivary and lacrimal glands resulting in oral and ocular dryness and the production of autoantibodies (anti-Ro or anti-Sjögren syndrome-related antigen A, anti-La, or anti-Sjögren syndrome-related antigen B). Similar visceral involvement and vasculitis may produce arthritis, atrophic gastritis, sclerosis cholangitis, pancreatitis, renal tubular acidosis, vaginitis, bronchitis, or interstitial pneumonitis.[21] Sjögren's syndrome may present in isolation (primary Sjögren syndrome), or with other systemic autoimmune phenomena in a mixed connective tissue disorder. Neurological involvement occurs in 20–25% of cases with the PNS and CNS involved equally.[22,25] Seizures occur in 3% of cases; the exact pathophysiological mechanism underlying primary Sjögren syndrome and epilepsy is unknown.[22,26]

Scleroderma

Scleroderma is a rare immune-mediated connective tissue disease characterized by diffuse fibrosis, inflammation, and vascular abnormalities involving the skin, muscles, and various internal organs (particularly the gastrointestinal tract, lung, heart, and kidneys). Limited cutaneous scleroderma, also known as CREST syndrome (i.e. Calcinosis, Raynaud's phenomenon, oesophageal dysmotility, Sclerodactyly, and Telangiectasia) is associated with anticentromere antibodies while diffuse cutaneous scleroderma is associated with antibodies to topoisomerase 1 and RNA polymerase.[21] Both the PNS and CNS may be affected. A systematic review of neurological involvement in scleroderma[27] demonstrated that epilepsy was the most frequently reported neurological condition in localized scleroderma, and less commonly observed in systemic scleroderma. The pathogenesis of epilepsy in systemic scleroderma is undetermined but inflammatory and vasculitic processes have been posited. Cases of focal epilepsy occur with linear scleroderma en coup de sabre, a localized form of scleroderma, associated with underlying cortical atrophy that is usually ipsilateral to the cutaneous lesion (up to 73%).[28] Epilepsy onset may precede the diagnosis of linear scleroderma en coup de sabre.

Ehlers–Danlos syndrome

Ehlers–Danlos syndrome (EDS) is an inherited connective tissue disorder affecting the synthesis and structure of collagen types I, II, and VI, characterized clinically by joint hypermobility, skin hyperextensibility and fragility, delayed wound healing, and easy bruising. There are 13 subtypes, distinguished by phenotype, mode of inheritance, and underlying genetic defects.[29] EDS is commonly associated with a wide range of neurological features such as headache, chronic pain, fatigue, cerebrovascular disorders, peripheral neuropathy, plexopathy, and epilepsy. While the association between epilepsy and EDS has been reported frequently, the exact incidence is unknown due to the heterogeneity of studies conducted so far. A variety of focal and generalized seizure types have been reported. The underlying pathological mechanism linking epilepsy and EDS is unclear. Association with polymicrogyria and periventricular heterotopia has been described and hypothesized to be related to biochemical and genetic abnormalities of connective tissue, thereby causing anomalous cellular migration.[29,30]

Systemic vasculitides

Systemic vasculitides are multiorgan diseases characterized by inflammation of the blood vessel wall. Resultant tissue damage is invariably caused by ischaemia.

Wegener's granulomatosis (granulomatosis with polyangiitis)

Wegner's granulomatosis, or granulomatosis with polyangiitis, is a necrotizing granulomatous vasculitis that primarily affects the respiratory tract and kidneys. The vasculitis affects medium- and small-diameter arteries and is often associated with the classical antineutrophil cytoplasmic antibody (c-ANCA). Up to 54% of patients may develop neurological involvement, with more frequent involvement of the PNS as a result of vasculitis. Central nervous system (CNS) involvement is much less common (4–8%), and may be due to granuloma formation, or extension of granulomas from primary sites in the ears or nasopharynx.[21,31,32] Epilepsy is uncommon, affecting approximately 10% of patients with neurological involvement; seizures are rarely observed as a primary presenting sign of Wegener's granulomatosis.[32]

Behçet's disease

Behçet's disease is an autoimmune, multisystem, vasculitic disorder characterized by recurrent oral and genital ulcers, uveitis, iritis, retinal vasculitis, thrombophlebitis, and arthritis.[21,31] The disease is associated with human leucocyte antigen B51. Neurological manifestations, usually affecting the brain, are seen in up to 10% of patients. Neurological involvement is an immune-mediated vascular inflammatory CNS disease with focal or multifocal parenchymal (intra-axial) involvement, often presenting as a brainstem syndrome or meningoencephalitis. Non-parenchymal (extra-axial) involvement is vascular, and commonly exemplified by cerebral venous sinus thrombosis with associated intracranial hypertension. Involvement of the spine or peripheral nervous system (PNS) is rare. Epilepsy occurs in 2.2–16.7% of patients, with one study suggesting an association between seizures and cerebral venous thrombosis.[33] Generalized tonic–clonic seizures occur most commonly, followed by focal seizures; status epilepticus and epilepsia partialis continua have been reported but are rare.

Diabetes mellitus

Diabetes mellitus is a complex metabolic disorder primarily characterized by hyperglycaemia. The two types of diabetes are principally distinguished by their response to insulin and by the underlying mechanism. Type 1 diabetes mellitus

(T1DM) is an autoimmune disorder resulting in the selective destruction of β cells. The mechanism underlying type 2 diabetes mellitus is an initial state of insulin resistance compensated by β-cell hypersecretion of insulin followed by β-cell dysfunction in genetically susceptible individuals. There is increasing evidence of a higher incidence of epilepsy in T1DM.

Type 1 diabetes mellitus

T1DM is characterized by the immune-mediated destruction of insulin-producing pancreatic β cells resulting in the loss of insulin production and life-long dependence on exogenous insulin. Both humoral and cellular immunity is involved in the pathogenesis of T1DM.[34] The comorbidities associated with T1DM have been well established and include cardiovascular, renal, and severe metabolic disorders due to vascular and nonvascular causes.

As previously described, seizures may be provoked acutely in the setting of metabolic derangements, such as hyper- and hypoglycaemia, both of which are hallmarks of T1DM. However, recent population-based studies[35–37] have demonstrated that patients with T1DM have up to a three times greater risk of developing epilepsy compared to matched controls. The mechanism of association between T1DM and epilepsy is unclear. Currently, multiple mechanisms have been proposed, such as enduring cortical damage resulting from metabolic abnormalities or cerebrovascular injury. Autoimmune factors have also been proposed. In particular, anti-glutamic acid decarboxylase (GAD) antibodies have been associated with T1DM (80%) and various neurological conditions, including epilepsy (6%).[35–38] Improved understanding of an underlying autoimmune mechanism has potential therapeutic implications, with the possibility of adjunctive therapy with immunosuppressive therapy.[38]

Cardiovascular disease

Multiple studies have shown that people with epilepsy have a higher prevalence of cardiovascular disease. The relationship between epilepsy and cardiovascular disease is complex and may be due to shared genetics and shared aetiological factors.[39]

People with epilepsy are potentially more likely to be obese, sedentary, and smokers, and have a worse cardiovascular risk profile (hypertension, hypercholesterolaemia, stroke) than the general population.[39,40] The use of ASMs may play a role: sodium channel blockers can produce conduction irregularities or arrhythmias, and enzyme-inducing agents may result in accelerated atherosclerosis by elevating serological vascular risk markers. Some ASMs are associated with weight gain, thereby increasing the risk of developing metabolic syndrome and, subsequently, cardiovascular risk[41–43] (see Chapter 3).

Various arrhythmias have been observed in the setting of seizures. Sinus tachycardia is very commonly associated with seizures and is often imperceptible.[44] Ictal asystole, bradycardia, and atrioventricular block have been described, most often in people with temporal lobe epilepsy; ictal asystole can be associated with physical injuries as a result of seizure-induced syncope.[39] Postictal asystole, ventricular tachycardia, and ventricular fibrillation are rare phenomena but of particular interest given their possible role in sudden unexpected death in epilepsy (SUDEP, see Chapter 9). There is a growing list of genes expressed in both the brain and heart that may provide a link between epilepsy and cardiac arrhythmias such as *SCN1A*, *SCN5A*, *SCN8A*, *KCNQ1*, and *KCNH2*.[39] Recurrent seizures may result in myocardial pathology through massive autonomic activation and resultant acute and chronic sympathetic overstimulation or subendocardial ischaemia.[41]

Predisposition to cerebrovascular disease

The presence of cardiovascular disease can potentially, through indirect mechanisms, cause epilepsy because of the predisposition to stroke. Post-stroke epilepsy accounts for 11% of all cases of adult epilepsy and occurs as a result of sustained alterations in neuronal excitability from gliotic scarring. This is particularly true in the setting of ischaemic strokes with cortical involvement, cerebral haemorrhage, and a history of early post-stroke seizures.[45] Small vessel disease, often caused by arteriosclerosis, may be present in people with epilepsy: subcortical white matter abnormalities on neuroimaging (leukoaraiosis) are frequently noted in adult patients with new-onset epilepsy but the epileptogenic role of leukoaraiosis must be further elucidated.

Conclusion

The burden of comorbid systemic disease and epilepsy is high and an understanding and appreciation of the incidence and clinical significance of these comorbidities is of paramount importance (Table 8.1). The presence of systemic disease must inform therapeutic decisions; comorbid illness can affect drug metabolism, drug–drug interactions, and can directly influence seizure control and quality of life.[47] The heterogeneous presentations and milieus of epilepsy promote the evolving concept of epilepsy as part of a spectrum of disorders that share a predisposition or tendency towards epileptic seizures.[47,48]

Table 8.1. Epilepsy and systemic disease

Systemic Disease	Aetiology	Common Clinical Characteristics	Frequency of Epilepsy	Mechanism of Epilepsy	Other Neurological or Neuropsychiatric Comorbidities	Treatment
Tuberous Sclerosis Complex	Neurocutaneous disorder Genetic: mutations in TSC1, TSC2; AD inheritance	Facial angiofibromas, hypomelanotic macules, shagreen patches, ungula fibromas, cardiac rhabdomyomas, renal angiomyolipomas, cortical tubers, SEN, SEGA	70–90%	Dysregulation of mTOR signalling pathway resulting in cortical dysplasia, abnormal vasculature, hyperexcitable neuronal circuits	Intellectual disability, learning disability, autism, attention deficits, mood disorder	Conventional ASM, ketogenic diet, VNS, epilepsy surgery (tuber resection), everolimus
Sturge-Weber Syndrome	Neurocutaneous disorder Genetic: mosaic mutation in GNAQ; sporadic	Port-wine facial birthmark, leptomeningeal vascular malformation, ocular angiomas, cortical malformation	72% with unilateral cerebral involvement, >90% of those with bilateral involvement	Abnormal vasculature, cerebral calcifications, and associated cortical malformations.	Intellectual disability, migraine headaches, focal neurologic deficits (hemiparesis)	Conventional ASM (topiramate used with caution), epilepsy surgery (focal resection, hemispherectomy)
Neurofibromatosis Type 1	Neurocutaneous disorder Genetic: mutation in NF1; AD	Café au lait macules, cutaneous/subcutaneous neurofibromas, axillary/groin freckling, optic pathway gliomas, Lisch nodules	6-10%	Cortical dysgenesis	Cognitive deficits, sleep disorders, mood disorders, migraine headache	Conventional ASM

(continued)

Table 8.1. Continued

Systemic Disease	Aetiology	Common Clinical Characteristics	Frequency of Epilepsy	Mechanism of Epilepsy	Other Neurological or Neuropsychiatric Comorbidities	Treatment
Systemic Lupus Erythematosus	Connective tissue disease Autoimmune	Arthritis, pericarditis, nephritis, photosensitivity, malar rash	6–51%	Antibody-mediated thrombotic occlusion associated with antiphospholipid antibodies; autoantibody-mediated inflammatory neuronal injury	Cognitive dysfunction, encephalopathy, psychosis, mood disorder, aseptic meningitis, cerebrovascular disease, myelopathy, neuropathy, myopathy, autonomic dysfunction	Conventional ASM; adjunct corticosteroid and/or immunosuppressive agent in setting of acute flare
Sjögren's Syndrome	Connective tissue disease Autoimmune	Xerostomia, xerophthalmia, arthritis, atrophic gastritis, sclerosis cholangitis, pancreatitis, renal tubular acidosis, vaginitis, bronchitis or interstitial pneumonitis	3%	Unknown	Myelopathy, optic neuropathy, aseptic meningitis, neuropathy (including cranial and autonomic neuropathy)	Conventional ASM
Scleroderma	Connective tissue disease Autoimmune	CREST syndrome (Calcinosis, Raynaud's phenomenon, oEsophageal dysmotility, Sclerodactyly, and Telangiectasia)	Up to 73% of patients with LSCS	Uncertain in systemic scleroderma, possibly due to inflammatory and/or vasculitic processes; underlying cortical atrophy observed in cases of LSCS	Neuropathy, psychosis, plexopahty, radiculopathy, myelopathy	Conventional ASM

Disease	Category	Clinical features	Neurological association	Neurological manifestations	Treatment
Ehlers-Danlos Syndrome	Connective tissue disease Genetic: AD, AR, x-linked recessive, with numerous genetic defects implicated	Joint hypermobility, skin hyperextensibility and fragility, delayed wound healing, easy bruisability	Unknown	Uncertain; association with polymicrogyria and periventricular heterotopia has been described	Headache, chronic pain, fatigue, cerebrovascular disorders, peripheral neuropathy, plexopathy,	Conventional ASM
Wegener's Granulomatosis	Vasculitis Autoimmune	Rhinosinusitis, purulent/bloody nasal discharge, oral/nasal ulcers, pulmonary consolidation, pleural effusion, glomerulonephritis, pericarditis, myocarditis	10% of patients with neurological involvement (4–8%)	Cerebral granulomatous involvement	Sensorineural hearing loss, mononeuritis multiplex, cranial neuropathy, CNS mass lesions (granuloma)	Conventional ASM; adjunct corticosteroid and/or immunosuppressive agent
Behçet's Disease	Vasculitis Autoimmune	Oral and genital ulcers, uveitis, iritis, retinal vasculitis, thrombophlebitis, and arthritis	2.2–16.7%	Immune-mediated vascular inflammatory CNS disease; association between seizures and cerebral venous thrombosis has been described	Brainstem syndrome and meningioencephalitis (intra-axial NBD), cerebral venous sinus thrombosis and intracranial hypertension (extra-axial NBD)	Conventional ASM

(continued)

Table 8.1. Continued

Systemic Disease	Aetiology	Common Clinical Characteristics	Frequency of Epilepsy	Mechanism of Epilepsy	Other Neurological or Neuropsychiatric Comorbidities	Treatment
Type 1 Diabetes Mellitus	Metabolic disorder Autoimmune	Polydipsia, polyuria, weight loss with hyperglycemia and ketonemia	Frequency unknown; up to 3-fold increased risk of developing epilepsy	Uncertain, but cortical damage from metabolic abnormalities, cerebrovascular injury, or autoimmune mechanisms been proposed	Peripheral neuropathy, cardiovascular autonomic neuropathy	Conventional ASM
Cardiovascular Disease	ASM-induced Genetic mutation Shared health behaviours	Certain ASMs may cause arrhythmias and elevate serological vascular risk markers; weight gain/obesity may lead to metabolic syndrome	Variable	Mutations in genes expressed in heart and brain (e.g. SCN1A, SCN5A, SCN8A, KCNQ1, KCNH2)	Neurological and neuropsychiatric comorbidities are variable, and may be dependent on presence of comorbid cerebrovascular disease	Conventional ASM. Cardiac pacemaker when appropriate.
		Ictal asystole, bradycardia, AV block. Rarely post-ictal asystole, VT, VF Cardiac ischemia, impaired heart rate variability		Predisposition to cerebrovascular disease may result in post-stroke epilepsy		

AD, autosomal dominant; AR, autosomal recessive; SEN, subependymal nodule; SEGA, subependymal giant cell astrocytoma; ASM, antiseizure medication; VNS, vagus nerve stimulator; LSCS, localized scleroderma *en coup de sabre*; CNS, central nervous system; NBD, neurologic manifestation in Behçet's disease; AV, atrioventricular; VT, ventricular tachycardia; VF, ventricular fibrillation

References

1. **Eisenschenk S, Cibula J, Gilmore R.** Seizures associated with nonneurologic medical conditions. In: **Wyllie E, Cascino G, Gidal B, Goodkin H,** eds. Wyllie's treatment of epilepsy: principles and practice, 5th ed. Philadelphia, PA: Lippincott Williams & Wilkins; 2011:438–50.

2. **Messing R, Simon R.** Seizures as a manifestation of systemic disease. Neurol Clin. 1986;**4**(3):563–84.

3. **Keezer M, Sisodiya S, Sander J.** Comorbidities of epilepsy: current concepts and future perspectives. Lancet Neurol. 2016;**15**(1):106–15.

4. **Seindenberg M, Pulsipher DT, Hermann B.** Association of epilepsy and comorbid conditions. Future Neurol. 2009;**4**(5):663–68.

5. **Gaitatzis A, Sisodiya S, Sander J.** The somatic comorbidity of epilepsy: a weighty but often unrecognized burden. Epilepsia. 2012;**53**(8):1282–93.

6. **Selassie A, Wilson D, Martz G, Smith G, Wagner J, Wannamaker B.** Epilepsy beyond seizure: a population-based study of comorbidities. Epilepsy Res. 2014;**108**(2):305–15.

7. **Hasbani DM, Crino PB.** Tuberous sclerosis complex. Handb Clin Neurol. 2018;**148**:813–22.

8. **Jeong A, Wong M.** Systemic disease manifestations associated with epilepsy in tuberous sclerosis complex. Epilepsia. 2016;**57**(9):1443–49.

9. **Northrup H, Krueger DA; International Tuberous Sclerosis Complex Consensus Group.** Tuberous sclerosis complex diagnostic criteria update: recommendations of the 2012 International Tuberous Sclerosis Complex Consensus Conference. Pediatr Neurol. 2013;**49**(4):243–54.

10. **Stafstrom C, Staedtke V, Comi A.** Epilepsy mechanisms in neurocutaneous disorders: tuberous sclerosis complex, neurofibromatosis type 1, and Sturge–Weber syndrome. Front Neurol. 2017;**8**:87.

11. **Mohamed AR, Bailey CA, Freeman JL, Maixner W, Jaxkson GD, Harvey AS.** Intrinsic epileptogenicity of cortical tubers revealed by intracranial EEG monitoring. Neurology. 2012;**79**(23):2249–57.

12. **Curatolo P.** Mechanistic target of rapamycin (mTOR) in tuberous sclerosis complex-associated epilepsy. Pediatr Neurol. 2015;**52**(3):281–89.

13. **Feliciano DM, Lin TV, Harman NW,** et al. A circuitry and biochemical basis of tuberous sclerosis symptoms: from epilepsy to neurocognitive deficits. Int J Dev Neurosci. 2013;**31**(7):667–78.

14. **Ruppe V, Dilsiz P, Reiss CS,** et al. Developmental brain abnormalities in tuberous sclerosis complex: a comparative tissue analysis of cortical tubers and perituberal cortex. Epilepsia. 2014;**55**(4):539–50.

15. **Bollo RJ, Kalhorn SP, Carlson C, Haegeli V, Devinsky O, Weiner HL.** Epilepsy surgery and tuberous sclerosis complex: special considerations. Neurosurg Focus. 2008;**25**(3):E13.

16. **Elliott RE, Carlson C, Kalhorn SP,** et al. Refractory epilepsy in tuberous sclerosis: vagus nerve stimulation with or without subsequent resective surgery. Epilepsy Behav. 2009;**16**(3):454–60.

17. **French JA, Lawson JA, Yapici Z, et al.** Adjunctive everolimus therapy for treatment-resistant focal-onset seizures associated with tuberous sclerosis (EXIST-3): a phase 3, randomised, double-blind, placebo-controlled study. Lancet. 2016;**388**(10056):2153–63.

18. **Comi AM.** Sturge–Weber syndrome. Handb Clin Neurol. 2015;**132**:157–68.

19. **Sebold AJ, Day AM, Ewen J, et al.** Sirolimus treatment in Sturge–Weber syndrome. Pediatr Neurol. 2021;**115**:29–40.

20. **Ferner RE, Huson SM, Thomas N, et al.** Guidelines for the diagnosis and management of individuals with neurofibromatosis 1. J Med Genet. 2007;**44**(2):81–88.

21. **Streifler J, Molad Y.** Connective tissue disorders: systemic lupus erythematosus, Sjögren's syndrome, and scleroderma. Handb Clin Neurol. 2014;**119**:463–73.

22. **Devinsky O, Schein A, Najjar S.** Epilepsy associated with systemic autoimmune disorders. Epilepsy Curr. 2013;**13**(2):62–68.

23. **Bruns A, Meyer O.** Neuropsychiatric manifestations of systemic lupus erythematosus. Joint Bone Spine. 2006;**73**(6):639–45.

24. **Karaaslan Z, Ekizoğlu E, Tektürk P, et al.** Investigation of neuronal auto-antibodies in systemic lupus erythematosus patients with epilepsy. Epilepsy Res. 2017;**129**:132–37.

25. **Moreira I, Texeira F, Martins Silva A, et al.** Frequent involvement of central nervous system in primary Sjögren syndrome. Rheumatol Int. 2015;**35**(2):289–94.

26. **Harboe E, Tjensvoll AB, Maroni S, Goransson LG, Greve OJ, Beyer MK, et al.** Neuropsychiatric syndromes in patients with systemic lupus erythematosus and primary Sjögren syndrome: a comparative population-based study. Ann Rheum Dis. 2009;**68**(10):1541–46.

27. **Amaral TN, Peres FA, Lapa AT, Marques-Neto JF, Appenzeller S.** Neurologic involvement in scleroderma: a systematic review. Semin Arthritis Rheum. 2013;**43**(3):335–47.

28. **Kister I, Inglese M, Lazer R, Herbert J.** Neurologic manifestations of localized scleroderma. Neurology. 2008;**71**(19):1538–45.

29. **Cortini F, Villa C.** Ehlers–Danlos syndromes and epilepsy: an updated review. Seizure. 2018;**57**:1–4.

30. **Verrotti A, Monacelli D, Castagnino M, Villa MP, Parisi P.** Ehlers–Danlos syndrome: a cause of epilepsy and periventricular heterotopia. Seizure. 2014;**23**(10):819–24.

31. **Moore P, Calabrese.** Neurologic manifestations of systemic vasculitides. Semin Neurol. 1994;**14**(4):300–306.

32. **Moore BM, Rothman SM, Brent Clark H, Vehe R, Laguna T.** Epilepsy: an anticipatory presentation of pediatric Wegener's granulomatosis. Pediatr Neurol. 2010;**43**(1):49–52.

33. **Kutlu G, Semercioglu S, Ucler S, Erdal A, Inan L.** Epileptic seizures in neuro-Behçet disease: why some patients develop seizure and others not? Seizure. 2015;**26**:32–35.

34. **Zaccardi F, Webb D, Yates T, Davies M.** Pathophysiology of type 1 and type 2 diabetes mellitus: a 90-year perspective. Postgrad Med J. 2016;**92**(1084):63–69.

35. **Chou IC, Wang CH, Lin WD, Tsai FJ, Lin CC, Kao CH.** Risk of epilepsy in type 1 diabetes mellitus: a population-based cohort study. Diabetologia. 2016;**59**(6):1196–203.

36. **Keezer MR, Novy J, Sander JW.** Type 1 diabetes mellitus in people with pharmacoresistant epilepsy: prevalence and clinical characteristics. Epilepsy Res. 2015;**115**:55–57.

37. Dafoulas CE, Toulis KA, McCorry D, et al. Type 1 diabetes mellitus and risk of incident epilepsy: a population-based, open-cohort study. Diabetologia. 2017;**60**(2):258–61.

38. Sander JW, Novy J, Keezer MR. The intriguing relationship between epilepsy and type 1 diabetes mellitus. Diabetologia. 2016;**59**(7):1569–70.

39. Shmuely S, van der Lende M, Lamberts RJ, et al. The heart of epilepsy: current views and future concepts. Seizure. 2017;**44**:176–83.

40. Kobau R, Zahran H, Thurman DJ, et al. Epilepsy surveillance among adults—19 states, Behavioral Risk Factor Surveillance System, 2005. MMWR Surveill Summ. 2008;**57**(6):1–20.

41. Schuele SU. Effects of seizures on cardiac function. J Clin Neurophyisiol. 2009;**26**(5):302–308.

42. Brodie MJ, Mintzer S, Pack AM, et al. Enzyme induction with antiepileptic drugs: cause for concern? Epilepsia. 2013;**54**(1):11–27.

43. Katsiki N, Mikhailidis DP, Nair DR. The effects of antiepileptic drugs on vascular risk factors: a narrative review. Seizure. 2014;**23**(9):677–84.

44. Van der Lende M, Surges R, Sander JW, et al. Cardiac arrhythmias during or after epileptic seizures. J Neurol Neurosurg Psychiatry. 2016;**87**(1):69–74.

45. Hassani M, Cooray G, Sveinsson O, et al. Post-stroke epilepsy in ischemic stroke cohort—incidence and diagnosis. Acta Neurol Scand. 2020;**141**(2):141–47.

46. Ferlazzo E, Gasparini S, Beghi, E, et al. Epilepsy in cerebrovascular disease: review of experimental and clinical data with meta-analysis of risk factors. Epilepsia. 2016;**57**(8):1205–14.

47. Keezer MR, Sisodiya SM, Sander JW. Comorbidities of epilepsy: current concepts and future perspectives. Lancet Neurol. 2016;**15**:106–13.

48. Institute of Medicine. Epilepsy across the spectrum: promoting health and understanding. Washington, DC: National Academies Press; 2012.

Chapter 9

Epilepsy and mortality

Rohit Shankar, Lance Watkins,
Samantha Ashby, and Jane Hanna

The context

National figures indicate that there are over 1000 epilepsy-related deaths each year in the UK.[1-3] Standardized mortality ratios (SMRs) for people with epilepsy are consistently two to three times higher than the general population, and there may be a 24-fold increase in the risk of *sudden* death.[4] Approximately half of the people with epilepsy in the UK are symptomatic, and for this population life expectancy may be up to 10 years lower than the general population.[5]

Comparing mortality rates of health-related causes across the population in the UK (2001–2014) suggests that for people with a neurological condition there is an alarming rise in age-standardized mortality rates (39%) versus a 6% decrease in all causes of death.[6] More concerning still is a 70% increase in epilepsy-related deaths, with an upward trend.[6] These findings are consistent with other national death registry data suggesting that rates of potentially avoidable deaths in epilepsy are higher than in other chronic conditions (such as asthma).[1] Even more concerning is a 69% increase in epilepsy-related deaths in people with epilepsy (2004–2014) identified within general practitioner data.[7]

A primary care population-based study found seizure freedom was linked to a lower risk of death for all age groups. Identified common risk factors include emergency visits and/or emergency admissions; prescription of more than one antiseizure medication (ASM), which indicates more difficult-to-control epilepsy; status epilepticus; and injuries in the group who died.[7] Other factors include missed ASMs and treatment for depression and alcohol misuse.[8] A national audit[9] found that 42% of epilepsy-related deaths were potentially avoidable with improved risk management and communication of risk.

By 2021, there was evidence that potential avoidable risk was much greater.[10] Where there are national surveillance studies, stark outcomes have shown a doubling of maternal deaths,[11] most of which were potentially avoidable, and worsening trends in learning disabilities.[12] A systematic review by the Mortality

Task Force of the International League Against Epilepsy (ILAE) also identified that many of the direct causes of death were potentially preventable. The most common attributable causes included status epilepticus, accidental fatal injury, suicide, and sudden unexpected death in epilepsy (SUDEP). SMRs were higher in people with treatment-resistant epilepsy, convulsive seizures, structural/metabolic causes of epilepsy, and those under 50 years of age.[13] Where there is a lack of access to medical facilities and treatment, there is also a significant increase in mortality rates.[14] There is emerging evidence that people with epilepsy have been at increased risk due to the impact that the coronavirus disease 2019 (COVID-19) pandemic has had on epilepsy services and the wider community.[15]

Epilepsy mortality risk factors

In order to identify and manage risk, everyone with epilepsy needs a quality-assured robust assessment.[16] The importance of identifying *and* communicating individual risks with patients has been highlighted in a UK study of epilepsy deaths.[17] It found that 80% of people with epilepsy who died suddenly had not engaged with specialist services in the year prior to their death. Of these deaths, 90% occurred in people with tonic–clonic seizures that had increased in frequency in the previous 3–6 months.[17] Despite this potential to identify risk factors and intervene, effective communication of such risks has not been consistent.[18-21]

Sudden unexpected death in epilepsy

An important cause of death in epilepsy is SUDEP. Current incidence and prevalence data are likely significant underestimations of the actual risk.[22] A systematic review of the literature estimates an annual incidence rate of 1.16 cases per 1000 person-years.[23] If we consider this in the context of the UK, 500–600 people die from SUDEP every year. Increased awareness and the unified definition of SUDEP should help identify cases and standardize research methodology in the future.[24]

When SUDEP data are pooled we start to observe associations, which help identify risk factors (Box 9.1).[17,25] Incidence rates of SUDEP are highest in people with complex treatment-resistant epilepsy, experiencing nocturnal convulsive seizures.[26] A retrospective review of definite and probable SUDEP cases under monitoring at the time of death identified a centrally mediated compromise in respiratory and cardiac functioning following a convulsive seizure.[27]

Efforts are ongoing to better appreciate the mechanisms that lead to SUDEP and our understanding is likely to develop in coming years. The seminal

Box 9.1 Mortality risk factors in epilepsy (including SUDEP)

- Active seizures.
- Injury.
- Generalized tonic–clonic seizures.
- Nocturnal seizures or seizures when asleep.
- Lack of night-time surveillance/supervision.
- Status epilepticus/prolonged seizures.
- Poor medicines adherence.
- Medication changes (frequent changes of ASM dosage compared with no change found to be associated with increased SUDEP risk).
- Alcohol/substance misuse.
- Depression or other psychiatric disorder.
- Intellectual disability.
- Pregnancy.
- Young adult age (20–40 years peak age range shown in research).
- Earlier age of epilepsy onset (before 16 years of age).
- Longer duration of epilepsy.
- Symptomatic epilepsy.
- Male sex.

MORTEMUS investigation of SUDEP cases demonstrated a pattern of terminal apnoea followed by asystole.[27] From these observations, a range of risk factors have been identified including considering the role of centrally impaired carbon dioxide retention, ictal laryngospasm, and cardiac arrhythmia.

There is a remarkable relationship between epilepsy and cardiac function. Seizures have a direct impact upon cardiac physiology and anatomy in the short and long term. Ictal events are associated with changes in heart rate, heart rate variability, ischaemia, and output. Comorbid epilepsy also increases mortality risk for genetic variants of long QT syndrome. There is ongoing work to develop biomarkers that may in the future help predict SUDEP risk. One example of many is that all of the SUDEP cases in the MORTEMUS study were associated with postictal generalized electroencephalogram suppression, although this has not been consistently found in case–control studies since. Postictal generalized electroencephalogram suppression was significantly associated with the presence of a tonic phase during seizure, duration of hypoxaemia, and older age. All of these factors may indicate severity of seizure but to date have not been proven to have a direct correlation with SUDEP risk.

Children with epilepsy are also at an increased risk of death compared to the general population. Most premature mortality in children with epilepsy is not seizure related; rather, it is often caused by respiratory illness in association with severe neurological disability, and comorbid conditions.[28] SUDEP is the most common cause of seizure-related death in children with epilepsy with incidence rates ranging from 0.2 to 0.3 per 1000 children with epilepsy per year. The evidence base has suggested that the incidence of SUDEP in children was significantly lower than in adults; however, we are now observing that there has likely been an underestimation in the paediatric population.[29]

In the UK, the National Institute for Health and Care Excellence (NICE) guideline NG217 highlights key aspects of epilepsy risk management and emphasizes the importance of communicating SUDEP risk factors with patients and families or carers.[30] The American Academy of Neurology practice guidelines also make evidence-based recommendations to help reduce mortality risk.[31] These recommendations focus on:

- Providing information on the level of risk and associated risk factors
- Optimizing therapeutic management to reduce the frequency of generalized tonic–clonic seizures
- Advocating night-time surveillance for those with nocturnal generalized tonic–clonic seizures
- Highlighting the benefits of seizure freedom and its impact on reducing risk.

However, there is recognition that uptake of such guidelines is variable and inconsistent. At present, there is no systematic plan on how to deliver discussion about SUDEP and assess risk in a person-centred way.[20]

Suicide

A population-based case–control study in Denmark (21,169 cases, 423,128 controls) found the risk of suicide in epilepsy to be around three times higher than for those without epilepsy. The highest risk of suicide was associated with comorbid psychiatric illness (13.7; $p < 0.0001$). The data also demonstrated an increased risk of suicide in the first 6 months after a diagnosis of epilepsy was made, particularly in those with a history of comorbid psychiatric illness (rate ratio 29.2; 95% confidence interval (CI) 16.4–51.9; $p < 0.0001$).[32]

In 2008, the US Food and Drug Administration issued an alert regarding suicidal ideation and behaviour in association with ASMs. In response, the Task Force on Therapeutic Strategies of the ILAE Commission on Neuropsychobiology produced an expert consensus statement. The review of the evidence suggests that suicidality in epilepsy is complex and multifactorial and should be considered on an individual basis. There may be an association between some ASMs and treatment of emergent psychiatric symptoms including suicidality, but the level of evidence available is limited. The risk of withholding ASM treatment or stopping ASM treatment is far higher and includes risk of death.[33]

There is some evidence to suggest a possible common pathogenic pathway between epilepsy and suicidality or suicide completion. People with a history of suicidality have a higher risk of receiving a diagnosis of epilepsy in the future. In the UK, a population-based retrospective study of 14,059 cases (56,184 matched controls) found the risk of first suicide attempt was almost three times higher in individuals who later went on to be diagnosed with epilepsy, independent of any comorbid psychiatric illness.[34]

Before initiating treatment with ASMs it is essential that a full psychiatric history and family history of mental illness is acquired (Box 9.2).[33] The emergence of psychiatric symptoms with ASM treatment is more likely in individuals with a history of psychiatric illness. Patients (and families or carers) should be advised to report any changes of mood or suicidal ideation to their specialist or general practitioner as soon as possible. Where there are treatment-emergent psychiatric symptoms that do not respond readily to changes in ASMs or

---

Box 9.2 Past psychiatric history—important risk factors

- Postictal suicidal ideation.
- Past history of mood disorder or anxiety disorder.
- Previous suicidal ideation or suicide attempts.
- Comorbid serious and enduring mental illness (major depressive disorder, bipolar affective disorder, schizophrenia).
- Family history of serious and enduring mental illness.
- Family history of completed suicide.
- Limited Social circumstances and lack of protective factors.

dosage, or there is evidence of an enduring mental illness, there needs to be a mechanism to involve the support of specialist psychiatrist services.[35]

Pregnancy

In the UK, maternal deaths are monitored under the Mothers and Babies: Reducing Risk through Audit and Confidential Enquiries or MBRRACE-UK auditing and enquiry system. Each year approximately 2500 women with epilepsy become pregnant, and there is an increased risk of mortality both during and after pregnancy (see Chapter 11). Between 2009 and 2012, 10 of 14 deaths identified in pregnant women with epilepsy may have been preventable.[36] These figures align with international data that suggest 1 in 1000 women with epilepsy die each year during or shortly after pregnancy.[37] Factors that are thought to have contributed to these deaths include reduced medication adherence, suboptimal ASM regimes, sleep deprivation, and risk-taking behaviours.[36] The Centre for Child and Maternal Death Enquiries highlighted in 2012 how women with epilepsy were not receiving risk information and that the clinical understanding of how to manage risk was low. In the report, many of the women who died from epilepsy stopped taking their medication out of fear that their medication would harm their unborn child. The deaths identified are often associated with complex social factors and comorbidities, a lack of preconception counselling, and no specialist epilepsy review during pregnancy.[38,39]

Epilepsy and pregnancy toolkit

- Designed for use before, during, and following pregnancy to help with decision-making, choice, risk reduction strategies, safety measures, and empowerment to help women with epilepsy become an equal partner in their epilepsy maternity healthcare.[40]
- This resource has been developed by an epilepsy specialist nurse/midwife from the experience of supporting women with epilepsy and healthcare professionals over the last 18 years. It showcases the latest evidence-based research and guidelines and links with epilepsy and pregnancy support groups. It is regularly updated to reflect opinions of women with epilepsy and health professionals.
- See www.womenwithepilepsy.co.uk for the latest version.

The teratogenic risks associated with the use of ASMs in pregnancy must be considered in context, and alongside the risk of uncontrolled seizures in pregnancy—including the risk of death to both the mother and unborn child. Generalized tonic–clonic seizures are associated with hypoxia and lactic acidosis, which can result in asphyxiation and death of the unborn child.[41] For the mother, uncontrolled generalized tonic–clonic seizures in pregnancy are associated with significantly increased mortality rates (ten times higher compared to women without epilepsy), the majority of which are due to SUDEP.[42]

Box 9.3 Factors that may improve outcomes for women with epilepsy in pregnancy

◆ Proactive preconception counselling.

◆ Good ASM adherence.

◆ Appropriate monitoring of serum ASM levels (owing to pharmacokinetic changes as pregnancy progresses). A baseline level is required for any interpretation and comparison.

◆ Regular specialist review.

◆ Coordinated communication between patient, neurologist, obstetrician and other relevant specialist teams.

The ILAE Task Force on Women and Pregnancy provides recommendations on management strategies at each stage in pregnancy, from preconception to postpartum, which are associated with better outcomes in terms of seizure control, malformations, and adverse effects from ASMs (Box 9.3).[43]

For women with epilepsy there are established benefits to an integrated planned approach to pregnancy. However, many pregnancies are unplanned. The UK Epilepsy Mortality Group highlights four 'golden moments' when there is an opportunity for healthcare interventions to help improve the outcome for women with epilepsy who become pregnant: preconception, pregnancy confirmation, later in pregnancy, and postpartum.[44]

Status epilepticus

A comprehensive systematic review of 22 population-based studies on the epidemiology of status epilepticus identified incidence rates of 1.29–73.7 per 100,000 adults (95% CI 76.6–80.3). The reason for such varying results is likely due to heterogeneity in study design and status epilepticus definition. The studies included suggest that there is a peak in incidence in the initial years after diagnosis, followed by a progressive increase over the lifespan.[45] Status epilepticus is often the first presentation of seizure activity in older adults (≥65 years of age; see Chapter 10) and can be associated with a mortality rate as high as one in four.[45]

Accidental fatal injury

When data are pooled, in people with epilepsy there is a significant increase in risk of death from all causes of injuries considered. People with epilepsy are at particular risk of death from drowning with adjusted odds ratio of 7.7 (95% CI 4.7–12.7) and SMR of 18.7 (95% CI 15–23.1).[46,47] There is also a statistically significant increased risk of death from falls in people with epilepsy (SMR 4.6; 95% CI 3.5–5.8).[47]

A prospective population-based cohort study from Sweden found that epilepsy was associated with increased injury and accident with a hazard ratio (HR) of 1.71 (95% CI 1.60–1.83).[48] However, the risk was lower when comorbidities were considered (HR 1.30). The risk of accident or injury was highest in the first 2 years after diagnosis and the highest HRs were observed for drowning, poisoning, and severe traumatic brain injury. The risk of injury or accident was not increased in children less than 15 years of age (possibly due to increased supervision).[48]

Preventing epilepsy deaths—how action can be taken to save lives

Risk should be considered an integral part of epilepsy assessment and management and should be monitored strategically with the support of evidence-based tools. Each risk discussion should be individualized, and personalized, considering the wider context and impact of epilepsy on quality of life and the influence of other comorbidities (Figure 9.1). The approach to epilepsy care can be considered in four broad domains that all influence each other:

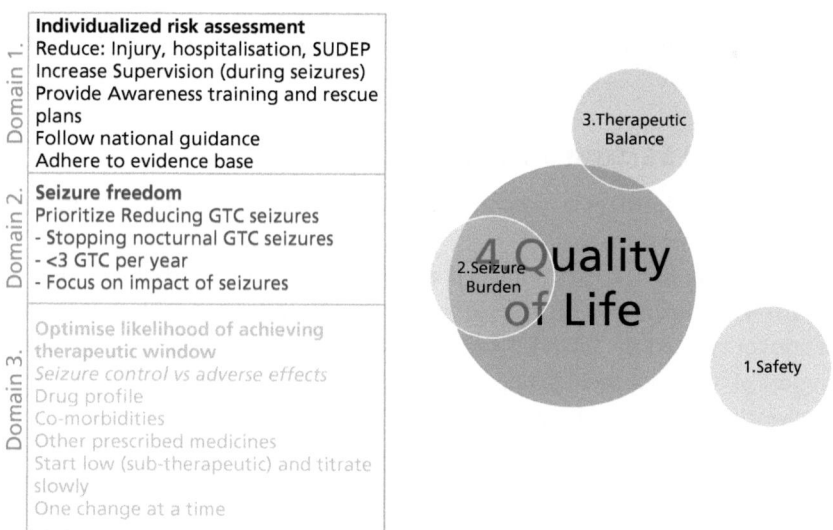

Figure 9.1 How to reduce risk—a domain approach.

1. *Safety*—individualized risk assessment.
2. *Seizure burden*—aim for seizure freedom.
3. *Therapeutic balance*—achieve therapeutic window (efficacy and adverse effect equilibrium).
4. *Quality of life*—influenced by all domains and central to any decision-making.

The role of communication between healthcare professionals, the person with epilepsy, family, or carers, and other aligned professionals is fundamental to effective risk management. This will help people with epilepsy make informed choices about their care—a lack of which is attributable to many potentially avoidable epilepsy deaths. Such approaches have proved positive in other long-term conditions such as asthma, diabetes, and stroke, where initiatives are supported by the health services to identify individuals at risk and tackle premature mortality.[49,50] The National Institute for Health and Care Excellence quality standard QS211[51] states that people with epilepsy should have a comprehensive epilepsy care plan that will include information about the individual, their specific epilepsy, management plans, and risk. This care plan should be available to all persons involved in the individual's healthcare, including primary and secondary care, social care professionals, and other social provision where appropriate.[52] The importance of taking a risk management approach to epilepsy mortality has been highlighted in the NHS Rightcare Epilepsy Toolkit[53] which provides best practice resources to support health service providers, health professionals, and people with epilepsy to tackle risk. Two such examples are shared in 'Prevention case study 2': the SUDEP and Seizure Safety Checklist[27,54–56] and EpSMon.[57]

SUDEP and Seizure Safety Checklist

Following the death of a young student nurse, Katie, SUDEP Action and Cornwall Partnership

NHS Foundation Trust completed a 9- year population study into epilepsy deaths, which led to the identification of core SUDEP risk factors.17 SUDEP Action formalized the 'SUDEP and Seizure Safety Checklist' in 2015 with the support of a development group of leading UK experts. The Checklist undergoes yearly literature and content updates.

Completion of the Checklist enables discussion around risk modification and management. It provides a standardized approach, supporting individualized discussions on risk and appropriate actions to reduce them.

The tool is now used by clinicians across the UK in varied clinical and community settings by a wide range of professionals. It is also available in Australia via a collaboration with Epilepsy Action Australia. See https://www.youtube.com/watch?v=Sz5BoejqdII.

EpSMon: Epilepsy Self-Monitor

This digital app is based upon the SUDEP and Seizure Safety Checklist, bringing epilepsy risk information to the fingertips of people living with epilepsy and helping them to monitor their risks in between health appointments so they can take actions to reduce them (e.g. see their clinician earlier or adapt lifestyle). By providing simple information on risk, it demonstrates the importance of risk awareness and empowers people with epilepsy to take action and advocate for the care and services they need to reduce their risks. See https://www.youtube.com/watch?v=wQ56a1g9CbY.

Both the SUDEP and Seizure Safety Checklist and the EpSMon app are recognized as best practice tools by NHS RightCare,[53] and in MBRRACE and LeDeR national mortality reports.[11,12]

Recent evidence from EpSMon highlighted the challenges faced in communication of risk.[58] An analysis over 5.5 years of a prospective real-world cohort of 2158 women with epilepsy of childbearing age revealed a preliminary risk awareness of 25.3% for pregnancy-related issues and 54.1% for SUDEP. Repeated EpSMon use increased SUDEP awareness but not awareness of pregnancy risks. It suggests that risk communication needs to be personalized with respect to the situation and the need. However, this is unlikely in current conventional clinical models. It is thus important to focus on digital solutions, which at present hold promise, but require work to raise implementation and acceptability.

The social impact of epilepsy mortality

The tragedy of an epilepsy death impacts the immediate family and extends beyond to friends, work colleagues, the community, and associated health professionals.[59,60] The consequence of this traumatic event is often transformative and lifelong. Early intervention can be helpful in reducing associated morbidity for any sudden unexpected death.[61]

As we have discussed, a large proportion of epilepsy deaths are unexpected and may have been avoidable. A lack of awareness of the risk of death, including SUDEP may exacerbate trauma.[52] The aggravation of grief for families who lacked information before a SUDEP death was a point of harm identified by the Scottish Public Services Ombudsman[62] during an inquiry:

> [H]ow they might have altered the outcome if they had only known this information. Mrs C accepted that Miss C may still have died even if they had known about SUDEP, but because there is the suggestion of the chance she might not have, they are not able to find any peace.

Epilepsy guidelines in the UK recommend that health professionals contact families to offer their condolences, invite them to discuss the death, and offer referral to bereavement counselling and a SUDEP support group.[63]

Case study 1

Fatal accident enquiry

The deceased was due to leave home for the university when she was diagnosed with tonic–clonic seizures and prescribed antiepileptic drugs following a nocturnal seizure. On a second review 5 months later, no further seizures were reported, and the medication was reduced because of concerns about side effects.

The family had reason to be concerned that she was not adhering to treatment following her move to the university. The deceased died suddenly in her sleep shortly after, and toxicology testing at post-mortem showed no evidence of antiepileptic drugs. (The Judge, Sheriff Alastair Duff, August 2011)[64]

The framework of services at SUDEP Action has been developed to support person-centred normalization and self-validation of expression of grief, whatever that is, with the centrality of the bereaved person recognized in every part of the service. The care pathway uses a triage service to enable each person to access relevant support (https://sudep.org/). Over 900 families have participated in an international research register which provides learnings from deaths and is partially cathartic.[65]

Notably, a survey of families through the COVID-19 pandemic found that 86% of those suddenly bereaved by epilepsy felt their mental health had been negatively impacted by the pandemic and the government's lockdown response, with 60% experiencing increased isolation and 51% experiencing distressing flashbacks.[57]

Medico-legal aspects and clinical governance

National and international guidelines all encourage the communication of risk as good practice as part of access to good epilepsy services.[30,31] This aligns with professional guidance supporting the benefits of working in partnership with patients to explore the benefits, risks, and burdens of treatment and non-treatment (General Medical Council). This position is reinforced by the Supreme Court in the *Montgomery* v *Lanarkshire Health Board* case (2015 UKSC 11).[66] A clinician cannot wait to ask about risk, nor assume that the patient does not need to know or would not attach significance to a risk. The assessment and communication of risk must be based on meaningful dialogue.

Medical Defence Union case summary

The UK Supreme Court judgment[66] further strengthens the position of judicial rulings in fatal accident inquiries in the UK since 2002, which found significant failings, and emphasized that the risk of SUDEP should be communicated to most people on or soon after diagnosis of epilepsy. These enquiries have pointed to the importance of personal care plans and support for families as lifesaving, endorsing the view that deaths may be avoided.

The complexity of medico-legal issues related to epilepsy mortality vary across different policy and country settings.[67,68] Space precludes more detailed analysis of this, but the complexities and challenges in this field have been significant over decades.[27,69]

Case study 2

A state report into the sudden death of a young man with learning disability found SUDEP and epilepsy risk was not understood as part of multisystemic failures across health and care or by the family of the deceased who had lived with epilepsy for decades and was at high risk.

The professionals involved in the investigation of death did not use national guidance on investigating a sudden death in a person with epilepsy and the death was recorded as cardiac related. The legal teams were also unaware of SUDEP and epilepsy risk.

The report, released 5 years after the deceased's death, recommended the SUDEP and Seizure Safety Checklist and EpSMon app as standardized good practice, and that national coronial and pathology systems consider how to improve investigation and recording of epilepsy-related deaths.

Conclusion

Epilepsy-related deaths pose a unique challenge and opportunity. Good practice models for supporting families use a holistic model to tackle systemic issues.[27,53,57] Bereaved families who are signposted early to SUDEP Action are offered specialist support with a range of practical options as part of a support and counselling service. The Epilepsy Deaths Register has been found to be cathartic and a valuable repository of learnings from deaths both relating to events leading up to a death and events in the aftermath.[65] The Register informs families that there is no system to inform all health professionals involved in care of a sudden death and offers facilitation. People seeking answers to questions or learnings are supported by a case worker who helps vulnerable families through highly complex medico-legal investigations after a sudden death and as and when needed through a lifetime living with grief.[70]

Other families will seek to be active and activities are offered within a structured support service co-designed by families and health professionals that recognizes and responds to needs including safeguarding.

Rising epilepsy-related deaths in the UK and wide-ranging systemic issues relating to these have promoted a good practice model led by families and clinicians to tackle inequalities. These strategies can now be deployed globally. Support for families and health professionals includes specialist support services and transformative research and innovation. One such innovation has been developing a validated tool to use when surveying attitudes of epilepsy clinicians towards SUDEP.[71] The pandemic has exposed pre-existing inequalities and has worsened them alongside opportunities for learning from deaths and change.

Epilepsy mortality has been recognized by the World Health Organization as an urgent public health problem: there is opportunity and every reason for rapid change in outlook and practice to reduce epilepsy risk and deaths.

References

1. **Office for National Statistics**. Death registrations in England and Wales summary tables: 2016. Deaths by age, sex, and underlying cause. 2018. Available at: https://www.ons.gov.uk/

2. **National Records of Scotland**. Deaths by sex and cause 2008–2018. 2019. Available at: https://www.nrscotland.gov.uk/

3. **Northern Ireland Statistics and Research Agency**. Registrar General annual report 2018: cause of death. 2019. Available at: https://www.nisra.gov.uk/publications/registrar-general-annual-report-2018-cause-death

4. **Ficker DM**. Sudden unexplained death and injury in epilepsy. Epilepsia. 2000;**41**(Suppl 2):7–12.

5. **Gaitatzis A, Johnson AL, Chadwick DW, Shorvon SD, Sander JW**. Life expectancy in people with newly diagnosed epilepsy. Brain. 2004;**127**(11):2427–32.

6. **Public Health England**. Deaths associated with neurological conditions in England 2001 to 2014: data analysis report. 2018. Available at: https://www.gov.uk/government/publications/deaths-associated-with-neurological-conditions

7. **Wojewodka G, Gulliford MC, Ashworth M**, et al, Epilepsy and mortality: a retrospective cohort analysis with a nested case–control study identifying causes and risk factors from primary care and linkage-derived data. BMJ Open. 2021;**11**:e052841.

8. **Ridsdale L, Charlton J, Ashworth M, Richardson MP, Gulliford MC**. Epilepsy mortality and risk factors for death in epilepsy: a population-based study. Br J Gen Pract. 2011;**61**(586):e271–78.

9. **Hanna N, Black M, Sander J**, et al. The National Sentinel Clinical Audit of Epilepsy-Related Death: epilepsy—death in the shadows. London: Stationery Office; 2002.

10. **Mbizvo GK, Schnier C, Simpson CR, Chin RFM, Duncan SE**. A national study of epilepsy-related deaths in Scotland: trends, mechanisms, and avoidable deaths. Epilepsia. 2021;**62**(1):2667–84.

11. **Knight M, Nair M, Tuffnell D, Shakespeare, J, Kenyon S, Kurinczuk JJ**, eds. Saving lives, improving mothers' care: lessons learned to inform maternity care from the UK and Ireland Confidential Enquiries into Maternal Deaths and Morbidity 2013–15. Oxford: National Perinatal Epidemiology Unit, University of Oxford; 2017.

12. **The Learning Disabilities Mortality Review (LeDeR)**. Annual report 2019. 2019. Available at: http://www.bristol.ac.uk/media-library/sites/sps/leder/LeDeR_2019_annual_report_FINAL2.pdf

13. **Thurman DJ, Logroscino G, Beghi E,** et al. The burden of premature mortality of epilepsy in high-income countries: a systematic review from the Mortality Task Force of the International League Against Epilepsy. Epilepsia. 2017;**58**(1):17–26.

14. **Levira F, Thurman DJ, Sander JW,** et al. Premature mortality of epilepsy in low- and middle-income countries: a systematic review from the Mortality Task Force of the International League Against Epilepsy. Epilepsia. 2017;**58**(1):6–16.

15. **Thorpe J, Ashby S, Hallab S,** et al. Evaluating risk to people with epilepsy during the COVID-19 pandemic: preliminary findings from the COV-E study. Epilepsy Behav. 2021;**115**:107658.

16. **Ridsdale L.** Avoiding premature death in epilepsy. Br Med J. 2015;**350**:h718.

17. **Shankar R, Jalihal V, Walker M,** et al. A community study in Cornwall UK of sudden unexpected death in epilepsy (SUDEP) in a 9-year population sample. Seizure. 2014;**23**(5):382–85.

18. **Ross D, Waddell B, Heath C.** Discussing SUDEP: have we improved? A retrospective case note analysis. Epilepsia. 2015;**56**(4):e33–35.

19. **Shankar R, Donner EJ, McLean B, Nashef L, Tomson T.** Sudden unexpected death in epilepsy (SUDEP): what every neurologist should know. Epileptic Disord. 2017;**19**(1):1–9.

20. **National Institute for Health and Care Excellence.** The epilepsies: the diagnosis and management of the epilepsies in adults and children in primary and secondary care. NICE guideline [CG137]: measuring the use of this guidance. 2015. https://www.nice. org.uk/guidance/CG137/uptake

21. **Devinsky O, Spruill T, Thurman D, Friedman D.** Recognizing and preventing epilepsy-related mortality: a call for action. Neurology. 2016;**86**(8):779–86.

22. **Sander JW, Bell GS.** Reducing mortality: an important aim of epilepsy management. J Neurol Neurosurg Psychiatry. 2004:**75**:349–51.

23. **Thurman DJ, Hesdorffer DC, French JA.** Sudden unexpected death in epilepsy: assessing the public health burden. Epilepsia. 2014;**55**(10):1479–85.

24. **Nashef L, So EL, Ryvlin P, Tomson T.** Unifying the definitions of sudden unexpected death in epilepsy. Epilepsia. 2012;**53**(2):227–33.

25. **Tomson T, Nashef L, Ryvlin P.** Sudden unexpected death in epilepsy: current knowledge and future directions. Lancet Neurol. 2008;**7**(11):1021–31.

26. **Ryvlin P, Nashef L, Lhatoo SD,** et al. Incidence and mechanisms of cardiorespiratory arrests in epilepsy monitoring units (MORTEMUS): a retrospective study. Lancet Neurol. 2013;**12**(10):966–77.

27. **SUDEP Action.** SUDEP and Seizure Safety Checklist. n. d. Available at: www.sudep.org/ checklist

28. **Shankar R, Donner EJ, McLean B, Nashef L, Tomson T.** Sudden unexpected death in epilepsy (SUDEP): what every neurologist should know. Epileptic Disord. 2017;**19**(1):1–9.

29. **Cross JH.** SUDEP and children: implications for clinical practice. In: **Hanna J, Panelli R, Jeffs T, Chapman D,** eds. Continuing the global conversation. SUDEP Action, SUDEP Aware & Epilepsy Australia; 2014. Available at: www.sudepglobalconversation.com.

30. **National Institute for Health and Care Excellence.** Epilepsies in children, young people and adults. NICE guideline [NG217]. 2022. Available at: https://www.nice.org.uk/guida nce/ng217

31. Harden C, Tomson T, Gloss D, et al. Practice guideline summary: sudden unexpected death in epilepsy incidence rates and risk factors: report of the guideline development, dissemination, and implementation Subcommittee of the American Academy of Neurology and the American Epilepsy Society. Neurology. 2017;**88**(17):1674–80.

32. Christensen J, Vestergaard M, Mortensen PB, Sidenius P, Agerbo E. Epilepsy and risk of suicide: a population-based case–control study. Lancet Neurol. 2007;**6**(8):693–98.

33. Mula M, Kanner AM, Schmitz B, Schachter S. Antiepileptic drugs and suicidality: an expert consensus statement from the Task Force on Therapeutic Strategies of the ILAE Commission on Neuropsychobiology. Epilepsia. 2013;**54**(1):199–203.

34. Hesdorffer DC, Ishihara L, Webb DJ, Mynepalli L, Galwey NW, Hauser WA. Occurrence and recurrence of attempted suicide among people with epilepsy. JAMA Psychiatry. 2016;**73**(1):80–86.

35. Watkins LV, Pickrell WO, Kerr MP. Treatment of psychiatric comorbidities in patients with epilepsy and intellectual disabilities: is there a role for the neurologist? Epilepsy Behav. 2019;**98**:322–27.

36. Kelso A, Wills A. Learning from neurological complications. In: Knight M, Kenyon S, Brocklehurst P, Neilson J, Shakespeare J, Kurinczuk JJ, eds. Saving lives, improving mothers' care: lessons learned to inform future maternity care from the UK and Ireland Confidential Enquiries into Maternal Deaths and Morbidity, 2009–2012. Oxford: National Perinatal Epidemiology Unit, University of Oxford; 2014:45–55.

37. Nashef L. SUDEP and pregnancy. In: Hanna J, Panelli R, Jeffs T, Chapman D, eds. Continuing the global conversation. SUDEP Action, SUDEP Aware & Epilepsy Australia; 2014. Available at: www.sudepglobalconversation.com

38. Centre for Maternal and Child Enquiries (CMACE). Saving mothers' lives: reviewing maternal deaths to make motherhood safer: 2006–2008. The eighth report of the confidential enquiries into maternal deaths in the United Kingdom. BJOG. 2011;**118**(Suppl 1):1–203.

39. Knight M, Nair M, Tuffnell D, Shakespeare J, Kenyon S, Kurinczuk JJ, eds. Saving lives, improving mothers' care: lessons learned to inform maternity care from the UK and Ireland Confidential Enquiries into Maternal Deaths and Morbidity 2013–15. Oxford: National Perinatal Epidemiology Unit, University of Oxford; 2017.

40. Morley K. Improving care for women with epilepsy. Br J Midwifery. 2008;**16**(10):649–55.

41. Hiilesmaa VK, Teramo KA. Fetal and maternal risks with seizures. In: Harden C, Thomas SV, Tomson T, et al., eds. Epilepsy in women. New York: Wiley; 2013:115–27.

42. Edey S, Moran N, Nashef L. SUDEP and epilepsy-related mortality in pregnancy. Epilepsia. 2014;**55**(7):e72–74.

43. Tomson T, Battino D, Bromley R, et al. Management of epilepsy in pregnancy: a report from the International League Against Epilepsy Task Force on Women and Pregnancy. Epileptic Disord. 2019;**21**(6):497–517.

44. Leach JP, Smith PE, Craig J, et al. Epilepsy and pregnancy: for healthy pregnancies and happy outcomes. Seizure. 2017;**50**:67–72.

45. Kim DW, Oh J. Comparison of new-onset and persistent epilepsy in the elderly. Acta Neurol Scand. 2019;**139**(4):395–98.

46. Bell GS, Gaitatzis A, Bell CL, Johnson AL, Sander JW. Drowning in people with epilepsy: how great is the risk? Neurology. 2008;**71**(8):578–82.

47. **Thurman DJ, Logroscino G, Beghi E**, et al. The burden of premature mortality of epilepsy in high-income countries: a systematic review from the Mortality Task Force of the International League Against Epilepsy. Epilepsia. 2017;**58**(1):17–26.

48. **Mahler B, Carlsson S, Andersson T, Tomson T.** Risk for injuries and accidents in epilepsy: a prospective population-based cohort study. Neurology. 2018;**90**(9):e779–89.

49. **Scott S.** Asthma; a reinvigorated interest in an old problem. Br J Health Care Manag. 2015;**21**(6):260–63.

50. **NHS.** NHS Health Check. n. d. Available at: https://www.nhs.uk/conditions/nhs-health-check/what-is-an-nhs-health-check-new/#more-information

51. **National Institute for Health and Care Excellence.** Epilepsy in adults. Quality standard [QS211]. 2023. Available at: https://www.nice.org.uk/guidance/qs211

52. **Kennelly C, Riesel J.** Sudden death and epilepsy: the views and experiences of bereaved relatives and carers. Wantage: Epilepsy Bereaved; 2002.

53. **NHS England.** Epilepsy toolkit. n. d. Available at: https://www.england.nhs.uk/rightcare/products/pathways/epilepsy-toolkit/

54. **Shankar R, Henley W, Boland C**, et al. Decreasing the risk of sudden unexpected death in epilepsy: structured communication of risk factors for premature mortality in people with epilepsy. Eur J Neurol. 2018;**25**(9):1121–27.

55. **Shankar R, Ashby S, McLean B, Newman C.** Bridging the gap of risk communication and management using the SUDEP and Seizure Safety Checklist. Epilepsy Behav. 2020;**103**(Pt B):106419.

56. **Newman C, Ashby S, McLean B, Shankar R.** Improving epilepsy management with EpSMon: a Templar to highlight the multifaceted challenges of incorporating digital technologies into routine clinical practice. Epilepsy Behav. 2020;**103**(Pt B):106514.

57. **SUDEP Action.** EpSMon: epilepsy self-monitoring. n. d. Available at: www.sudep.org/epsmon

58. **Zhou SM, McLean B, Roberts E**, et al. Analysing patient-generated data to understand behaviours and characteristics of women with epilepsy of childbearing years: a prospective cohort study. Seizure. 2023;**108**:24–32.

59. **Donner EJ, Waddell B, Osland K**, et al. After sudden unexpected death in epilepsy: lessons learned and the road forward. Epilepsia. 2016;**57**:46–53.

60. **Hanna J, Ashby S.** Lives cut short: a report on urgent measures to tackle deaths in epilepsy and support the bereaved during the Covid-19 pandemic. SUDEP Action; November 2020. Available at: https://sudep.org/lives-cut-short

61. **Yates DW, Ellison G, McGuiness S.** Care of the suddenly bereaved. BMJ. 1990;**301**(6742):29.

62. <Details TBC for 'Scottish Public Services Ombudsman, 2009'>

63. **NICE Quality Standards.** End of life care; quality standard 14, care after a death: bereavement support. 2017. Available at: https://www.nice.org.uk/guidance/qs13/chapter/quality-statement-14-care-after-death-bereavement-support

64. <Details TBC for 'The Judge, Sheriff Alastair Duff, August 2011'>

65. **The Epilepsy Deaths Register.** Available at: www.epilepsydeathsregister.org

66. <Details TBC for '*Montgomery* v *Lanarkshire Health Board* (2015 UKSC 11).'>

67. **Wannamaker BB, Hanna J.** SUDEP and legal issues. In: **Hanna J, Panelli R, Jeffs T, Chapman D,** eds. Continuing the global conversation. SUDEP Action & SUDEP Aware; 2018. Available at: www.sudepglobalconversation.com

68. **Stirling J, Hanna J, Wannamaker BB.** Judicial reports on avoidable deaths. In: **Hanna J, Panelli R, Jeffs T,** eds. Continuing the global conversation. SUDEP Action & SUDEP Aware; 2019. Available at: www.sudepglobalconversation.com

69. **Hanna J, Panelli R.** Challenges in overcoming ethical, legal and communication barriers in SUDEP. In: **Lathers C, Shraeder PL, Bunge M, Leesma JE,** eds. Sudden death in epilepsy: forensic and clinical issues. Boca Raton, FL: CRC Press; 2010:915–36.

70. **Cowdry T, Stirling J.** Learnings from supporting traumatic grief in the aftermath of sudden epilepsy deaths. Epilepsy Behav. 2020;**103**:106416.

71. **Watkins LV, Ashby S, Hanna J, Henley W, Laugharne R, Shankar R.** An evidence-based approach to provide essential and desirable components to develop surveys on sudden unexpected death in epilepsy (SUDEP) for doctors: a focused review. Seizure. 2023;**106**:14–21.

Section 4

Epilepsy-related comorbidity in special groups

Chapter 10

Epilepsy in older people

Emma Torzillo, Arjune Sen, and
Steven C. Schachter

Introduction

Epilepsy is one of the most common neurological diseases worldwide and the lifetime risk of epilepsy increases dramatically from later adulthood to older age, doubling from age 50 to age 80 years.[1,2] Globally, the population is ageing in almost all countries, with up to one in six people expected to be aged over 65 years in 2050, with the rate of increase three times higher in lower- and middle-income countries (LMIC) compared to higher-income countries.[3] The number of people aged over 80 years is growing fastest[3] and the number of cases of epilepsy will rise sharply as populations age. Older people with epilepsy comprise both those with earlier-onset epilepsy, living into older age, and those with late-onset epilepsy (increasingly defined as onset after the age of 50 years). Older people with epilepsy experience unique physical, social, and economic challenges, and require specific approaches to their treatment.

Despite this growing area of need, research looking specifically at the needs of older people with epilepsy is limited. Many large trials have only small numbers of older people or exclude them all together—in part owing to comorbidities, including cognitive impairment. This means it is difficult to be confident that the evidence we have for the effectiveness of treatments applies to older people with epilepsy in the same way that it applies to younger people.

In the UK, care of older people with epilepsy is primarily performed by the general practitioner (GP, or primary healthcare physician; 91%) and to a lesser degree by neurologists, rather than geriatricians.[4] Two-thirds of those who had poorly controlled epilepsy were managed solely by the GP. These are clinically complex individuals with refractory epilepsy, who have geriatric issues compounded by seizures, epilepsy comorbidities, and medication effects. More information, education, and support are therefore needed to assist healthcare workers to care for this group of patients.

In this chapter we will examine:

◆ The epidemiology of epilepsy in older people

◆ The presentation of seizures in older people

◆ Investigations for a first seizure in an older person

◆ The aetiology of epilepsy in older people

◆ The prognosis and treatment of epilepsy in older people

◆ Refractory epilepsy

◆ Mortality and morbidity

◆ Older people with epilepsy—their views and experiences.

We have included a number of real-life clinical cases to highlight practical lessons and illustrate the complexity of epilepsy in older people.

Epidemiology of epilepsy in older people

The highest incidence of epilepsy, that is, the occurrence of new cases, occurs in younger children and older age.[5,6] This 'U-shaped' curve is best demonstrated in studies in higher-income countries. There may be more limited case ascertainment in older people in LMICs, owing to under-reporting and early mortality,[5–7] though a recent burden of disease study found a similar age-related bimodal prevalence of epilepsy globally.[8] In older people, the incidence increases over the decades, with the highest incidence of epilepsy being in those aged over 75 years. The most common type of epilepsy also changes with age, with focal epilepsy representing a much higher proportion of cases in older people.[2] The highest prevalence, or total number of people living with epilepsy, is also in older people.[5,9] This is higher still in nursing home residents, with a seven- to eightfold increased prevalence of epilepsy compared to community-dwelling older people.[10]

Changes in global demographics mean that older people are an increasingly large part of our population. Though the proportion of older people in the population is greatest in high-income countries, the pace of this growth has been most pronounced in South and South-East Asia, Latin America, and the Caribbean.[3] In addition to this rapidly changing demographic, incidence rates of epilepsy in LMICS (138.99 per 100,000 person years; 95% confidence interval (CI) 69.45–278.16) are more than double that of high-income countries (48.86 per 100,000 person years; 95% CI 39.05–61.13).[11] A number of earlier studies posited that this significant difference may be due to a higher rate of infectious disease as a cause of epilepsy, particularly neurocysticercosis, malaria, and HIV. More recent data, however, suggest that stroke is a very common aetiology in LMICS as well as in resource-rich settings, accounting for more than 50% of new-onset epilepsy in adults.[12,13]

Within higher-income countries, rates of epilepsy are stratified across different sections of the older population. A review of older Medicare beneficiaries in the US found the highest rates of epilepsy in older people aged over 85 years. Also, incidence increased in those with lower incomes, and those from Native American and Black communities.[9] The effect of sex differences on epilepsy rates is variable across global demographics. Studies in the US have had mixed results, with some suggesting that epilepsy may be more prevalent in men, and others showing no difference.[9,14] Sex differences have not been associated with significant differences in prevalence of epilepsy across age groups in Asia.[12] However, studies in sub-Saharan Africa have measured an increased prevalence of epilepsy in men, and postulated that this may relate to an increased risk of head injury in this group, as well as under-reporting of epilepsy by women due to stigma.[15]

Presentation of seizures in older people

Seizures in older people may present in unusual or atypical ways including falls, confusional states, memory difficulties, hallucinations, focal neurological symptoms, or sleep disorders.[16] Compared to epilepsy in younger age groups, new-onset epilepsy in older people is more likely to present with focal impaired awareness seizures lasting between 30 seconds to 3 minutes, and with only subtle clinical features, such as blank staring, loss of awareness, confusion, and memory problems. There is less frequent progression to bilateral tonic clonic seizures (Table 10.1).[17,18]

A seizure is often considered in the differential diagnosis of collapse presenting to primary care or the emergency department, and the distinction between seizure and syncope remains difficult. Syncope is the sudden and transient loss of consciousness and postural tone owing to cerebral hypoperfusion. The primary causes of syncope in older adults are neural-mediated syncope (including orthostatic hypotension), carotid sinus hypersensitivity, and dysrhythmias.[19] Despite a number of attempts to create scoring systems and define 'rule in, rule out' historical features, differentiating between syncope and seizure remains difficult owing to clinical crossover, particularly in older people.[20] Cardiogenic syncope and seizures can both involve loss of consciousness, injury, tongue biting, incontinence, and convulsive movements. Convulsive syncope has been

	New-onset epilepsy in the elderly (age ≥60 years)	Chronic epilepsy in the elderly (onset in childhood or middle age)	Epilepsy in young age groups (<18 years)
Most common type	Focal epilepsy or status epilepticus[a]	Generalized and focal epilepsies	All types but in particular epilepsy syndromes, developmental and epileptic encephalopathies
Most common characteristic of seizures	Short duration focal seizures (30 s to 2–3 min) with *subtle* clinical features: • Blank stare • Loss of awareness • Confusion • Memory problems	• Tonic–clonic seizures (jerking and muscle stiffening) with loss of awareness • Short duration focal seizures (30 s to 2–3 min)	• Tonic–clonic seizures (jerking and muscle stiffening) with loss of awareness • Cluster seizures (repetitive seizures which start and stop but occur in groups) • In severe developmental encephalopathies, seizures can last longer than 5 min • Seizure duration of approximately 10 s (focal epilepsy with loss of awareness) to 2–3 min (generalized) with clearer clinical features
Features of the postictal period	Long postictal confusion period (up to 2 weeks) Easily misdiagnosed as delirium or patient experiencing a "funny turn"	Both short and long postictal confusion period Fatigue	Short postictal confusion period (up to a few hours) Fatigue

[a]Status epilepticus can present as confusion without clear generalized tonic–clonic activity (a seizure lasting longer than 5 min and seizures closely follow one another without recovery of awareness between them for at least 30 min)

Figure 10.1 New-onset epilepsy presentation in different patient groups

Table taken from a recent review of epilepsy in older people, undertaken by Australian neurologists Vu et al. New-onset epilepsy in the elderly. British Journal of Clinical Pharmacology. 2018;84:2208–2217.

documented to occur in up to 42% of people who do not have epilepsy in tilt table test centres and blood donor facilities. Most commonly this manifests in the form of brief myoclonic jerks, but may also present as focal jerking or tonic–clonic convulsions.[21] A history of prolonged standing prior to the collapse, or of proceeding straining, micturition, or coughing can point to reflex or vasovagal syncope as the cause of recurrent events. Orthostatic hypotension is common in older people with a prevalence of 16.4% in the community and up to 50% in institutionalized individuals. Checks of postural blood pressures are therefore an important test to perform in this age group.

If elicited, a definite history of focal symptoms at the onset of collapse is helpful in suggesting a seizure aetiology, particularly psychic/olfactory/abdominal sensations or aphasia.[22] Though there is typically a rapid cognitive recovery following syncope, in older people this can be more prolonged, and up to 40% of older patients may have complete amnesia of a syncopal event.[19,23] Pre-existing heart disease is an independent predictor of a cardiac cause of syncope, and important to elicit in the history. Performing an electrocardiogram in all people presenting with seizures is vital, given there is such significant clinical crossover in these presentations, and a baseline electrocardiogram is the best initial test in the diagnosis of a number of life-threatening dysrhythmias.[24]

Cerebrovascular disease is common in older people, and there are a number of situations where the diagnosis of seizures versus transient ischaemic attack (TIA) may be confused, missing an opportunity for early investigation and treatment. Recurrent events of neurological disturbance that are stereotyped are more likely to be focal seizures, while TIAs typically affect different vascular territories causing varied symptoms. A caveat is that critical stenotic disease, particularly of the large cervical vessels, can cause recurrent transient events that are stereotyped because they affect a single vascular territory, either via hypoperfusion or embolism. Another differential is of 'amyloid spells', transient neurological events in the setting of amyloid angiopathy. This pathology is more common in older people, and in a minority of those affected produces recurrent stereotyped neurological events that typically have 'positive' symptoms such as spreading sensory change, though both negative and positive symptoms can occur.[25] While symptoms in seizures tend to occur over 1–2 minutes, amyloid spells have a more 'migraine-like' presentation with sensory spread over 10–15 minutes. TIAs typically produce 'negative' symptoms of weakness and loss of sensation or speech, which are unusual in a seizure. Transient unilateral paralysis is more likely to represent TIA than a mimic such as seizure or migraine.[26] Some exceptions to this rule include the postictal phenomena of 'Todd's paresis' which can involve a limb or speech, and is thought to be more common in older people.[27,28] 'Limb shaking' can also be an unusual presentation of cerebrovascular disease, typically as a result of a critical stenosis resulting in hypoperfusion, and recognition of this phenotype and investigation with carotid imaging is crucial.[29] TIA/minor stroke generally should not cause impairment of consciousness or amnesia, though a subtle aphasia owing to a left hemisphere cortical infarct can be mistaken for confusion and requires careful attention.

Postictal confusion can be prolonged in older people and cause a fluctuating delirium or be mistaken for a symptom of dementia.[30] Witness description of the onset of confusion and any pre-existing cognitive dysfunction can be particularly difficult to ascertain. In community-dwelling adults aged over 65 years recently surveyed in the UK, over 20% of men and over 35% of women were living alone.[31] Even in those adults receiving full-time care in nursing homes, shift work and staff turnover can make adequate collateral history difficult and time-consuming to obtain.

Transient global amnesia is a disease of older people that can be misdiagnosed as epilepsy, while at the same time epileptic events presenting as periodic memory disturbance or 'transient epileptic amnesia' (TEA) can be missed, and the event assumed to represent transient global amnesia (see Chapter 5). Transient global amnesia is characterized by anterograde amnesia without clouding of consciousness or loss of personal identity, with prominent repetitive questioning. It is most common in the seventh decade.[32] Acute magnetic resonance imaging (MRI) can show mesial temporal lobe changes.[33] The disturbance of memory typically lasts between 4 and 6 hours, though can last up to 24 hours, and it is most commonly an isolated event. Transient epileptic amnesia typically lasts less than 1 hour and can be associated with other impairments of cognition. It also presents in older adults, though the mean age of onset is slightly younger at 57 years.[34] Transient epileptic amnesia is predominantly a postictal phenomenon but may be ictal.[34] Useful clinical differentiators between the two are the shorter duration, and the repetitive episodes associated with transient epileptic amnesia.[35]

Clinical case

A 60-year-old man, with a background of idiopathic cardiomyopathy, presented with recurrent episodes of transient amnesia and emotionality associated with headache, occurring over 2 years. MRI was normal. Electroencephalography (EEG) showed rare right frontotemporal sharp waves. Autoantibodies were negative. The initial diagnosis was transient global amnesia and subsequently migraine following repeated attacks. The gentleman then had two convulsive seizures in the neurology waiting room, suggesting that the underlying diagnosis was focal epilepsy. He was commenced on levetiracetam and remains free of all events at 1 year.

Status epilepticus may be a more common presentation of epilepsy in older people and may carry a higher mortality rate.[36] *De novo* non-convulsive status epilepticus can present as a confusional state or delirium without any previous history of seizures, and this diagnosis can be difficult. If another cause is not revealed after initial investigations, including baseline bloods and brain imaging, up to 16% of patients with confusion of unknown origin may have non-convulsive status identified on EEG.[37] Given the subtle presentation, it is probable that rates of non-convulsive status epilepticus are underestimated in older people. In a study of patients aged over 60 years presenting with confusion of unknown cause to the emergency department, acute onset of the confusion (over <24 hours), female sex and an inability to respond to very simple commands were predictors of non-convulsive status, later confirmed on EEG.[37] Other important clinical signs to look for in the confused older person are subtle motor signs of rhythmic twitching or myoclonus, automatisms, and ocular movement abnormalities including hippus. These can, however, all be present in delirium or metabolic encephalopathy, emphasizing the importance of performing an EEG in these individuals.[38] Important features to explore in a patient's history are recent use/cessation of benzodiazepines, newly prescribed medications (such as antipsychotics or antibiotics) which may lower seizure threshold, and a history (even distant) of brain pathology or epilepsy, both of which increase the risk of occult status epilepticus.

Clinical case

A 78-year-old woman, with a background of cerebrovascular disease, was hospitalized with pneumonia and commenced on an intravenous cephalosporin antibiotic. She developed a persistent delirium despite improving inflammatory markers, and no other cause was identified. EEG revealed status epilepticus. Antibiotic therapy was changed and she commenced levetiracetam. Her level of consciousness improved over 24 hours, and subsequent EEG showed resolution of seizures.

Movement disorders can resemble seizures in older people. New-onset myoclonus, particularly when associated with encephalopathy, can be a manifestation of myoclonic status, due to either an underlying epilepsy or an acute toxic-metabolic state. Performing an EEG is important in this setting to exclude cortical discharges associated with the movements, as this may require treatment with antiseizure medications (ASMs). Epilepsia partialis continua, often associated with cerebrovascular disease or tumour in adults, can be mistaken for a tremor or new-onset weakness or ataxia.[39] Faciobrachial dystonic seizures in LGI1 antibody-associated encephalitis are frequent, brief, uni- or bilateral movements involving the face, arm, and sometimes the leg, and these too are commonly missed or misdiagnosed.[40] Early recognition and treatment of faciobrachial dystonic seizures can prevent cognitive decline.[41] Periodic limb movements during sleep can mimic focal seizures and occasionally require further investigation with video EEG.[39]

Psychogenic non-epileptic attacks, or dissociative seizures, also occur in older people. In a retrospective review of people admitted for video telemetry at the US Cleveland Clinic Foundation, 39 individuals over 60 years of age were identified, and of those, one-third were diagnosed with psychogenic seizures.[42] The predominant clinical presentation was with simple motor activity such as tremor, shaking, stiffening, and jerking, though there were also more complex motor movements with semi-purposeful behaviour, orobuccal movements initially diagnosed as automatisms, and hyperventilation. Four of the patients had loss of responsiveness, with episodes of lying still with eyes closed, as the predominant symptom. Of note, a small number of these patients had both non-epileptic attacks and epileptic seizures. Misdiagnosis of non-epileptic attacks can lead to inappropriate and potentially harmful treatment with ASMs, as well as a delay in psychiatric care.

Investigation of the first seizure in older people

Evaluation of possible seizures in older people begins with the history. Collateral history from a witness or carer is crucial and can often be the most important part of the assessment. Home video of attacks on mobile phones is increasingly possible, and it is useful to ask if any episodes have been, or can in the future be, captured when taking the history. Videos can then be shared with clinicians for review.

Blood tests to exclude infection, endocrinological or metabolic disturbance are important in new-onset seizures. An electrocardiogram is particularly important in older people when recurrent attacks of collapse could represent syncope due to cardiac arrhythmia in over 30% of patients.[19] Computed tomography of the brain is helpful to exclude an acute haemorrhage, traumatic injury, or large lesion (particularly when contrast is administered) in the setting of an acute seizure. However, it is not sensitive enough to exclude ischaemic, infective, inflammatory, or malignant lesions, and an MRI of the brain should be performed in the medium term.

MRI is a helpful test to investigate the cause of epilepsy in older people. A consecutive cohort study in Lebanon, prospectively analysing 104 people with new-onset epilepsy over the age of 60 years, found that 67% had an epileptogenic lesion on a 1.5-Tesla or 3-Tesla MRI brain scan.[43] The authors only included lesions that were concordant with seizure semiology and likely to be epileptogenic, and excluded findings of isolated global atrophy, small vessel disease, or postoperative encephalomalacia in the absence of cortical gliosis. Of all patients scanned, 32% had a vascular abnormality, the vast majority of which was a prior ischaemic insult; 20% had a tumour, of which metastases were more common than primary brain tumours; and 13% had evidence of previous traumatic brain injury. However, it is important to note that MRIs may be overly sensitive in older epilepsy. White matter changes and atrophy are more common in older people, and these should not be overinterpreted in diagnosing epilepsy, particularly in the setting of a single event.

EEG requires cautious interpretation in older people. EEG has a relatively low sensitivity in epilepsy, between 25% and 56%, and a moderate specificity, between 78% and 98%.[44] Older adults may be more likely to have both an increased rate of non-specific as well as epileptiform findings. An interesting study of 16 healthy adults aged over 90 years of age found 83% had abnormal EEGs, primarily due to generalized or temporal slowing.[45] Three of these adults, with no evidence of epilepsy, had definite epileptiform abnormalities.[45] Non-specific EEG abnormalities have been found to be high in patients presenting with syncope, a common differential in older people with epilepsy.[46] The incidence of epileptiform abnormalities measured in healthy adults, approximately 0.5%, increases to up to 30% in adults with structural abnormalities, which themselves increase in older people due to a rise in cerebrovascular lesions, tumours, and neurodegenerative processes.[44] On the other hand, in the right clinical setting, the EEG can provide supportive evidence for the diagnosis of epilepsy in older people, and facilitate the commencement of appropriate treatment.

Causes of seizures and epilepsy in older people

There are many potential causes of new-onset seizures in older people. Older people may be more at risk of acute symptomatic seizures due to polypharmacy and increased susceptibility to metabolic disturbance due to physiological changes of ageing. Like younger people with epilepsy, traditional risk factors such as previous head injury, meningoencephalitis, and complications of prematurity and birth trauma should be investigated when taking the history. Family history may be less relevant in older people, although rarely a latent genetic generalized epilepsy may become symptomatic for the first time in later adulthood, particularly in the setting of sleep deprivation or polypharmacy.

Similarly, those with childhood-onset epilepsy who have been in remission for many years may become symptomatic again in older age. People with genetic generalized epilepsies, as well as those with epileptic and developmental encephalopathies, are living longer and transitioning to adult and older aged care services.

The most commonly identified cause of late-onset epilepsy is cerebrovascular disease, which accounts for more than a third of identified causes. However, the aetiology remains unknown in up to 50% of late-onset epilepsy.[47,48] A single-centre cohort study in China found that over 50% of the 104 consecutive patients over the age of 50 years had 'symptomatic epilepsy', or epilepsy due to a structural or metabolic brain disease.[49] The most frequent cause was cerebrovascular disease, followed by primary or metastatic disease and traumatic brain injury. A large cohort study of veterans aged 66 years and over showed that people with any central nervous system insult, be it stroke, dementia, brain tumour, or other abnormality, were more likely to experience new-onset epilepsy, though cerebrovascular disease and dementia had the strongest relationship with new-onset epilepsy.[50] Interestingly, statin therapy, older age, hypercholesterolaemia, and obesity were associated with a reduced likelihood of developing epilepsy.

Both Alzheimer's disease and vascular dementia increase the risk of developing epilepsy.[51] In Han Chinese individuals, the risk of developing seizures was increased in those with Alzheimer's disease compared to controls (hazard ratio 1.58; 95% CI 1.09–2.28), with the mean time from the diagnosis of dementia until first seizure being 3.6 years.[52] People with Alzheimer's disease and a single seizure have a more than 70% risk of further seizures, suggesting that a diagnosis of epilepsy should be made and treatment considered after the first seizure in people with Alzheimer's disease.[53]

A number of midlife risk factors for the development of late-onset epilepsy have been identified in a large US cohort study. Hypertension, diabetes mellitus, smoking history, alcohol use, and APOE ε4 status were associated with an increased risk of developing epilepsy after the age of 60 years, even after accounting for the confounding presence of stroke and dementia.[54] Exercise was found to be protective and the real importance of this work is the suggestion that modifying risk factors in mid-life may prevent later-onset epilepsy.

Less common but important causes of new-onset epilepsy include the autoimmune encephalidities, typically presenting in association with rapid cognitive or behavioural change. Antibodies to LGI1, CASPR2, GABA, and AMPA receptors are most likely in the older population. Rarely, genetic metabolic causes such as mitochondrial disease can present in older age.

Clinical case

A 75-year-old man, with a background of type 2 diabetes, chronic renal failure, and recurrent abdominal pain, presented with new-onset focal status epilepticus. His family history was significant for a sister with epilepsy who died in childhood. MRI revealed increased T2 signal and oedema over the left temporoparietal region. EEG showed multifocal clinical and subclinical seizures. The patient required intubation and sedation to manage his level of consciousness and seizures. After an apparent improvement with commencement of ASMs, he deteriorated, and MRI showed new increased T2 signal and oedema over the right temporal region. He developed acute-on-chronic renal failure as well as ischaemic colitis and passed away. Urinary metabolic analysis revealed a diagnosis of the rare genetic disorder, MELAS (Mitochondrial encephalopathy, Lactic acidosis, and Stroke-like episodes).

Comorbidities

Cognitive impairment

An association between epilepsy and cognitive impairment has been established in multiple studies (see Chapter 5). Difficulty remains in teasing out how the two are related. A number of groups have found that older people with epilepsy, without a formal diagnosis of dementia, have cognitive impairment on formal testing when compared to healthy controls, across multiple domains of verbal and visual memory, executive function, attention, and language.[55,56] Total number of ASMs and comorbid anxiety predicted poor cognitive performance in those with epilepsy. The total number of ASMs with known effects on cognition was not associated with poorer performance, raising the possibility that this was in fact a marker for severity of epilepsy.[55]

The contribution of ASMs to cognitive impairment in older people with epilepsy is difficult to ascertain. Studies of older people with new-onset epilepsy prior to commencement of ASMs have confirmed that over 50% had objective impairment in executive function at this early stage, though a much smaller number reported subjective cognitive concerns or functional impairments.[57]

Dementia

There is emerging evidence of a bidirectional association between epilepsy and dementia (see Chapter 5). Not only is dementia associated with an increased risk of developing epilepsy, there is some evidence that people with epilepsy have an increased risk of dementia. This may be due to pathological changes in the brain driven by seizures, or it may be that both diseases have common underlying mechanisms. In a number of studies, people with new-onset epilepsy had a 1.5–1.89 increased relative risk of developing dementia within

7 years.[58,59] Some possible explanations of this risk include imaging findings of increased cerebrovascular disease in older people with childhood-onset epilepsy, positron emission tomography evidence of increased prefrontal amyloid deposition in people with epilepsy, and aggregations of tau protein and amyloid precursor protein (forming beta amyloid), found in tissue of individuals with focal cortical dysplasia and temporal lobe epilepsy.[51]

Stroke

Cerebrovascular disease is a common cause of epilepsy, has an increased prevalence in older people and is a common comorbidity in people with epilepsy. While seizures in the acute period after stroke (up to 7 days) are typically viewed as provoked and less likely to recur, later-onset (remote) seizures following stroke have a high likelihood of recurrence at over 70%.[60] Important considerations in those with stroke and epilepsy are the increased risk of bleeding following seizures in people who are taking anticoagulation, as well as potential medication interactions with ASMs, particularly enzyme-inducing medications such as carbamazepine, which may increase the metabolism, and thus decrease the efficacy, of anticoagulation.[60]

Mood disorders

Adults with epilepsy are more than twice as likely to have a diagnosis of anxiety or depression compared to people without epilepsy, and mood disorders are present in over 20% of adults with epilepsy[61,62] (see Chapter 6). Mood disorders have historically been under-recognized in older people and have a poor prognosis, with almost half of all patients remaining clinically depressed at 1-year follow-up, and a higher risk of recurrence compared to people in middle age.[63,64] Patient and practitioner concerns regarding medication side effects and the overemphasis on potential proconvulsant activity of antidepressants can lead to undertreatment of mood disorders. Current evidence suggests that, in fact, most antidepressants are safe in people with epilepsy. With selective serotonin reuptake inhibitors and serotonin–noradrenaline (norepinephrine) reuptake inhibitors the risk of exacerbating seizures is very small, and these drugs should be confidently used as first-line treatment.[65] Bupropion, clomipramine, amoxapine, and maprotiline, however, should be avoided or used with caution.[65] In older individuals with multiple comorbidities, prescription must be balanced against the risks associated with polypharmacy; however, given the potential benefits, antidepressant medication should not be withheld if there is evidence of a mood disorder and more severe depression.[66]

Rarely, a new mood disturbance or rapidly progressive cognitive impairment at the time of, or preceding, a first seizure, can herald a wider neurological process such as an autoimmune encephalitis.

Clinical case

A 72-year-old man, previously well, though depressed since the death of his mother 2 months prior, presented with five convulsive seizures over 3 weeks, with incomplete recovery between events, appearing 'vague' and confused interictally. A low sodium concentration of 123 nmol/L was noted. MRI was normal. Cerebrospinal fluid constituents were normal. EEG revealed non-convulsive status epilepticus. The patient had a prolonged intensive care admission with status epilepticus. He was found to have high $GABA_B$ and GAD antibody positivity in serum and cerebrospinal fluid. A positron emission tomography scan revealed prostatic cancer, which was histologically confirmed as a rare small cell tumour. The patient received surgery and chemotherapy, and was seizure free at 1 year on two ASMs.

Prognosis and treatment

In assessing and treating people with seizures, it is important to make the diagnosis of epilepsy where appropriate, and thus to start treatment. Epilepsy is a disease diagnosed in three clinical circumstances: (1) two unprovoked seizures occurring greater than 24 hours apart, (2) a single seizure and a high probability of a second seizure, or (3) a recognizable epilepsy syndrome.[67] This second description is most relevant in older people. When investigating the cause of a single seizure, the finding of a structural lesion such as a previous stroke, or the recognition of an important comorbidity such as Alzheimer's disease, suggest a high probability that further seizures will occur. If this is estimated to be approximately 60% (i.e. greater than the background recurrence risk after a first seizure), then the diagnosis of epilepsy can be made, and commencing medications to reduce risk should be strongly considered.

New-onset epilepsy in older people may be more responsive to medical therapy than epilepsy occurring at a younger age. A review of four studies of older people with new-onset seizures reported seizure freedom with the use of ASMs in 60–92% of patients.[18] In a Japanese cohort of patients aged over 65 years in a specialist epilepsy clinic, over 95% were seizure free at 1-year follow-up, the majority treated with ASM monotherapy.[48]

In the longer term, though many patients may be in remission from seizures on treatment, the risk of recurrent seizures after withdrawing treatment may be higher in older people even if they have been seizure free for some time.[68] Also, the risks of having even a single seizure may be higher in older people owing to fracture risk, social isolation, and comorbidities. Changing long-term medications in older people with epilepsy must therefore be done cautiously. Reduction in long-standing medications such as phenytoin, phenobarbitone, and clonazepam, even if the dose appears to be low or the serum level is apparently 'subtherapeutic', can lead to a recurrence of seizures in older people who have been seizure free. The role of EEG in this decision-making process is complex, as there is no uniform relationship between interictal discharges or non-specific abnormalities and risk of future seizures. However, EEG may reveal important diagnostic patterns, such as generalized discharges in older people with long-standing epilepsy, and a very active interictal EEG may suggest that ASM therapy needs to be continued, even in those who are seizure free.

Clinical case

An 82-year-old woman with absence epilepsy, on long-term phenobarbitone, presented with increased falls and forgetfulness over 1 week. A recent phenobarbitone level performed in the community had been high, and her dose had been reduced 2 weeks prior to presentation. EEG revealed absence status epilepticus. Appreciating that it is not a drug of choice in modern epilepsy prescribing, Phenobarbitone dosage was increased and acute treatment with benzodiazepine was commenced. Symptoms improved over 48 hours.

Choosing the right ASM in older people can be difficult (see Chapter 3). Physiological changes associated with ageing, such as reduced renal clearance and hepatic enzymatic function, can increase the risk of adverse events. Older people are often taking other medications, and polypharmacy increases the risk of side effects. There have been some trials that have looked specifically at ASMs in this demographic. Lamotrigine, gabapentin, and carbamazepine were compared in a multicentre randomized control trial for new-onset epilepsy in older people.[69] The investigators found no difference in seizure control at 12 months, but a significant difference in retention rates, primarily due to side effects, with lamotrigine being the best tolerated, followed by gabapentin then carbamazepine.[69] A European study comparing levetiracetam, lamotrigine, and carbamazepine found similar efficacy in seizure control after 12 months, but significantly better retention rates with levetiracetam compared to carbamazepine, with over 30% of patients withdrawing from carbamazepine due to adverse events.[70] Importantly, the median daily dose of carbamazepine in this study was relatively low, at 380.0 mg/day, and despite this the withdrawal rate was high. The median dose of lamotrigine (95 mg/day) and of levetiracetam (950 mg/day) were also on the lower side, and no difference in dose was found between those who remained seizure free and those who continued to have seizures. This finding supports an approach of initiating these medications in low doses, titrating cautiously, and perhaps expecting seizure control at lower doses than in younger people.

Carbamazepine and its derivatives (oxcarbazepine, eslicarbazepine) are associated with an increased risk of hyponatraemia. In a large cohort study in Ontario, Canada, carbamazepine use in older people (median age 76 years) significantly increased the risk of hospitalization with hyponatraemia within 30 days of initiation, with a relative risk of 8.20 (95% CI 5.40–12.46), compared to matched non-users.[71] In carbamazepine users, older age, cancer, a history of previous hyponatraemia, and diuretic use were all identified as significant risk factors for symptomatic hyponatraemia, with co-administration of a diuretic increasing the relative risk to 14 (95% CI 8.82–28).[71]

ASMs with enzyme-inducing properties, particularly carbamazepine, have also been shown to alter lipid levels, likely due to their effect on the cytochrome P450 system, and that effect is maintained in the long term.[72] Switching people to non-enzyme-inducing drugs such as levetiracetam or lamotrigine, results in significant reductions in total cholesterol, low-density lipoprotein, triglyceride, and C-reactive protein levels in the short term.[73] The clinical relevance of these changes are not clear. There is some evidence of an increased rate of myocardial infarction (rate ratio 1.16; 95% CI 1.02–1.33) in those on enzyme-inducing ASMs, particularly in those taking the medication for more than 24 months, though this would translate to a relatively small number of additional events and may have only a small clinical impact.[74]

People with epilepsy have an increased risk of fractures, which is particularly pertinent in older people. This is due to an increased risk of traumatic injury due to seizures, poorer bone health, and medication side effects.[75,76] There is now a wealth of evidence that ASMs, particularly the enzyme-inducing drugs and sodium valproate, disturb bone health and contribute to osteoporosis.[77] The exact mechanisms remain unclear; however, increased metabolism of vitamin D and vitamin K, and increased synthesis of calcitonin, have all been postulated.[78] Some studies have suggested levetiracetam may also negatively affect bone mineral density (BMD), though the mechanism is not known, and gabapentin use was associated with reduced BMD and increased fracture risk in one study.[78,79] Overall, however, non-enzyme-inducing ASMs appear to have the best profile in bone health and increasingly levetiracetam and lamotrigine are considered the initial ASMs of choice in older people with epilepsy.

Treatment with vitamin D increases 25-OH-vitamin D and calcium levels in people with epilepsy, although a definite effect on BMD at standard doses was not demonstrated in a recent systematic review, likely due to heterogeneous study methodologies.[80] Though the role of vitamin D and calcium supplementation in preventing osteoporosis and fractures has not been fully established in epilepsy, the risk of harm from vitamin D is likely to be low.[81] The addition of a bisphosphonate in individuals with epilepsy with a normal BMD appears to significantly slow BMD reduction over time, and reduces the risk of fractures.[82] Overall, though there are no disease-specific guidelines for the investigation and management of osteoporosis in people with epilepsy, given the multiple potential causes in this population, it may be best to proactively assess all older people with epilepsy for fracture risk and optimize their utilization of preventative treatments.[83]

Refractory epilepsy in older people

When epilepsy is refractory to standard treatment in older people, a number of possibilities should be considered. Firstly, the diagnosis should be revisited, and the following questions asked: is this truly epilepsy? Could these events be cardiac, metabolic, or ischaemic in origin? Could these be psychogenic non-epileptic attacks?

Secondly, medication adherence should be considered and confirmed as much as is possible. Almost half of older people with epilepsy may be non-adherent with their ASM treatment, owing to side effects and poor tolerance, particularly in the setting of higher rates of cognitive disturbance and fatigue, as well as misconceptions about potential adverse effects, complexity of ASM dosing regimens, and medication costs.[84,85]

Finally, if the diagnosis is focal epilepsy, and adherence has been confirmed, then the clinician should consider referral to a tertiary epilepsy service to investigate whether epilepsy surgery would be of benefit (see Chapter 4).

Epilepsy surgery can provide approximately 70% seizure-free rates in appropriately selected patients, with just under 50% of patients remaining seizure free at 5 years.[86–88] Growing evidence suggests that older adults have the same seizure-related outcomes as younger people following epilepsy surgery. They may, however, be at risk of poorer cognitive outcomes. The majority of studies assessing epilepsy surgery in older people have examined groups with a mean age in the mid 50s.[89–92] The largest investigation into the surgical outcome in those over 60 years of age reviewed 64 consecutive cases of older adults undergoing epilepsy surgery at a single centre.[93] The median age was 65 years, and the median duration of epilepsy was 22 years, with the most common pathology being mesial temporal sclerosis. The older people with epilepsy had a later age of seizure onset than a control group of younger adults though a longer duration of epilepsy, and they were three times more likely to have a lesional finding on MRI than younger people. There was no difference in seizure-free outcome between the younger and older group, which was 60–80%, and there was no difference in major adverse events.[93] In the older group, the adverse events included four postoperative subdural hygromas requiring drainage. However, there was a significantly increased risk of a postoperative decline in confrontational naming in the older group. There was no difference in anxiety or depression scores pre or post surgery.

A recent study of 119 consecutive patients in a German centre looked more closely at cognitive outcomes after epilepsy surgery.[94] They noted that older patients had high levels of cognitive dysfunction prior to surgery, with 93% having impaired to severely impaired performance in at least one domain on formal testing.[94] Even with this high preoperative morbidity, there was a measurable decline in verbal memory postoperatively, and this was significantly worse after left-sided resection. Importantly, there was an improvement in quality of life in the whole cohort postoperatively, underscoring the patient reported benefits of surgery, despite these neuropsychological deficits.

Subgroups of older people require more invasive investigation and monitoring prior to epilepsy surgery. Intracranial EEG can provide further information to localize focal epilepsy and improve the chance of seizure freedom after surgery.[95–97] Surgical techniques have improved significantly over the last 30 years, and the use of stereo EEG, using thin, flexible electrodes inserted via burr holes, has been associated with improved seizure freedom and reduced complication rates compared to subdural grids.[98] A small cohort study demonstrated that this can be a useful adjunctive test in older people, though it is not without risk.[99] Similarly, as they become more widely available, newer techniques such as laser ablation may become the treatment modality of choice in older people with epilepsy given a lower propensity to adverse events and reduced neurocognitive effects[100] (see Chapter 4).

Epilepsy morbidity and mortality

Overall mortality is increased in epilepsy, across the age groups[101,102] (see Chapter 9). In population-based studies of epilepsy in higher-income countries, the standardized mortality ratio (SMR) ranges from 1.8 to 4.1[103] (SMRs are calculated by comparing the mortality in the studied population of people with epilepsy with the number of 'expected deaths' calculated from a reference population. If there is an excess of recorded deaths, the ratio is >1). Prevalence and mortality of epilepsy is higher still in LMIC.[1] In a UK longitudinal study, the major causes of death were cancers (including lung cancer), cerebrovascular disease, pneumonia, and ischaemic heart disease.[104] This was despite the fact that the majority of people in the cohort, originally identified by GPs as those presenting with new-onset seizures, were in remission from epilepsy (free of seizures for >5 years) by this stage of follow-up. The reasons for this increased mortality are not clear. The SMR is also increased in selected populations of people with epilepsy, such as hospitalized patients, suggesting that mortality is related to seizure frequency and severity, as well as comorbidity.[103] There is some evidence that mortality rates are increased in those with poor medication adherence.[101]

Though the majority of older people with epilepsy may obtain seizure freedom, mortality in this group remains higher than in younger adults. Most studies have found the SMR is highest in younger age groups, reflecting the low overall mortality in this reference age group, as well as the increased mortality in children with epilepsy and global deficits.[105] However, the excess mortality is greatest in the elderly, at 47 per 1000 in those 75 years and older, up to eight times higher than in children.[103] Even in those who are predominantly seizure free, mortality rates were as high as 45% in the 2 years following diagnosis.[18] The majority of these deaths appear to be from non-neurological disease, and the reasons for these being higher in this group are unclear. While, for example, the high rate of death from pneumonia has been presumed to be due to aspiration following a seizure, this increased risk persists even in those who are in complete remission from seizures.[104] It appears that a new diagnosis of epilepsy is a marker of increased risk, and clinicians should be particularly alert to addressing risk factors and comorbidities in this group.

Though the prevalence of sudden unexpected death in epilepsy (SUDEP) in the general epilepsy population may be more than 1 in 1000 people with epilepsy, the highest rates are seen in the third and fourth decade, rather than in older people with epilepsy.[106] This may be due to an undercounting of SUDEP which preferentially affects the older age strata due to a larger number of potential confounding causes of death due to comorbidities, as well as the reduced rate of autopsy.[107]

Older people's views and experiences

The diagnosis of epilepsy can be difficult and delayed in older people, for all of the reasons discussed in this chapter. How, though, does this affect older people themselves? A qualitative study from 2014 of 20 adults over 60 years of age found over half reported that they had experienced a delay in diagnosis, on average between 12 and 18 months.[108] This delay was particularly prominent in

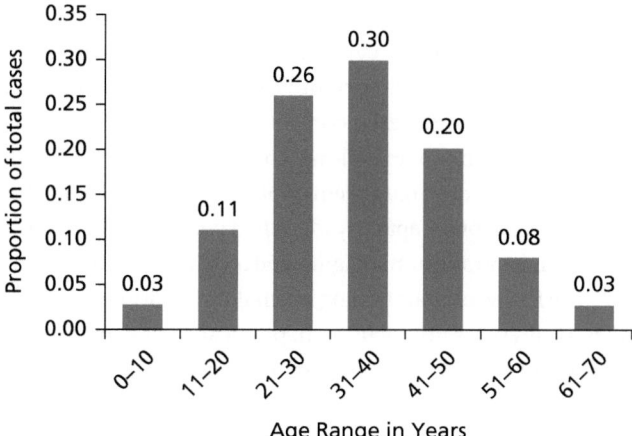

Figure 10.2 Distribution of SUDEP cases across the age groups separated by decile. Data taken from four population studies demonstrated that the highest proportion of SUDEP cases were in the third and fourth decades.
From Thurman et al. Sudden unexpected death in epilepsy: assessing the public health burden. Epilepsia. 2014;55(10):1479–1485.

women, who experienced a delay in diagnosis even when they presented with convulsions, while men experienced a delay only when they presented with more difficult-to-interpret focal seizures. In some cases this was due to an initial misdiagnosis of the events as transient ischemic attacks (TIAs) or other recurrent attacks. Both men and women reported that some of this delay was due to their own hesitation in informing a medical practitioner of their symptoms, sometimes due to embarrassment, a desire to keep working, or fear of a more serious diagnosis. Both men and women reported a prolonged period before referral to a neurologist as another cause of the diagnostic delay. A number of women in the study expressed that they felt their concerns were not taken seriously by care providers, a concern that was not expressed by any of the male participants. These findings emphasize the importance of careful attention to the history of older people, particularly women, with recurrent attacks and of always considering the diagnosis of epilepsy in this patient group. Prompt onward referral to specialist services is essential.

Quality of life in older people with epilepsy is affected by the broad range of physical, psychological, and social aspects of the condition. Low energy levels or fatigue due to epilepsy have been highlighted as among the most important issues identified by older people themselves in a number of studies.[109] A survey of older adults with focal epilepsy found that the two most common concerns reported were driving and medication side effects.[110] In contrast, seizure frequency was identified as the strongest predictor of quality of life in a recent systematic review, with moderate evidence to suggest that comorbidities and depressive symptoms were also important.[109] It is clear that, at times, clinicians may be focused on improving seizure control, while patients may feel that their major problem is fatigue, not being allowed to drive (see Chapter 14), or other comorbidities. These concerns may seem contradictory to both parties.

Older people with new-onset epilepsy identified two major outcomes they considered to be most important in managing epilepsy, in a small qualitative study from the US.[111] The first was 'maintaining normalcy', including being able to continue their roles as carers for grandchildren, physical health, and life satisfaction. The second important message was 'we want to be involved', with the majority of participants expressing that they wanted to be more included in the treatment of their epilepsy, with a strong feeling that they lacked control over their treatment. They also expressed that they would like to integrate their epilepsy care with the management of their individual comorbidities. In this study there was a sense from some participants that seizures were in some ways 'the easy part' and that being able to go about their normal life was their primary focus, and sometimes they felt this was a different focus to that of their caregivers.

Conclusion

Providing the best care for older people with epilepsy requires keeping an open mind in a broad range of settings where the presentation of seizures may be subtle or unexpected. Investigations must consider both common and rare aetiologies, while interpretation of tests requires an understanding that MRI and EEG may reveal a number of incidental findings in older people. Treatment must account for comorbid conditions which may associate with epilepsy or influence drug choice, exacerbate potential side effects of medications, and contribute to long-term complications. Older people with epilepsy express a strong desire for maintaining their important roles in both work and family life, which require better control of seizures. Also, older people also want to be more involved in decision-making in partnership with clinicians, so that not just their epilepsy, but their overall health and quality of life are addressed.

References

1. **World Health Organization**. Epilepsy: a public health imperative. 2019. Available at: https://www.who.int/publications/i/item/epilepsy-a-public-health-imperative
2. **Hauser WA, Annegers JF, Kurland LT.** Incidence of epilepsy and unprovoked seizures in Rochester, Minnesota: 1935–1984. Epilepsia. 1993;34(3):453–68.

3. United Nations Department of Economic and Social Affairs Population Division. World population ageing 2019. 2020. Available at: https://www.un.org/en/development/desa/population/publications/pdf/ageing/WorldPopulationAgeing2019-Report.pdf

4. Bagshaw J, Crawford P, Chappell B. Care in people 60 years of age and over with chronic or recently diagnosed epilepsy: a note review in United Kingdom general practice. Seizure. 2009;18(1):57–60.

5. Banerjee PN, Filippi D, Allen Hauser W. The descriptive epidemiology of epilepsy—a review. Epilepsy Res. 2009;85(1):31–45.

6. Forsgren L, Beghi E, Oun A, Sillanpää M. The epidemiology of epilepsy in Europe—a systematic review. Eur J Neurol. 2005;12(4):245–53.

7. Edwards T, Scott AG, Munyoki G, et al. Active convulsive epilepsy in a rural district of Kenya: a study of prevalence and possible risk factors. Lancet Neurol. 2008;7(1):50–56.

8. GBD 2016 Epilepsy Collaborators. Global, regional, and national burden of epilepsy, 1990–2016: a systematic analysis for the Global Burden of Disease Study 2016. Lancet Neurol. 2019;18(4):357–75.

9. Ip Q, Malone DC, Chong J, Harris RB, Labiner DM. An update on the prevalence and incidence of epilepsy among older adults. Epilepsy Res. 2018;139:107–12.

10. Birnbaum AK, Leppik IE, Svensden K, Eberly LE. Prevalence of epilepsy/seizures as a comorbidity of neurologic disorders in nursing homes. Neurology. 2017;88(8):750–57.

11. Fiest KM, Sauro KM, Wiebe S, et al. Prevalence and incidence of epilepsy: a systematic review and meta-analysis of international studies. Neurology. 2017;88(3):296–303.

12. Mac TL, Tran DS, Quet F, Odermatt P, Preux PM, Tan CT. Epidemiology, aetiology, and clinical management of epilepsy in Asia: a systematic review. Lancet Neurol. 2007;6(6):533–43.

13. Thurman DJ, Begley CE, Carpio A, et al. The primary prevention of epilepsy: a report of the prevention task force of the International League Against Epilepsy. Epilepsia. 2018;59(5):905–14.

14. Tang DH, Malone DC, Warholak TL, et al. Prevalence and incidence of epilepsy in an elderly and low-income population in the United States. J Clin Neurol. 2015;11(3):252–61.

15. Wagner RG, Ngugi AK, Twine R, et al. Prevalence and risk factors for active convulsive epilepsy in rural Northeast South Africa. Epilepsy Res. 2014;108(4):782–91.

16. Brodie MJ, Elder AT, Kwan P. Epilepsy in later life. Lancet Neurol. 2009;8(11):1019–30.

17. Chen L-A, Cheng S-J, Shuo-Bin J. Epilepsy in the elderly. Int J Gerontol. 2012;6(2):63–67.

18. Vu LC, Piccenna L, Kwan P, O'Brien TJ. New-onset epilepsy in the elderly. Br J Clin Pharmacol. 2018;84(10):2208–17.

19. Hogan TM, Constantine ST, Crain AD. Evaluation of syncope in older adults. Emerg Med Clin North Am. 2016;34(3):601–27.

20. Sheldon R, Rose S, Ritchie D, et al. Historical criteria that distinguish syncope from seizures. J Am Coll Cardiol. 2002;40(1):142–48.

21. Sheldon R. How to differentiate syncope from seizure. Cardiol Clin. 2015;33(3):377–85.

22. McKeon A, Vaughan C, Delanty N. Seizure versus syncope. Lancet Neurol. 2006;5(2):171–80.

23. Tallis R, Boon P, Perucca E, Stephen L. Epilepsy in elderly people: management issues. Epileptic Disord. 2002;4(Suppl 2):S33–39.

24. White JL, Hollander JE, Pines JM, Mullins PM, Chang AM. Electrocardiogram and cardiac testing among patients in the emergency department with seizure versus syncope. Clin Exp Emerg Med. 2019;6(2):106–12.

25. Andreas C, Peeters A, Fox Z, et al. Spectrum of transient focal neurological episodes in cerebral amyloid angiopathy. Stroke. 2012;43(9):2324–30.

26. Amort M, Fluri F, Schäfer J, et al. Transient ischemic attack versus transient ischemic attack mimics: frequency, clinical characteristics and outcome. Cerebrovasc Dis. 2011;32(1):57–64.

27. Xu SY, Li ZX, Wu XW, Li L, Li CX. Frequency and pathophysiology of post-seizure Todd's paralysis. Med Sci Monit. 2020;26:e920751.

28. Theodore WH. Effects of age and underlying brain dysfunction on the postictal state. Epilepsy Behav. 2010;19(2):118–20.

29. Schulz UG, Rothwell PM. Transient ischaemic attacks mimicking focal motor seizures. Postgrad Med J. 2002;78(918):246–47.

30. Godfrey JBW. Misleading presentation of epilepsy in elderly people. Age Ageing. 1989;18(1):17–20.

31. Sanchez Santos MT, Williamson E, Bruce J, et al. Cohort profile: Oxford Pain, Activity and Lifestyle (OPAL) Study, a prospective cohort study of older adults in England. BMJ Open. 2020;10(9):e037516.

32. Spiegel DR, Smith J, Wade RR, et al. Transient global amnesia: current perspectives. Neuropsychiatr Dis Treat. 2017;13:2691–703.

33. Lee HY, Kim JH, Weon YC, et al. Diffusion-weighted imaging in transient global amnesia exposes the CA1 region of the hippocampus. Neuroradiology. 2007;49(6):481–87.

34. Butler CR, Zeman A. The causes and consequences of transient epileptic amnesia. Behav Neurol. 2011;24(4):299–305.

35. Hommet C, Mondon K, Camus V, De Toffol B, Constans T. Epilepsy and dementia in the elderly. Dem Geriatr Cogn Disord. 2008;25(4):293–300.

36. Lv RJ, Wang Q, Cui T, Zhu F, Shao XQ. Status epilepticus-related etiology, incidence and mortality: a meta-analysis. Epilepsy Res. 2017;136:12–17.

37. Veran O, Kahane P, Thomas P, Hamelin S, Sabourdy C, Vercueil L. De novo epileptic confusion in the elderly: a 1-year prospective study. Epilepsia. 2010;51(6):1030–35.

38. Woodford HJ, George J, Jackson M. Non-convulsive status epilepticus: a practical approach to diagnosis in confused older people. Postgrad Med J. 2015;91(1081):655–61.

39. Freitas ME, Ruiz-Lopez M, Dalmau J, et al. Seizures and movement disorders: phenomenology, diagnostic challenges and therapeutic approaches. J Neurol Neurosurg Psychiatry. 2019;90(8):920–28.

40. Irani SR, Stagg CJ, Schott JM, et al. Faciobrachial dystonic seizures: the influence of immunotherapy on seizure control and prevention of cognitive impairment in a broadening phenotype. Brain. 2013;136(10):3151–62.

41. Thompson J, Bi M, Murchison AG, et al. The importance of early immunotherapy in patients with faciobrachial dystonic seizures. Brain. 2018;141(2):348–56.

42. Kellinghaus C, Loddenkemper T, Dinner DS, Lachhwani D, Lüders HO. Non-epileptic seizures of the elderly. J Neurol. 2004;**251**(6):704–709.

43. Arabi M, Dirani M, Hourani R, et al. Frequency and stratification of epileptogenic lesions in elderly with new onset seizures. Front Neurol. 2018;**9**:995.

44. Smith SJM. EEG in the diagnosis, classification, and management of patients with epilepsy. J Neurol Neurosurg Psychiatry. 2005;**76**(Suppl 2):ii2–7.

45. Peltz CB, Kim HL, Kawas CH. Abnormal EEGs in cognitively and physically healthy oldest-old: findings from the 90+ Study. J Clin Neurophysiol. 2010;**27**(4):292–95.

46. Fattouch J, Di Bonaventura C, Strano S, et al. Over-interpretation of electroclinical and neuroimaging findings in syncopes misdiagnosed as epileptic seizures. Epileptic Disord. 2007;**9**(2):170–73.

47. Hernández-Ronquillo L, Adams S, Ballendine S, Téllez-Zenteno JF. Epilepsy in an elderly population: classification, etiology and drug resistance. Epilepsy Res. 2018;**140**:90–94.

48. Tanaka A, Akamatsu N, Shouzaki T, et al. Clinical characteristics and treatment responses in new-onset epilepsy in the elderly. Seizure. 2013;**22**(9):772–75.

49. Tian HJ, Wang XQ, Shi XB, Lang SY. Evaluation of clinical features of elderly epilepsy in China. Int J Clin Exp Med. 2015;**8**(2):2399–404.

50. Pugh MJV, Knoefel JE, Mortensen EM, Amuan ME, Berlowitz DR, Van Cott AC. New-onset epilepsy risk factors in older veterans. J Am Geriatr Soc. 2009;**57**(2):237–42.

51. Sen A, Capelli V, Husain M. Cognition and dementia in older patients with epilepsy. Brain. 2018;**141**(6):1592–608.

52. Cheng C-H, Liu CJ, Ou SM, et al. Incidence and risk of seizures in Alzheimer's disease: a nationwide population-based cohort study. Epilepsy Res. 2015;**115**:63–66.

53. Vöglein J, Ricard I, Noachtar S, et al. Seizures in Alzheimer's disease are highly recurrent and associated with a poor disease course. J Neurol. 2020;**267**(10):2941–48.

54. Johnson EL, Krauss GL, Lee AK, et al. Association between midlife risk factors and late-onset epilepsy: results from the Atherosclerosis Risk in Communities Study. JAMA Neurol. 2018;**75**(11):1375–82.

55. Miller LA, Galioto R, Tremont G, et al. Cognitive impairment in older adults with epilepsy: characterization and risk factor analysis. Epilepsy Behav. 2016;**56**:113–17.

56. Martin RC, Griffith HR, Faught E, Gilliam F, Mackey M, Vogtle L. Cognitive functioning in community dwelling older adults with chronic partial epilepsy. Epilepsia. 2005;**46**(2):298–303.

57. Witt JA, Werhahn KJ, Krämer G, Ruckes C, Trinka E, Helmstaedter C. Cognitive-behavioral screening in elderly patients with new-onset epilepsy before treatment. Acta Neurol Scand. 2014;**130**(3):172–77.

58. Breteler MMB, de Groot RR, van Romunde LK, Hofman A. Risk of dementia in patients with Parkinson's disease, epilepsy, and severe head trauma: a register-based follow-up study. Am J Epidemiol. 1995;**142**(12):1300–305.

59. Keret O, Hoang TD, Xia F, Rosen HJ, Yaffe K. Association of late-onset unprovoked seizures of unknown etiology with the risk of developing dementia in older veterans. JAMA Neurol. 2020;**77**(6):710–15.

60. Zelano J, Holtkamp M, Agarwal N, Lattanzi S, Trinka E, Brigo F. How to diagnose and treat post-stroke seizures and epilepsy. Epileptic Disord. 2020;**22**(3):252–63.

61. **Tellez-Zenteno JF, Patten SB, Jetté N, Williams J, Wiebe S.** Psychiatric comorbidity in epilepsy: a population-based analysis. Epilepsia. 2007;**48**(12):2336–44.

62. **Scott AJ, Sharpe L, Hunt C, Gandy M.** Anxiety and depressive disorders in people with epilepsy: a meta-analysis. Epilepsia. 2017;**58**(6):973–82.

63. **Cole MG, Bellavance F, Mansour A.** Prognosis of depression in elderly community and primary care populations: a systematic review and meta-analysis. Am J Psychiatry. 1999;**156**(8):1182–89.

64. **Mitchell AJ, Subramaniam H.** Prognosis of depression in old age compared to middle age: a systematic review of comparative studies. Am J Psychiatry. 2005;**162**(9):1588–601.

65. **Landmark CJ, Henning O, Johannessen SI.** Proconvulsant effects of antidepressants— what is the current evidence? Epilepsy Behav. 2016;**61**:287–91.

66. **Kok RM, Reynolds CF.** Management of depression in older adults: a review. JAMA. 2017;**317**(20):2114–22.

67. **Fisher RS, Acevedo C, Arzimanoglou A,** et al. ILAE official report: a practical clinical definition of epilepsy. Epilepsia. 2014;**55**(4):475–82.

68. **Lamberink HJ, Otte WM, Geerts AT,** et al. Individualised prediction model of seizure recurrence and long-term outcomes after withdrawal of antiepileptic drugs in seizure-free patients: a systematic review and individual participant data meta-analysis. Lancet Neurol. 2017;**16**(7):523–31.

69. **Rowan AJ, Ramsay RE, Collins JF,** et al. New onset geriatric epilepsy: a randomized study of gabapentin, lamotrigine, and carbamazepine. Neurology. 2005;**64**(11):1868–73.

70. **Werhahn KJ, Trinka E, Dobesberger J,** et al. A randomized, double-blind comparison of antiepileptic drug treatment in the elderly with new-onset focal epilepsy. Epilepsia. 2015;**56**(3):450–59.

71. **Gandhi S, McArthur E, Mamdani MM,** et al. Antiepileptic drugs and hyponatremia in older adults: two population-based cohort studies. Epilepsia. 2016;**57**(12):2067–79.

72. **Isojärvi JI, Pakarinen AJ, Myllylä VV.** Serum lipid levels during carbamazepine medication. a prospective study. Arch Neurol. 1993;**50**(6):590–93.

73. **Mintzer S, Skidmore CT, Abidin CJ,** et al. Effects of antiepileptic drugs on lipids, homocysteine, and C-reactive protein. Ann Neurol. 2009;**65**(4):448–56.

74. **Renoux C, Dell'Aniello S, Saarela O, Filion KB, Boivin JF.** Antiepileptic drugs and the risk of ischaemic stroke and myocardial infarction: a population-based cohort study. BMJ Open. 2015;**5**(8):e008365.

75. **Persson HBI, Alberts KA, Farahmand BY, Tomson T.** Risk of extremity fractures in adult outpatients with epilepsy. Epilepsia. 2002;**43**(7):768–72.

76. **Sheth RD, Gidal BE, Hermann BP.** Pathological fractures in epilepsy. Epilepsy Behav. 2006;**9**(4):601–605.

77. **Diemar SS, Sejling AS, Eiken P, Andersen NB, Jørgensen NR.** An explorative literature review of the multifactorial causes of osteoporosis in epilepsy. Epilepsy Behav. 2019;**100**(Pt A):106511.

78. **Miziak B, Chrościńska-Krawczyk M, Czuczwar SJ.** An update on the problem of osteoporosis in people with epilepsy taking antiepileptic drugs. Expert Opin Drug Saf. 2019;**18**(8):679–89.

79. **Arora E, Singh H, Gupta YK.** Impact of antiepileptic drugs on bone health: need for monitoring, treatment, and prevention strategies. J Fam Med Prim Care. 2016;5(2):248–53.

80. **Fernandez H, Mohammed HT, Patel T.** Vitamin D supplementation for bone health in adults with epilepsy: a systematic review. Epilepsia. 2018;59(4):885–96.

81. **Espinosa PS, Perez DL, Abner E, Ryan M.** Association of antiepileptic drugs, vitamin D, and calcium supplementation with bone fracture occurrence in epilepsy patients. Clin Neurol Neurosurg. 2011;113(7):548–51.

82. **Lazzari AA, Dussault PM, Thakore-James M, et al.** Prevention of bone loss and vertebral fractures in patients with chronic epilepsy—antiepileptic drug and osteoporosis prevention trial. Epilepsia. 2013;54(11):1997–2004.

83. **Dobson R, Yarnall A, Noyce AJ, Giovannoni G.** Bone health in chronic neurological diseases: a focus on multiple sclerosis and Parkinsonian syndromes. Pract Neurol. 2013;13(2):70–79.

84. **Zeber JE, Copeland LA, Pugh MJV.** Variation in antiepileptic drug adherence among older patients with new-onset epilepsy. Ann Pharmacother. 2010;44(12):1896–904.

85. **Ettinger AB, Baker GA.** Best clinical and research practice in epilepsy of older people: focus on antiepileptic drug adherence. Epilepsy Behav. 2009;15(2 Suppl 1):S60–63.

86. **Wiebe S, Blume WT, Girvin JP, Eliasziw M.** A randomized, controlled trial of surgery for temporal-lobe epilepsy. N Engl J Med. 2001;345(5):311–18.

87. **Mohan M, Keller S, Nicolson A, et al.** The long-term outcomes of epilepsy surgery. PLoS One. 2018;13(5):e0196274.

88. **Téllez-Zenteno JF, Dhar R, Wiebe S.** Long-term seizure outcomes following epilepsy surgery: a systematic review and meta-analysis. Brain. 2005;128(5):1188–98.

89. **Ichikawa N, Fujimoto A, Okanishi T, Sato K, Enoki H.** Efficacy and safety of epilepsy surgery for older adult patients with refractory epilepsy. Ther Clin Risk Manag. 2020;16:195–99.

90. **He X, Zhou J, Guan Y, Zhai F, Li T, Luan G.** Prognostic factors of postoperative seizure outcomes in older patients with temporal lobe epilepsy. Neurosurg Focus. 2020;48(4):E7.

91. **Bialek F, Rydenhag B, Flink R, Malmgren K.** Outcomes after resective epilepsy surgery in patients over 50 years of age in Sweden 1990–2009—a prospective longitudinal study. Seizure. 2014;23(8):641–45.

92. **Srikijvilaikul T, Lerdlum S, Tepmongkol S, Shuangshoti S, Locharernkul C.** Outcome of temporal lobectomy for hippocampal sclerosis in older patients. Seizure. 2011;20(4):276–79.

93. **Punia V, Abdelkader A, Busch RM, et al.** Time to push the age limit: epilepsy surgery in patients 60 years or older. Epilepsia Open. 2018;3(1):73–80.

94. **Delev D, Taube J, Helmstaedter C, et al.** Surgery for temporal lobe epilepsy in the elderly: improving quality of life despite cognitive impairment. Seizure. 2020;79:112–19.

95. **Peedicail JS, Almohawes A, Hader W, et al.** Outcomes of stereoelectroencephalography exploration at an epilepsy surgery center. Acta Neurol Scand. 2020;141(6):463–72.

96. **Cardinale F, Rizzi M, Vignati E, et al.** Stereoelectroencephalography: retrospective analysis of 742 procedures in a single centre. Brain. 2019;142(9):2688–704.

97. Dührsen L, Sauvigny T, Ricklefs FL, et al. Decision-making in temporal lobe epilepsy surgery based on invasive stereo-electroencephalography (SEEG). Neurosurg Rev. 2020;43(5):1403–408.

98. Yan H, Katz JS, Anderson M, et al. Method of invasive monitoring in epilepsy surgery and seizure freedom and morbidity: a systematic review. Epilepsia. 2019;60(9):1960–72.

99. Punia V, Bulacio J, Gonzalez-Martinez J, et al. Extra operative intracranial EEG monitoring for epilepsy surgery in elderly patients. Epilepsy Behav Case Rep. 2018;10:92–95.

100. Youngerman BE, Save AV, McKhann GM. Magnetic resonance imaging-guided laser interstitial thermal therapy for epilepsy: systematic review of technique, indications, and outcomes. Neurosurgery. 2020;86(4):E366–82.

101. Ridsdale L, Charlton J, Ashworth M, Richardson MP, Gulliford MC. Epilepsy mortality and risk factors for death in epilepsy: a population-based study. Br J Gen Pract. 2011;61(586):e271–78.

102. Tian N, Croft JB, Kobau R, Zack MM, Greenlund KJ. CDC-supported epilepsy surveillance and epidemiologic studies: a review of progress since 1994. Epilepsy Behav. 2020;109:107123.

103. Forsgren L, Hauser WA, Olafsson E, Sander JW, Sillanpää M, Tomson T. Mortality of epilepsy in developed countries: a review. Epilepsia. 2005;46(Suppl 11):18–27.

104. Neligan A, Bell GS, Johnson AL, Goodridge DM, Shorvon SD, Sander JW. The long-term risk of premature mortality in people with epilepsy. Brain. 2011;134(2):388–95.

105. Trinka E, Bauer G, Oberaigner W, Ndayisaba JP, Seppi K, Granbichler CA. Cause-specific mortality among patients with epilepsy: results from a 30-year cohort study. Epilepsia. 2013;54(3):495–501.

106. Einarsdottir AB, Sveinsson O, Olafsson E. Sudden unexpected death in epilepsy. a nationwide population-based study. Epilepsia. 2019;60(11):2174–81.

107. Thurman DJ, Hesdorffer DC, French JA. Sudden unexpected death in epilepsy: assessing the public health burden. Epilepsia. 2014;55(10):1479–85.

108. Miller WR, Buelow JM, Bakas T. Older adults and new-onset epilepsy: experiences with diagnosis. J Neurosci Nurs. 2014;46(1):2–10.

109. Baranowski CJ. The quality of life of older adults with epilepsy: a systematic review. Seizure. 2018;60:190–97.

110. Martin R, Vogtle L, Gilliam F, Faught E. What are the concerns of older adults living with epilepsy? Epilepsy Behav. 2005;7(2):297–300.

111. Miller WR. Patient-centered outcomes in older adults with epilepsy. Seizure. 2014;23(8):592–97.

Chapter 11

Teratogenic risk and aspects of epilepsy relating to women's health

John Craig and Michael Kinney

Introduction

Many improvements have been seen in the last three decades in the care of girls and women with epilepsy. Prior to this, little was understood about drug safety.

For many women, pregnancy is both a joyful time and potentially stressful time. Epilepsy can result in significant additional complexity, with often difficult decisions required about antiseizure medications (ASMs). Epilepsy can impact the life course of women in other ways—in relation to menses, menopause, bone health, contraception, and even marital relationships or dating (see Chapter 15).

Most pregnant women with epilepsy will achieve a successful outcome and have a healthy child. High-quality patient education, support, and timely access to individualized advice is vital. This chapter will outline the improvements which have occurred over the last 20 years alongside the factors considered to be best clinical care.

Teratogenic risk and other risks to the fetus

Seizures

There is limited evidence that focal, absence, or myoclonic seizures are harmful to the fetus. Bilateral tonic–clonic seizures have been linked to fetal bradycardia and miscarriage, with animal studies demonstrating neurological and psychological sequelae in offspring exposed to convulsive seizures *in utero*. For status epilepticus, the risks are higher, with data from EURAP, the

International Registry of Antiepileptic Drugs and Pregnancy, recording four adverse outcomes (one perinatal death and three major congenital malformations (MCMs)) in 21 cases of status epilepticus.[1] There is limited information on the impact of seizures on cognitive and neurobehavioural development; one study noted an association between tonic–clonic seizures and cognitive development.[2]

Seizures during pregnancy have been associated with preterm birth and offspring with low birth weight or who are small for gestational age.[3]

Risks of antiseizure medications

ASMs potentially affect all aspects of embryonic and fetal development. In recent years, the results of national and international pregnancy registers have defined the relative risks of ASMs, taken in monotherapy or polytherapy. There are, however, still significant delays obtaining safety information in pregnancy. While developmental concerns were noted within 10 years of valproate being available in the early 1970s, it is only several decades later that regulatory authorities have issued strict guidance on its use in women of childbearing years.[4]

ASMs are taken prepregnancy and are required to be continued through pregnancy in nearly all women with epilepsy. As such, there is the potential for there to be an impact on fetal growth, the occurrence of major and minor malformations, and cognitive and neurodevelopmental delay (Table 11.1).

The risks for pregnancy loss are somewhat conflicting, having been reported to be higher in unplanned pregnancies, where there is a parental history of MCMs and with the use of ASM polytherapy.[5]

Effect on fetal growth

ASMs taken in pregnancy have been reported to affect fetal growth. In one study, 11% of infants born to women with epilepsy who were taking ASMs were small for gestational age. This compared with 5% for infants of mothers with epilepsy who were not taking ASMs. The rate was similar for women with epilepsy who were taking ASMs and those taking ASMs for other indications.[6] In a recent registry study, rates of small-for-gestational-age outcomes were highest for topiramate-, phenobarbital-, and zonisamide-exposed infants.[6] Some conflicting results between different studies have been seen and further replication is required. Differences in head circumference have been reported, with reductions noted for carbamazepine and valproate.

Table 11.1 Major congenital malformation risks reported by large international registries: Key MCM outcome data from three of the large prospective pregnancy registries are illustrated. The highest frequency of registrations to these studies are for carbamazepine, lamotrigine, levetiracetam, and valproate and consequently more data are available for risk counselling for these drugs.

ASM	Number of MCMs in monotherapy exposures/total number of monotherapy exposures (MCM rate; 95% CI)		
	UK and Ireland Epilepsy and Pregnancy Register[7]	EURAP[8]	North American AED Pregnancy Registry[9]
Carbamazepine	43/1657 (2.6%; 1.9–3.5)	Dose ≤700 mg 58/1276 (4.5%; 3.5–5.8)	31/1033 (3.0%; 2.1–4.2)
		>700 mg 49/681 (7.2%; 5.4–9.4)	
Lamotrigine	49/2098 (2.3%; 1.8–3.1)	Dose ≤325 mg 46/1870 (2.5%;1.8–3.3)	31/1562 (2.0%;1.4–2.8)
		>325 mg 28/644 (4.3%; 2.9–6.2)	
Levetiracetam	2/304 (0.70%; 0.2–2.5)	17/599 (2.8%; 1.7–4.5)	11/450 (2.4%; 1.2–4.3)
Oxcarbazepine	Not reported	10/333 (3.0%; 1.4–5.4)	4/182 (2.2%; 0.6–5.5)
Phenobarbital	Not reported	19/294 (6.5%; 4.2–9.9)	11/199 (5.5%; 2.8–9.7)
Phenytoin	3/82 (3.7%; 1.3–10.2)	8/125 (6.4%; 2.8–12.2)	12/416 (2.9%; 1.5–5.0)
Topiramate	3/70 (4.3%; 1.7–13.3)	6/152 (3.9%;1.5–8.4)	15/359 (4.2% (2.4–6.8)
Valproate	82/1220 (6.7%; 5.5–8.3)	Dose ≤650 mg 38/600 (6.3%; 4.5–8.6)	30/323 (9.3%; 6.4–13.0)
		>650 to ≤1450 mg 75/666 (11.3%; 9.0–13.9)	
		>1450 mg 29/115 (25.2%; 17.6–34.2)	

Major congenital malformations

MCMs are malformations that require medical or surgical intervention (Table 11.1). The MCM risk is higher in ASM polytherapy,[10] increases with the number of ASMs used, and is ASM specific, with somewhat different types of MCM for each ASM. Valproate is associated with the highest teratogenic risk.[7-9]

The overall risk of an MCM with valproate exposure *in utero* is approximately 10%,[11] with the risk consistently being shown to be dose dependent.[7,8,12] Results from EURAP found a MCM rate of 5.6% in pregnancies exposed to less than 700 mg per day of valproate, 10.4% in those exposed to between 700 mg and 1500 mg per day, and 24.2% in those exposed to over 1500 mg per day.[12] This was replicated in further work from the same group.[8] The types of MCMs reported with valproate include neural tube defects, cardiovascular defects, genitourinary defects, in males in particular, facial clefts, and musculoskeletal defects.[7-9]

The risk of MCMs for phenytoin and phenobarbital have been quoted as 6% and 6–7%, respectively, in a recent review from the Medicines and Healthcare products and Regulatory Agency (MHRA) in the UK.[13] Results for carbamazepine are variable, with the UK and Ireland Epilepsy and Pregnancy Register and the North American AED Pregnancy Register reporting MCM rates just above background.[7,9] In contrast, EURAP reported a doubling of the MCM rate for carbamazepine and a measurable dose response, with a 4.5% MCM rate in those exposed to less than or equal to 700 mg per day, compared with 7.2% in those exposed to over 700 mg per day.[8] The MHRA has quoted a risk for carbamazepine of 4–5%.[13]

For more novel ASMs, the most information is available for lamotrigine[7-9,14] and levetiracetam,[7-9] where rates similar to background have been reported.[13] Based on currently available information, the risk of a MCM for topiramate is estimated to be 4–5%,[13] with an emphasis on clefting abnormalities. Less information is available for the other ASMs. Results for oxcarbazepine have been encouraging,[8] but there is very little information available for many other ASMs, including clobazam, zonisamide, pregabalin, gabapentin, lacosamide, eslicarbazepine acetate, perampanel, brivaracetam, cannabidiol and cenobamate.

Polytherapy results are much more difficult to interpret due to the number of potential combinations. While overall the risks for MCMs are higher for polytherapy,[7,10] recent studies demonstrate that medication regimens containing valproate and possibly topiramate confer the greatest risk. The North American AED Pregnancy Register showed a risk of MCMs of 9.1% among infants exposed to lamotrigine taken along with valproate as part of a polytherapy regimen, compared with 2.9% for lamotrigine plus any other ASM (1.5; 95% confidence interval (CI) 0.7–3.0).[15] This was also seen for carbamazepine, with risks of 15.4% when carbamazepine was used with valproate as part of a polytherapy regimen, compared to 2.5% when taken with any ASM other than valproate. For MCMs, there is some evidence that low-dose valproate taken as part of a polytherapy regimen may be safer with respect to MCMs than high-dose valproate taken as monotherapy.[16]

Cognitive and other neurodevelopmental effects

The risk of neurodevelopmental disability, including cognitive impairment, autistic spectrum disorder and autism, attention deficit hyperactivity disorder, and other behavioural problems is the subject of ongoing study. For the majority of ASMs the risks are largely unknown.[13] Studies have consistently shown that cognitive functioning is lower in children born to women with epilepsy exposed to valproate. The Neurodevelopmental Effects of Antiepileptic Drugs study found that at age 6 years mean IQ in those exposed to valproate is between 8 and 11 points lower than those exposed to other ASMs.[17] The risk was dose dependent with a mean IQ of 94 for those exposed to more than 1000 mg per day, compared with 104 for those exposed to less than 1000 mg per day.[17] *In utero* valproate exposure is associated with a wide range of other cognitive deficits, including reduced measures of verbal ability, non-verbal ability, memory, and executive function, which are dose related. For those with clinically confirmed fetal valproate syndrome the risks are higher, with an estimated 25% having intellectual disability. Other neurodevelopmental disorders such as autistic spectrum disorders and autism are increased for valproate, compared with other ASMs.[18] There is a two- to threefold increase in the subsequent risk of attention deficit hyperactivity disorder for those exposed to valproate *in utero* compared to other ASMs.[19] Considering all of the potential impacts of valproate on fetal brain development, it is estimated that 30–40% of all children exposed to valproate *in utero* will have lifelong neurodevelopmental disorders,[13] resulting in reduced educational attainment and the requirement for additional support.

Results for other ASMs, where available, are generally more favourable. The risks of neurodevelopmental delay and behavioural upset are lower with carbamazepine, although some studies have reported reduced IQ, non-verbal memory, and delayed language compared with background.[13] For lamotrigine, risks of neurodevelopmental delay closer to background have been reported.[13,17] For levetiracetam, results have not suggested an increased risk for neurodevelopmental delay[20]; however, this is based on a very limited number of cases. In contrast, in a recent report, behavioural problems and emotional difficulties were reported with *in utero* exposure to valproate, carbamazepine, lamotrigine, and levetiracetam.[21] For topiramate, preliminary published results are somewhat mixed.[13]

In summary, for most ASMs neurodevelopmental studies have only recruited small numbers and assessed outcomes at an early stage of development. Other than for valproate for which the evidence is strong, the impact of most ASMs on cognitive, neurodevelopmental, and behavioural outcomes is not fully understood.

Maternal considerations

Pregnancy and seizure control

For approximately two-thirds of women seizure control is unchanged during pregnancy.[1] For the other third, roughly equal proportions experience an improvement or deterioration in seizure control. Factors associated with the occurrence of seizures during pregnancy are multiple, including changes in adherence rates and altered pharmacokinetics of ASMs during pregnancy. A prospective, multicentre study compared seizure control between two epochs in women with epilepsy; pregnancy combined with the first 6 weeks postpartum was compared to the subsequent 7.5-month postpartum period. Women with epilepsy who did not become pregnant were controls.[22] Those women who became pregnant demonstrated a similar reduction in seizure control compared to the non-pregnant group. Notably, women who were pregnant did have significantly higher odds of dose alterations in medication (odds ratio 6.36; 95% CI 3.8–10.6), suggesting that careful management in pregnancy can reduce the risk of seizure control worsening. Risks vary by treatment, with seizures being more common for those taking two or more ASMs, those not on any treatment, and those prescribed lamotrigine and oxcarbazepine.[1] Seizures are more common in those with unplanned pregnancies and who have not received preconception counselling, and less likely in those who are seizure free before pregnancy.[1,22,23]

Maternal mortality

Women with epilepsy are between five and ten times more likely to die during pregnancy compared with all pregnancies (see Chapter 9) across the general population. This has been demonstrated consistently, including in a number of confidential enquiries into maternal deaths and morbidity in the UK. In the most recent report, most deaths were due to sudden unexpected death in epilepsy (SUDEP).[24] A case–control study has suggested a higher risk of SUDEP with lamotrigine although associations between SUDEP and specific ASMs remains controversial. The increased risk for maternal mortality extends up to 1 year postpartum.

Other pregnancy outcomes

Meta-analyses have demonstrated an increased risk for adverse obstetric outcomes such as pregnancy-induced hypertension, pre-eclampsia, antepartum and postpartum haemorrhage, labour induction, and caesarean sections.[25] Pregnant women with epilepsy have an increased rate of depression and other psychiatric disorders and have a greater risk for exacerbations of these conditions. Medications for psychiatric disorders have less safety information than is presently available for ASMs. Suicide risk should be considered, given its threefold increase in those with epilepsy, with urgent referral pathways in place for those requiring psychiatric input.

Minimizing the risks

A number of guidelines exist to inform the practitioner of the best management of women with epilepsy of childbearing years.

These have been developed nationally in the UK (National Institute for Health and Care Excellence, Scottish Intercollegiate Guidelines Network, Royal College of Obstetricians and Gynaecologists)[26–28] and internationally, including through the International League Against Epilepsy.[29] For valproate, in particular, regulations are increasingly proscriptive and include providing clear information on the risks of valproate in pregnancy, documentation of discussions and decisions reached, as well as agreement on a pregnancy prevention programme. Practical difficulties may occur for those who require valproate as an effective ASM option, for those who fail to comply with advice offered, and for those with intellectual disability, where enforcing a contraceptive choice may be considered inappropriate. Managing these and other difficulties is the focus of a recent multidisciplinary review.[30] Valproate guidance updated - please see attachments with this file https://www.gov.uk/guidance/valproate-use-by-women-and-girls

Preconception counselling should be available to all women with epilepsy considering pregnancy. This should start at the time of diagnosis or from adolescence onwards, whichever is earlier. Re-evaluation of the diagnosis, the need for ongoing treatment, and its appropriateness, including the dose of any ASMs taken, should be considered in all women and girls who are thinking of conceiving. For women who opt to stay on valproate this is difficult and trying to reduce the dose, as much as possible, should be discussed. Changing to the prolonged-release preparation and fractionating the dose might be considered, although outside of preclinical studies, these have not been shown to be beneficial. Identification of other risk factors to include smoking, alcohol, other drugs, and obesity should be explored.

Folic acid

Folic acid should be prescribed before conception (typically several months prior) and at least until the end of the first trimester[26] and arguably through the entire pregnancy. The optimum dosage remains undetermined, with community-based studies using dosages ranging from 0.5 to 4.0 mg daily. There is no evidence that folate supplementation confers additional protection against MCMs in the offspring of women using ASMs, beyond that which is seen with its protective effects in the general population. Studies have shown that preconceptual folic acid may protect against adverse ASM-associated cognitive and neurodevelopmental effects, including for valproate.[17] Such results have been seen with high-dose folic acid (5 mg) in the general population. Ensuring normal vitamin B_{12} and vitamin D levels is appropriate as part of good preparation for pregnancy and vitamin B_{12} levels should be checked prior to commencing folate replacement. Taking high doses of folate in the presence of relative vitamin B_{12} deficiency can precipitate subacute combined degeneration of the spinal cord.

Pregnancy

Fetal monitoring

Pregnancies in women with epilepsy should be supervised in obstetric units, with access to high-resolution ultrasound scanning and full access to all available prenatal tests. National Institute for Health and Care Excellence guidelines on the epilepsies and obstetric guidelines advocate high-resolution scanning for all at 18–20 weeks.[26,28]

Epilepsy monitoring during pregnancy

Women with epilepsy should have access to specialist care from neurologists, with epilepsy expertise, during pregnancy. For those taking valproate, urgent review of treatment should be arranged in cases of suspected or inadvertent pregnancy. Valproate withdrawal or switching to an alternative ASM during pregnancy can be practically difficult and have risks of worsening seizures. One study found bilateral tonic–clonic seizures were twice as common in those where valproate was withdrawn (33%; n = 93) or replaced (29%; n = 38) in pregnancy, compared with those maintained on it (16%; n = 1588).[31]

Therapeutic drug monitoring (TDM) in pregnancy is supported by the International League Against Epilepsy for lamotrigine, oxcarbazepine, gabapentin, topiramate, levetiracetam, and zonisamide.[29] In the UK, the MHRA recommends monitoring of lamotrigine before, during, and after pregnancy, with TDM of oxcarbazepine, levetiracetam, and phenytoin when felt to be clinically indicated.[32] The frequency of monitoring is less clear, with some advocating as frequent as monthly TDM. The only randomized controlled trial evidence for the effect of ASM TDM found no significant difference in the time to first seizure or deterioration in seizure control between those monitored clinically and in those having TDM to guide ASM dose escalation in pregnancy (EMPiRE study).[33] In contrast, as previously referred to in the section 'Pregnancy and seizure control', with careful monitoring and dose adjustment of ASMs, deterioration in seizure control might be minimized. Where ASM levels are available before pregnancy, it has been recommended to increase doses in those with falling serum levels to maintain the individualized prepregnancy target concentration.[29]

Labour and delivery

Most women with epilepsy will have an uncomplicated labour. Two to three per cent may have a seizure. It is essential that ASMs are continued during labour, with repetitive or prolonged seizures being managed as per usual practice, except in cases of eclampsia. Eclampsia is a life-threatening emergency where convulsive seizures occur in the setting of pre-eclampsia. Emergency treatment with magnesium sulfate is used to control seizures. It is recommended that labour should proceed in facilities equipped for maternal and neonatal resuscitation. Pethidine should be avoided as it may trigger seizures. The requirement for instrumental or assisted delivery is usually based on obstetric concerns rather than the underlying epilepsy.

Postpartum period

Breastfeeding is safe, although for some older ASMs such as phenobarbital and primidone, drug accumulation can occur in the neonate. Most ASMs are secreted in low levels in breast milk. Improved cognitive functioning has been found in breastfed children born to women with epilepsy, compared to those not breastfed.[34]

When ASM doses have been increased in pregnancy, serum ASM levels can rise quickly after delivery. While TDM might be considered, a steady state is not possible, due to the rapid changes in clearance in the early postpartum period. The rate of taper to avoid toxicity depends on the primary route of elimination for each ASM. For lamotrigine, empirical reductions every 2–3 days over the first few weeks has been advocated. A plan for tapering ASM doses that had risen during pregnancy to preconception levels should be agreed prior to delivery.

Information on safe infant handling, bathing, and feeding techniques should be imparted to protect the newborn. Reconsideration of ASM choices, contraceptive options, and planning for future pregnancies should be discussed and recorded.

Other aspects relating to women's health

Female hormones and seizure control

Catamenial epilepsy is the association of epileptic seizures at certain stages of the hormonal cycle: perimenstrual (most common), periovulatory, and the inadequate luteal phase.[35] An accurate seizure diary cross-referenced with the dates of menses is essential to diagnose a catamenial trigger. A proposed definition for catamenial epilepsy is an observed twofold increase in seizures at one of these particular stages, identified over a 2-month time period.[36] A mid-luteal (day 22 of cycle) progesterone level of less than 5 ng/mL is used to demonstrate an inadequate luteal phase.

The exact cause of catamenial clustering of seizures is not clearly understood. Multidian (multiday) rhythms of seizure exacerbation have been identified on long-term implanted intracranial electroencephalography, suggesting an association with hormonal rhythms, but the patterns appear to be even more complex, with other factors likely involved.[37] Good evidence for targeted treatment of seizures around the time of menses is lacking, with clobazam being a common choice for treating predictable clusters of seizures.

Epilepsy, antiseizure medications, and fertility

Few studies have robustly addressed the issue of fertility in women with epilepsy, and the existing evidence is conflicting, with some suggesting a lower fertility rate.[38] Proposed factors include hormonal issues, anovulatory cycles, irregular menses, amenorrhoea seen more commonly with certain ASMs (notably enzyme inducers which can increase sex hormone binding globulin, reducing the serum hormone levels), and polytherapy.[38] Temporal lobe epilepsy may result in hypothalamic–pituitary–gonadal axis disturbance. Valproate is associated with polycystic ovarian syndrome, which is linked to fertility issues.

Social isolation, mental health factors, and stigma could all limit meeting prospective partners, perhaps explaining a lower rate of marriage (see Chapter 15). Stigma associated with epilepsy may result in people with epilepsy not disclosing the diagnosis to prospective partners.[39] People with epilepsy may have high divorce rates,[39] and even well-controlled epilepsy can impact marriage. The effects of epilepsy on the spouse of a person with epilepsy should not be underestimated and they should be supported.

Antiseizure medications and contraception

Epilepsy specialists should be familiar with issues around contraception to help women make informed choices, relevant to their epilepsy. This should be in conjunction with the primary care doctor or family planning specialist. These

Table 11.2 Common contraceptive choices of specific importance to women with epilepsy

Contraceptive choice	Issues to consider
IUDs (copper IUD and Mirena®/levonorgestrel intrauterine system)	◆Highly efficacious ◆Considered an optimal method of contraception for women with epilepsy ◆Reversible non-oral long-term solution ◆Does not interact with ASMs
Depot medroxyprogesterone acetate (DPMA)	◆Depot injectable ◆Does not interact with ASMs
Oral contraception	◆Adherence is a key issue (consider cognitive comorbidities) ◆If ethinylestradiol hormonal contraception (combined oral contraceptives, patch, and vaginal ring) is added to lamotrigine it can result in a reduction in serum lamotrigine levels, predisposing to seizures. It is safest to avoid using ethinylestradiol hormonal contraception with lamotrigine. If, however, ethinylestradiol is used, omit the week-long break in ethinylestradiol—as there is a risk of fluctuating lamotrigine serum levels and drug toxicity ◆Enzyme-inducing ASMs (carbamazepine, eslicarbazepine, felbamate, oxcarbazepine, perampanel, phenobarbital, phenytoin, primidone, rufinamide, topiramate) can interact with hormonal contraception resulting in enhanced oestrogen and progesterone metabolism. To prevent contraceptive failure additional methods may be required such as barrier, or IUD). Changes to the dosing of ethinylestradiol can be considered under expert guidance from the family planning team. Changing the ASM may be possible, under specialist advice. Progesterone depot injections and the Mirena® coil can be used. ◆It is perhaps an oversimplification, but oestrogens have proconvulsant properties, and progesterone has anticonvulsant properties based on animal models. There is no applicable evidence base to justify not using ethinylestradiol or hormonal contraception on the grounds of aggravating seizures[42]
Emergency contraception choices	◆ Consider copper IUD and levonorgestrel (double dose, i.e. 3 mg total)

IUD, intrauterine device.

issues are outlined in Table 11.2. Contraception impacts on the choice of ASM and should be discussed at times of changes in ASMs. It is vital to be familiar with the bidirectional interactions between contraception and ASMs to prevent either contraceptive failure or unnecessary breakthrough seizures.[40] The full range of options should be made available where possible to allow girls and women to make the best choice depending on lifestyle and epilepsy factors after a holistic review.

Women with epilepsy have a high rate of unplanned pregnancies so it is useful to discuss contraception at transition between paediatric and adult care.[41] Highly effective contraception is mandated for women of reproductive years using sodium valproate (Valproate Pregnancy Prevention Programme).[4]

Epilepsy and the menopause

The menopause is important to consider with respect to epilepsy.[43] Menopause occurs in the general population on average at age 51 years and is defined as having no menses over a 12-month epoch. The hallmark of the perimenopausal years is inconsistent ovulation, elevation of the oestrogen:progesterone ratio, and variability in menses. Follicle-stimulating hormone and luteinizing hormone levels decrease with a rise in gonadotropin-releasing hormone levels after menopause. High seizure frequency has been associated with premature menopause.[44] A cross-sectional study suggests seizure control improves after menopause, particularly in those with catamenial epilepsy.[45]

The safety of hormone replacement therapy has not been fully established in women with epilepsy, with one prematurely terminated randomized trial of the brand Prempro* finding a dose-related increase in seizure frequency.[46] Serum lamotrigine levels can potentially be lowered by hormone replacement therapy preparations owing to oestrogen content. Further studies are required to guide safe prescribing. Another important consideration, which has an important bearing when approaching menopause, is the impact of ASMs on bone health, particularly enzyme-inducing ASMs and valproate.[47]

Women in comparison to men have a higher risk of low bone density and osteoporosis with consequent increased risk of fractures. For women with epilepsy, expert guidance recommends checking vitamin D levels[26] in those using enzyme-inducing ASMs or valproate (see Chapter 3). Good advice includes calculating daily dietary calcium intake and assessing the vitamin D level.[48] In certain cases, bone mineral density scanning and the opinion of a metabolic bone specialist may be needed.

Conclusion

Significant advances have been made in the care of women with epilepsy over the past several decades, yet there is no place for complacency. All clinicians and other professionals involved in the care of women and girls with epilepsy should strive to embed best practice in a quality-assured manner, within the framework of multidisciplinary team working.

References

1. **Battino D, Tomson T, Bonizzoni E,** et al. Seizure control and treatment changes in pregnancy: observations from the EURAP epilepsy pregnancy registry. Epilepsia. 2013;**54**(9):1621–27.
2. **Adab N, Kinu U, Vinten J,** et al. The longer term outcome of children born to mothers with epilepsy. J Neurol Neurosurg Psychiatry. 2004;**75**(11):1575–83.
3. **Chen Y-H, Chiou H-Y, Lin H-C, Lin H-L.** Effect of seizures during gestation on pregnancy outcomes in women with epilepsy. Arch Neurol. 2009;**66**(8):979–84.
4. **Medicines and Healthcare products Regulatory Agency.** Valproate use by women and girls. Available at: https://www.gov.uk/guidance/valproate-use-by-women-and-girls
5. **Tomson T, Battino D, Bonizzoni E,** et al. Anti-epileptic drugs and intrauterine death: a prospective observational study from EURAP. Neurology. 2015;**85**(7):580–88.
6. **Hernández-Díaz S, McElrath TF, Pennell PB,** et al. Fetal growth and premature delivery in pregnant women on antiepileptic drugs. Ann Neurol. 2017;**82**(3):457–65.
7. **Campbell E, Kennedy F, Russell A,** et al. Malformation risks of antiepileptic drug monotherapies in pregnancy: updated results from the UK and Ireland Epilepsy and Pregnancy Registers. J Neurol Neurosurg Psychiatry. 2014;**85**(9):1029–34.
8. **Tomson T, Battino D, Bonizzoni E,** et al. Comparative risk of major congenital malformations with eight different antiepileptic drugs: a prospective study of the EURAP registry. Lancet Neurol. 2018;**17**(6):530–38.
9. **Hernández-Díaz S, Smith CR, Shen A,** et al. North American AED Pregnancy Registry North American AED Pregnancy Registry. Comparative safety of antiepileptic drugs during pregnancy. Neurology. 2012;**78**(21):1692–99.
10. **Holmes LB, Harvey EA, Coull BA,** et al. The teratogenicity of anticonvulsant drugs. N Engl J Med. 2001;**344**(15):1132–38.
11. **Meador K, Reynolds MW, Crean S, Fahrbach K, Probst C.** Pregnancy outcomes in women with epilepsy: a systematic review and meta-analysis of published pregnancy registries and cohorts. Epilepsy Res. 2008;**81**(1):1–13.
12. **Tomson T, Battino D, Bonizzoni E,** et al. Dose-dependent risk of malformations with antiepileptic drugs: an analysis of data from the EURAP epilepsy and pregnancy registry. Lancet Neurol. 2011;**10**(7):609–17.
13. **Medicines and Healthcare products Regulatory Agency.** Public assessment report of antiepileptic drugs: review of safety of use in pregnancy. 7 January 2021. Available at: https://assets.publishing.service.gov.uk/government/uploads/system/uploads/attachment_data/file/950066/AED-PAR-PDF-FINAL-Jan21.pdf [accessed 16 December 2021].

14. **Cunnington MC, Weil JG, Messenheimer JA, Ferber S, Yerby, M, Tennis P.** Final results from 18 years of the International Lamotrigine Pregnancy Registry. Neurology. 2011;**76**(21):1817–23.

15. **Holmes LB, Mittendorf R, Shen A, Smith CR, Hernandez-Diaz S.** Fetal effects of anticonvulsant polytherapies: different risks from different drug combinations. Arch Neurol. 2011;**68**(10):1275–81.

16. **Tomson T, Battino D, Bonizzoni E,** et al. Dose-dependent teratogenicity of valproate in mono- and polytherapy: an observational study. Neurology. 2015;**85**(10):866–72.

17. **Meador KJ, Baker GA, Browning N.** Fetal antiepileptic drug exposure and cognitive outcomes at age 6 years (NEAD study): a prospective observational study. Lancet Neurol. 2013;**12**(3):244–52.

18. **Christensen J, Gronborg TK, Sorensen MJ,** et al. Prenatal valproate exposure and risk of autism spectrum disorders and childhood autism. JAMA. 2013;**309**(16):1696–703.

19. **Cohen MJ, Meador KJ, Browning N,** et al. Fetal antiepileptic drug exposure: motor, adaptive, and emotional/behavioral functioning at age 3 years. Epilepsy Behav. 2011;**22**(2):240–46.

20. **Bromley RL, Calderbank R, Cheyne CP,** et al. Cognition in school-age children exposed to levetiracetam, topiramate, or sodium valproate. Neurology. 2016;**87**(18):1943–53.

21. **Huber-Mollema Y, Oort FJ, Lindhout D, Rodenburg R.** Behavioral problems in children of mothers with epilepsy prenatally exposed to valproate, carbamazepine, lamotrigine or levetiracetam monotherapy. Epilepsia. 2019;**60**(6):1069–82.

22. **Pennell P, French JA, May RC,** et al. Changes in seizure frequency and antiepileptic therapy during pregnancy. N Engl J Med. 2020;**383**(26):2547–56.

23. **Thomas SV, Syam U, Devi JS.** Predictors of seizures during pregnancy in women with epilepsy. Epilepsia. 2012;**53**(5):e85–88.

24. **MBRRACE.** Saving lives, improving mothers' care: lessons learned to inform maternity care from the UK and Ireland Confidential Enquiries into Maternal Deaths and Morbidity 2016–18. 2020. Available at: https://hubble-live-assets.s3.amazonaws.com/birth-companions/file_asset/file/76/MBRRACE-UK_Maternal_Report_Dec_2020_v10.pdf [accessed 16 December 2021].

25. **Viale L, Allotey J, Cheong-See F,** et al. Epilepsy in pregnancy and reproductive outcomes: a systematic review and meta-analysis. Lancet. 2015;**386**(10006):1845–52.

26. **National Institute of Health and Care Excellence.** Epilepsies in children, young people and adults. https://www.nice.org.uk/guidance/ng217.

27. **Scottish Intercollegiate Guidelines Network (SIGN).** Diagnosis and management of epilepsy in adults (SIGN publication no. 143). Edinburgh: SIGN; 2015. Available at: https://www.sign.ac.uk/our-guidelines/epilepsies-in-children-and-young-people-investigative-procedures-and-management/ [accessed 15 December 2021].

28. **Royal College of Obstetricians and Gynaecologists.** Epilepsy in pregnancy (Green-top guideline 68). 2016. Available at: https://www.rcog.org.uk/en/guidelines-research-servi ces/guidelines/gtg68/ [accessed 16 December 2021].

29. **Tomson T, Battino D, Bromley R,** et al. Management of epilepsy in pregnancy: a report from the International League Against Epilepsy Task Force on Women and Pregnancy. Epileptic Disord. 2019;**21**(6):497–517.

30. **Shakespeare J, Sisodiya S.** Guidance document on valproate use in women and girls of childbearing years. 2020. Available at: https://www.gov.uk/guidance/valproate-use-by-women-and-girls [accessed 30 January 2024].

31. **Tomson T, Battino D, Bonizzoni E,** et al. Withdrawal of valproic acid treatment during pregnancy and seizure outcome: observations from EURAP. Epilepsia. 2016;**57**(8):173–77.

32. **Medicines and Healthcare products Regulatory Agency.** Antiepileptic drugs in pregnancy—update advice. 2021. Available at: https://www.gov.uk/drug-safety-update/antiepileptic-drugs-in-pregnancy-updated-advice-following-comprehensive-safety-rev iew [accessed 11 December 2021].

33. **Thangaratinam S, Marlin N, Newton S,** et al. AntiEpileptic drug Monitoring in PREgnancy (EMPiRE): a double-blind randomised trial on effectiveness and acceptability of monitoring strategies. Health Technol Assess. 2018;**22**(23):1–152.

34. **Birnbaum AK, Meador KJ, Karanam A,** et al. Antiepileptic drug exposure in infants of breastfeeding mothers with epilepsy. JAMA Neurol. 2020;**77**(4):441–50.

35. **Herzog AG, Klein P, Ransil BJ.** Three patterns of catamenial epilepsy. Epilepsia. 1997;**38**(10):1082–88.

36. **Herzog AG.** Catamenial epilepsy: definition, prevalence, pathophysiology and treatment. Seizure. 2008;**2**(2):151–59.

37. **Baud MO, Kleen JK, Mirro EA,** et al. Multi-day rhythms modulate seizure risk in epilepsy. Nat Commun. 2018;**9**(1):88.

38. **Sukumaran SC, Sarma PS, Thomas SV.** Polytherapy increases the risk of infertility in women with epilepsy. Neurology. 2010;**75**(15):1351–55.

39. **Kinariwalla N, Sen A.** The psychosocial impact of epilepsy on marriage: a narrative review. Epilepsy Behav. 2016;**63**:34–41.

40. **Faculty of Sexual and Reproductive Healthcare of the Royal College of Obstetricians and Gynaecologists.** FSRH guidelines & statements. Available at: www.fsrh.org/standa rds-and-guidance/current-clinical-guidance [accessed 5 December 2020].

41. **Herzog AG, Mandle HB, Cahill KE,** et al. Predictors of unintended pregnancy in women with epilepsy. Neurology. 2017;**88**(8):728–33.

42. **Reimers A, Brodtorb E, Sabers A.** Interactions between hormonal contraception and antiepileptic drugs: clinical and mechanistic considerations. Seizure. 2015;**28**:66–70.

43. **Sveinsson O, Tomson T.** Epilepsy and menopause: potential implications for pharmacotherapy. Drugs Aging. 2014;**31**(9):671–75.

44. **Harden CL, Koppel BS, Herzog AG,** et al. Seizure frequency is associated with age at menopause in women with epilepsy. Neurology. 2003;**61**(4):451–55.

45. **Harden CL, Pulver MC, Ravdin L,** et al. The effect of menopause and perimenopause on the course of epilepsy. Epilepsia. 1999;**40**(10):1402–407.

46. **Harden CL, Herzog AG, Nikolov BG,** et al. Hormone replacement therapy in women with epilepsy: a randomized, double-blind, placebo-controlled study. Epilepsia. 2006;**47**(9):1447–51.

47. **Medicines and Healthcare products Regulatory Agency.** Antiepileptics: adverse effects on bone. 2014. Available at: https://www.gov.uk/drug-safety-update/antiepileptics-adve rse-effects-on-bone [accessed 30 November 2021].

48. **Dobson R, Cock HR, Brex P,** et al. Vitamin D supplementation. Pract Neurol. 2018;**18**(1):35–42.

Section 5

The psychosocial impact of epilepsy

Chapter 12

Epilepsy and the impact on study, learning, and memory

Ian Brown

Introduction

For the majority of people with epilepsy, the seizure event only occupies a small proportion of their time and the majority of individuals (about two-thirds) become seizure free on antiseizure medications (ASMs). This, though, does not explain the cognitive and memory problems that can have a very significant effect on the quality and richness of the life of affected individuals. Such difficulties may have a significant impact on interactions with family, friends, and colleagues and may certainly affect performance at school, university, and the workplace. Such difficulties may be mistaken for carelessness or inattention, leading to frustration and possibly interpersonal conflict with colleagues and supervisors. It is interesting, and even surprising, that the extent of the memory difficulties, rather than the diagnosis of epilepsy itself or the overall intellectual functioning, appears to have the greatest association with the low socioeconomic status of people with epilepsy and this can result in a slowly increasing exclusion from family and interactive social life.[1] This aspect will be explored further in this chapter with some suggestions and strategies for minimizing the impact of this important, but currently poorly understood comorbidity.

Current empirical evidence on the impact

Baxendale[1] nicely explores the extent of the problem, and she makes the important distinction between subjective complaints and objective measures of impairment. Patient ratings of memory problems are closely related to measures of anxiety and depression but could also be a reflection of difficulties adjusting or coping with the condition[2,3] (see Chapter 6). Autobiographical memory problems can be a particular feature of frontal lobe epilepsy and in those who suffer with transient epileptic amnesia.[4] The term 'an awful memory' is often used by patients to represent a mixture of cognitive difficulties and can be associated with adjustment to the diagnosis and prevailing mood. Formal testing can sometimes overestimate or underestimate the extent of the problem but there is a general consensus that within the epilepsy population there exists a higher rate of memory and cognitive problems. The IQ of people with epilepsy (if you discount the group with underlying associated cerebral abnormalities and syndromic epilepsy) falls within the average range of normative healthy samples within a statistically 'normal' distribution,[5] but this is usually at the inception of the disorder and other factors such as ASMs and the incidence of status epilepticus may adversely affect this finding as time passes.

Children with epilepsy, but with no other comorbidities and of normal intelligence, may demonstrate lower academic achievement.[6] A recent systematic review study by Wo and colleagues indicated that in 14 studies (70% of total studies), children aged between 5 and 18 years with epilepsy were found to have lower academic achievements when compared with healthy controls, and these findings were stable over time (2–4 years).

Cognitive dysfunction is multifactorial and some of the dysfunction may be anatomical due to the pathology, some may be due to the course of the disease, and some may be due to treatment. The pathology cannot usually be altered, although surgery may be possible. The course of the disease can be influenced by non-surgical interventions, such as ASMs, but these may also have deleterious effects on cognition. It is interesting, though, that in neuropsychological testing of newly diagnosed patient's cognitive difficulties were often found *before* starting any form of treatment.[7]

The region of the pathology will often dictate the symptoms and the type of cognitive impairment. There are mechanistic explanations for these differences, which can even be elucidated at the cellular and biochemical level, and this will be discussed in greater detail in the next section ('Mechanisms for the impact'), but it is useful to understand the gross regional anatomy initially. Pathology of the temporal lobe, especially the mesial temporal structures, will damage the learning and consolidation of new material. Damage to the hippocampus and the anatomically related perirhinal cortex, as may occur in neonatal anoxia, will have a significant effect on the memory network and therefore people with temporal lobe epilepsy (TLE) are very likely to have abnormal memory function. Three distinct phenotypes of cognitive impairment were identified by Hermann and colleagues.[8] Almost half of the people with TLE (47%) were minimally impaired, 24% were impaired on memory measures, and the remaining

29% were impaired on a broader range of tasks including measures of memory, executive functions, and processing speed. These deficits were reflected in decreasing volume abnormalities of temporal and extratemporal lobe brain structures. This finding may have important implications for the treatment of people with TLE, especially the use of counselling, as cognition may further decline as time passes.

Frontal lobe pathology (epilepsy) presents a different picture where the problem is the temporal ordering of events and confabulation may be used to fill the gaps. Neuropsychological studies[9] found both TLE and frontal lobe epilepsy groups to be significantly impaired on memory tasks but both groups had executive functioning within normal limits (which was surprising for frontal lobe epilepsy). Impaired use of language was common to both groups.

The aetiology of a lesion also plays an important role in cognitive disturbance and this is almost certainly related to the early plasticity of cerebral functioning. Early developmental lesions are usually associated with little cognitive disturbance whereas fast-growing tumours in the adult brain can have a significant effect on cognitive function.

Other, more variable factors can also have a significant effect on cognitive function, especially memory, and the most significant of these is seizure control with seizure clusters causing reduced memory function and attention span although this is usually temporary.

Recent research has also revealed the significance of interictal discharges (IDs),[10] which may have deleterious effects on memory and cognition. Therefore, there is compelling evidence that IDs adversely influence ongoing cognitive processes. This effect is location specific in the sense that the function that is altered is the one supported by the structure where IDs occur. Thus, cortical neural systems of information processing can be disrupted at the time of the ID. Hippocampal IDs also affect cognitive processes. Using intracranial recordings in temporal lobe epilepsy, examining patient and animal models, Kleen et al.[11,12] showed that IDs significantly affect the recall of information in working memory when the ID event was at the precise time that information needed to be recalled from memory.

The relatively common epilepsy comorbidities of depression and anxiety will also reduce learning capacity and recall and this will complicate the picture and can be additive to poor seizure control. More than one-third of the variance in the self-perception of memory disturbance is the result of psychological factors.[13] Poor seizure control in epilepsy will affect cognition and memory: the poorer the control, the greater the deficit. Focal seizures appear to have the least effect. Generalized seizures with drop attacks (potentially causing head injury) and status epilepticus will have the most deleterious effects (with status epilepticus most harmful). The rate of age-related decline of cognitive function is not the same as that observed in the normal population[14] and people with epilepsy potentially start their decline from a lower level (perhaps because of the accumulation of beta amyloid) and will consequently become impaired at an earlier age, although sex and the location of the pathology will also play a part[15] (see Chapter 10).

Mechanisms for the impact

Effective control of seizures may well have an impact on cognition and as a general rule the cognitive problems usually increase with the increasing dose of medication and the number of different medications prescribed. Surgery (especially to the hippocampus) does not always mean postoperative decline in memory function,[16] with only one-third of patients experiencing a significant decline in memory and most remaining unchanged or even improved (20%) possibly due to the removal of the epileptogenic zone and elimination of subclinical seizure activity.

Potentially, the most deleterious outcome of surgery is a postoperative deterioration in memory and ongoing seizures. This may incur a lifetime risk of developing an amnestic syndrome and there have been a number of case studies where this has been the unfortunate outcome.[17] (The 'amnestic syndrome' is characterized by disorientation, particularly in time, impairment of immediate recall, loss of recent memory, retroactive memory loss of varying extent, and a tendency to confabulation.) The risk of developing amnestic syndrome following temporal lobe surgery is increased if the contralateral temporal lobe hippocampal structures become damaged following an episode of seizure clusters or status epilepticus.[17]

It is worth mentioning here the index case, patient HM, who underwent resective surgery of both hippocampi and some of the surrounding cortex of the temporal lobes in 1953 for drug-resistant (pharmacoresistant) epilepsy and thereafter suffered significant problems with his 'declarative' or 'explicit' long-term memory for facts and events. He had little problem with his 'non-declarative' or 'implicit' long-term memory for habits and skills, the storage of which is not principally within the temporal lobe. This patient was extensively studied, lived until 82 years of age, and gave neuroscientists major insights into the anatomical sites of specific types of memory storage.

Medication, which may be effective in controlling seizures, may also affect cognition. As a general rule, cognitive problems increase with increasing doses of medication and the number of different medications used, but the picture is far from clear and there is even some evidence of improved cognition with certain AEDs.[18] This is explored in more detail in Chapters 3 and 5, but in summary the older agents such as phenobarbital appear to have the greatest cognitive toxic potential, carbamazepine can sometimes impair motor speed, and phenytoin can impair visually guided motor functions. Based on the evidence reviewed,[18] levetiracetam and lamotrigine are the agents least likely to interfere with cognitive processes and levetiracetam may even have beneficial cognitive effects although it is difficult to disentangle these positive effects from simply better seizure control.

Mitigation strategies for minimizing the impact

One of the most important factors for minimizing the impact of epilepsy on study, learning, and memory is seizure control. Seizures will always disturb and potentially damage the cerebral network and reduce the quality of life of the individual. This will have an impact on work, relationships, learning, study, memory, and personal confidence. The aim for all clinicians treating epilepsy is to achieve good seizure control without significant medication side effects. This will always be challenging, but the range and specificity of ASMs has improved considerably since the introduction of phenobarbital in 1912—a medication which remains on the World Health Organization's 'Essential Medicines' list. It is also the least expensive anticonvulsant and is commonly used in Africa and many other areas of the world where cost is an important consideration. Achieving a balance of medication type, a minimum dosage to be effective, and minimization of side effects is the aim and monotherapy is always the best option. This though is not always possible and additional medication is added incrementally until the desired optimal result is achieved. Good seizure control is usually possible in around two-thirds of patients but one-third will remain pharmacoresistant and other strategies need to be considered to improve the quality of life. Multiple medications increase the risk of side effects, but with more complex regimens, medications may be forgotten and therefore adherence becomes an additional consideration. Medication choice is important for a number of reasons as all ASMs will affect the cerebral network to some extent (which is of course their purpose), but their individual effects on memory, study, and learning will be different.[16] This was briefly discussed in the preceding section with reference to a useful study by Eddy et al.[18] ('The cognitive impact of antiepileptic drugs') and the side effects of the drug, especially on cognition and memory, which need to be taken into account. Seizure control, though, generally *outweighs* all other considerations, even at the expense of using more than one anticonvulsant.

The choice of effective ASM has increased considerably since the early 1900s and the two most commonly prescribed anticonvulsant medications in hospital practice nowadays (levetiracetam and lamotrigine) have very favourable cognitive profiles.

Aldenkamp et al.[19] have usefully described a number of specific learning difficulties and associated these in part with anatomical sites and these are described below with some further explanation where appropriate:

- *Memory deficit*, which is associated with temporal lobe pathology and dysfunction, where short-term memory and memory span may be impaired.
- *Attentional deficit*, which can cause global academic difficulty and is often associated with primary generalized epilepsy and a higher frequency of tonic–clonic seizures.
- *Speed factor deficit*, where there is a slowing of information processing, especially when performing complex tasks, and is particularly demonstrated when undertaking mathematical activities.
- *Problem-solving deficit*, where there may be a disturbance of higher cognitive processing. This will potentially affect concept formation, decision-making, and verbal reasoning.

Summary and conclusions

Many authors describe the overall problem of cognitive deficit as 'the epilepsy factor' irrespective of the type of seizure. This may be a function of reduced alertness and reduced sustained attention but such a broad term is not particularly helpful. The above-mentioned characteristics may well be related to overall seizure control and therefore the medication regimen and what other measures have been taken to improve the clinical situation for that individual need to be considered. The introduction of non-medication interventions (such as surgery or vagus nerve stimulation) and/or an improved medication choice may be critical here and that will depend very much on the seizure type and its suspected or confirmed aetiology.

The narrative in this chapter and the many references to recent research have given a number of workable strategies for mitigating epilepsy from significantly disturbing the learning and memory requirements (or process) for study at any educational level. It is essential therefore that the very best mitigational opportunities are offered to the patient at the earliest possible time. Below I have constructed a checklist of what needs to be offered to ensure that an individual will achieve their estimated full potential. Although certain special, but usually available, resources are required, at a potentially increased cost to the health services, the longer-term savings to both health and social care will almost certainly outweigh this initial investment, although funding may still be a challenge.

Checklist for optimizing the learning, study, memory, and professional qualification opportunities for people with epilepsy

1. Above all other considerations, seizures are the most important single symptom to eliminate or mostly control, if at all possible. Even between seizures unwanted electrical activity may still occur in the form of IDs and these also can be controlled by a number of strategies, the most common of which is medication. Seizure control is therefore a major therapeutic aim as nothing is more disruptive and damaging to the cerebral network and the life of the individual than uncontrolled seizures.

2. Early intervention by a multidisciplinary epilepsy team is essential as this will allow the very earliest of clinical management interventions and the early recognition of poor epilepsy control; medication side effects; and changes in, or a steady deterioration of, behaviour, cognition, and academic performance. This strategy will be enhanced by the engagement of an expert in the comorbidities of epilepsy, working closely with the whole epilepsy service and especially the epilepsy specialist nurses.

3. Linking all the services together for the benefit of the individual from childhood, through the school years, and into tertiary education will optimize the person's potential and ensure that any deterioration of attainment is recognized early and explored. The specialist nurse team is best positioned to liaise with the educational facility (school, college, or university) and will also be able to provide specialist training on emergency care. This 'out-of-hospital' relationship of the nurse team will ensure that behavioural changes and variable performance are not overlooked and the person is quickly referred back to the epileptologist when necessary.

4. Fast track and easy access to clinical psychology and specialist psychiatric services are essential. It is well known that there is a reciprocal relationship between epilepsy and certain psychological disorders, and some may well predate the onset of epilepsy. This relationship is still being explored but it is clear that the psychological impact of epilepsy must never be neglected and special psychological care and support needs to be introduced at the earliest opportunity. This I found to my detriment some years ago when asked to give advice on a final year medical student who had suffered a seizure during clinical duties. A brief synopsis of the case history and the lesson I learnt is provided.

Case history

A very sad outcome and lesson learnt

Almost 20 years ago, I was asked by a teaching hospital trust to advise on a medical student in her final year who had suffered a primary generalized seizure while working and learning on a clinical ward. I arranged to see her in my Occupational Health clinic and in the meantime a colleague in the 'first fit clinic' saw her without delay. She was undergoing the usual battery of investigations and still attending clinical teaching, but suffered a further seizure when she was an observer in the operating theatre and this caused considerable disruption to the proceedings.

I brought my appointment forward but took the decision to suspend her from practical clinical training for the time being. She was aware that this suspension could possibly mean the year may need to be repeated and was very upset by this decision and questioning as to whether her future medical career was potentially compromised. While waiting for her to attend my clinic I was told that she had taken her own life in the student residence. This outcome was an insurmountable and terrible tragedy for us all, especially the patient, her parents, siblings, and friends.

The lesson I learnt and the mistake I will never make again

The seizure events were such a potentially significant threat to this student's career that I should have seen her without delay and out of clinic. I better understand how an individual initially contemplates the diagnosis of epilepsy, with most not appreciating that good control can be achieved in the majority and most jobs are possible and safe. We also now appreciate that psychological disturbance is often a comorbidity of the condition and can often predate the first seizure. This may well be additive to the probable acutely unsettled psychological state of the patient and may well lead to a crisis, as it did in this case. Immediate and skilled professional support was required but was delayed. The assessment was urgent and needed immediate attention!

This chapter though needs to be completed on an optimistic note and exploring the wealth of literature on study, learning, and memory points to three imperative strategies that need to be addressed to optimize the best outcome for people with epilepsy. These I have listed in order of priority:

1. The best seizure control possible using the lowest dose of medication and the minimum number of ASMs to achieve optimal control.

2. Continuing neurological and psychological support for the person with epilepsy, examining seizure control, educational progress, and changes in psychological state. This can be a mixture of specialist nurse, neuropsychologist, and epileptologist input.

3. An exploration of non-drug treatment strategies with an assessment for neurosurgery, especially with lesions in the temporal lobe where there has been considerable progress and many excellent outcomes.

The evidence for these three strategies has been explored in some depth within the preceding text and, in my view, should always be implemented by a multidisciplinary team for the best possible patient outcome.

References

1. **Baxendale S.** Epilepsy: cognition and memory in adults. In: **Shorvon S, Guerrini R, Cook M, Lhatoo S,** eds. Oxford textbook of epilepsy and epileptic seizures. Oxford: Oxford University Press; 2013:367–74.

2. **Rayner G, Wrench JM, Wilson SJ.** Differential contributions of objective memory and mood to subjective memory complaints in refractory epilepsy. Epilepsy Behav. 2010;**19**(3):359–64.

3. **Hall KE, Isaac CL, Harris P.** Memory complaints in epilepsy: an acute reflection of memory impairment or an indicator of poor adjustment? A review of the literature. Clin Psychol Rev. 2009;**29**(4):354–67.

4. **Zeman A, Butler C,** Transient epileptic amnesia. Curr Opin Neurol. 2010;**23**(6):610–16.

5. **Berg AT, Langfitt FM, Testa SR,** et al. Global cognitive function in children with epilepsy: a community based study. Epilepsia. 2008;**49**(4):608–14.

6. **Wo SW, Ong LC, Low WY, Lai PSM.** The impact of epilepsy on academic achievement in children with normal intelligence and without major comorbidities: a systematic review. Epilepsy Res. 2017;**136**:35–45.

7. **Taylor J, Kolamunnage-Dona, Marson AG, Smith PE, Aldencamp AP, Baker KA.** Patients with epilepsy: cognitively compromised before the start of antiepileptic drug treatment? Epilepsia. 2010;**51**(1):48–56.

8. **Hermann B, Seienberg M, Lee EJ, Chan F, Rutecki P.** Cognitive phenotypes in temporal lobe epilepsy. J Int Neuropsychol Soc. 2007;**13**(1):12–20.

9. **Cahn-Weiner DA, Wittenberg D, McDonald C.** Everyday cognition in temporal lobe and frontal lobe epilepsy. Epileptic Disord. 2009:**11**(3):222–27.

10. **Lenck-Santini PP, Scott RR.** Mechanisms responsible for cognitive impairment in epilepsy. Cold Spring Harb Perspect Med. 2015;**5**(10):a022772.

11. **Kleen JK, Scott RC, Holmes GL, Lenck-Santini PP.** Hippocampal interictal spikes disrupt cognition in rats. Ann Neurol. 2010;**67**(2):250–57.

12. **Kleen JK, Scott RC, Holmes GL,** et al. Hippocampal interictal epileptiform activity disrupts cognition in humans. Neurology. 2013;**81**(1):18–24.

13. **Salas-Puig J, Gil-Nagel A, Serratosa JM,** et al. Self-reported memory problems in everyday activities in patients with epilepsy treated with antiepileptic drugs. Epilepsy Behav. 2009;**14**(4):622–27.

14. **Romoli M, Sen A, Parnetti L,** et al. Amyloid-β: a potential link between epilepsy and cognitive decline. Nat Rev Neurol. 2021;**17**(8):469–85.

15. **Baxendale S, Heaney D, Thompson PJ, Duncan JS.** Cognitive consequences of childhood onset temporal lobe epilepsy across the adult lifespan. Neurology. 2010;**75**(8):705–11.

16. **Baxendale S, Thompson PJ, Duncan JS.** Improvements in memory function following anterior temporal lobe resection for epilepsy. Neurology. 2008;**71**(17):1319–25.

17. **Dietl T, Urbach H, Helmstaedter C,** et al. Persistent severe amnesia due to seizure recurrence after unilateral temporal lobectomy. Epilepsy Behav. 2004;**5**(3):394–400.

18. **Eddy CM, Rickards HE, Cavanna AE.** The cognitive impact of antiepileptic drugs. Ther Adv Neurol Disord. 2011;**4**(6):385–407.

19. **Aldenkamp AP, Weber B, Overweg-Plandsoen WC, Reijs R, Mil S.** Educational underachievement in children with epilepsy: a model to predict the effects of epilepsy on educational achievement. J Child Neurol. 2005;**20**(3):175–80.

Chapter 13

Epilepsy, employment, and work

Ian Brown

Introduction

Individuals with epilepsy are more than twice as likely to be unemployed, especially in areas of relatively high unemployment.[1] This situation has been recorded for at least 60 years and of all occupationally related health disorders 'unemployment' is possibly the most chronically damaging. Unemployment itself causes poor health and health inequalities, and this effect is still seen after adjustment for social class, poverty, age, and pre-existing morbidity. A person signed off work for 6 months has only a 50% chance of ever returning to employment.[2]

Considerable research has been undertaken on the employment of people with epilepsy and caution needs to be exercised when considering the data, as within the employment statistics there are a number of distinct categories where the prospects for long-term employment are much better than the overall blanket unemployment rate. Analysis within that variability allows for a much better understanding of the obstacles to employment and how many of these can be overcome. This will be the starting point for this chapter as an understanding of both intrinsic and extrinsic factors that can possibly be changed will offer the person with epilepsy a much greater chance of finding and keeping work, which represents an integral and important part of normal everyday life. Before this though, it is worth stating a few generalizations about the employment of individuals with epilepsy and variations throughout the globe.

The unemployment rate for people with epilepsy is two to three times that of the general population in the US. For those with uncontrolled seizure disorders, it may be as high as 50%. Furthermore, people with epilepsy who are gainfully employed tend to be effectively underemployed (less engaged than they would wish to be) or earn less than people who do not have epilepsy.[3] In the UK, the unemployment risk for people with epilepsy was roughly double for men and treble for women in a UK community study.[4] In the US, the unemployment prevalence was approximately five times that of the general US population[5] which contrasted significantly with Sweden, where the unemployment rates among people with epilepsy were hardly different to those of the population as a whole.[6]

These very contrasting figures perhaps give an indication of sociocultural differences, but studies that look at employment of people with epilepsy as an undifferentiated group will not give an indication of the excellent employment outcomes for people with well-controlled epilepsy, who are the majority.[7] The study outcomes of Jacoby[7] revealed similar employment rates as those of the general UK population. This result is mirrored in a number of other national studies where a major problem within poor employment prospects is (unsurprisingly) poorly controlled seizures—one of a number of obstacles influencing the employment of people with epilepsy.

A 2009 UK study on early epilepsy[8] throws more light on the situation. Employability was predicted by greater seizure frequency and poor personal health. Also, those in work at the start of the study tended to remain so, and similarly, those unemployed did not find work, which indicates a stagnation of mobility within the labour market. Employability is particularly poor for those long-term followed cohorts with childhood-onset epilepsy, with a seven-fold risk of unemployment compared to controls[9] and a significantly reduced earning potential.[10]

The factors that influence the employability of people with epilepsy

A most useful framework of the factors that could influence employment has been devised by Craig and Oxley[11] and they have suggested a broad dividing classification of 'intrinsic' and 'extrinsic' factors, further subdivided into 'covert' and 'overt' factors. This has been reproduced here in a modified form (with permission from Oxford University Press).

Covert extrinsic	Covert intrinsic
Attitude of employers	Fear of discrimination
Attitude of co-workers	Impaired self-image
Low expectations of significant others	Low personal expectations
Overt extrinsic	**Overt intrinsic**
Statutory employment limitations	Poor seizure control
Driving regulations	Cognitive impairment
	Low educational achievement

Covert extrinsic—the attitude of employers and the attitude of co-workers

Epilepsy has always been associated with stigma and there have been many studies that also give indications of attitudinal and institutional discrimination. A UK study[12] revealed that 84% of employers questioned stated that jobs existed in their organization suitable for a person with epilepsy, but only a quarter of these employers had ever knowingly employed a person with the disorder. A fifth of the employers thought that epilepsy would present a major employment issue and that absenteeism and workplace accidents would be higher despite no substantive evidence for this assumption. It is not surprising therefore that more than 50% of people with epilepsy do not disclose the condition to their employer.[13] If the employer has the benefit of an occupational health service, then the disclosure rate is usually higher as the information remains confidential and the employer–employee relationship is accommodating rather than restrictive, but this remains an assumption as there have not been any studies on the comparative disclosure numbers.

Nomenclature of the condition is also important, and an informative study was undertaken examining the effect of three different labels: 'epilepsy', 'seizure disorder', and 'seizure condition'.[14] Employers were asked to rank the likelihood of employing a person with each of these 'conditions'. Much to the surprise of the investigators, 'epilepsy' was more favourably judged than the other labels. Perhaps this was because the employer had a better understanding of this term rather than the other terms and this study indicates that labels are important. Other countries have also considered that nomenclature is important and a recent Korean study[15] explored using the term 'cerebroelectric disorder' rather than epilepsy to examine whether this would reduce stigma and discrimination but found that it only increased the knowledge and understanding of colleagues and had no effect on stigma (or concealment of the condition). I always point out that the term 'epileptic' is to be avoided as this defines the condition *as the person* and 'a person with epilepsy 'is a much-preferred description.

There is even bias against carers who have responsibility for a person with epilepsy (not other conditions such as asthma), and this is described as 'contamination by association'.[16] Epilepsy also appears to give concern to co-workers (if they are aware of the condition—see above), and this usually boils down to a lack of understanding of the condition and a failure of any educational communication.[17] There is therefore a vicious cycle of stigma, fear, and non-disclosure and each of these feeds into the next stage in the cycle which can only be broken by an educational programme for both employees and managers. Such training is essential, but often absent, for such a relatively common condition.

Covert intrinsic—the attitude of people with epilepsy towards themselves

People with epilepsy often strongly hold certain beliefs about themselves and these are often reinforced by their employment status. Fearing injury to themselves or colleagues was a strongly held belief by the unemployed and often reinforced (even more strongly) by their family. A seminal paper by Mogil on 'empathy' explored its useful and less useful characteristics.[18] This researcher found that an empathic response was revealed in rodents as well as primates, particularly humans. Such empathy may well be comforting to the sufferer but this response can also impede and discourage certain outgoing activities in human subjects and have an adverse effect on encouraging an individual with epilepsy to 'get out and about' and specifically explore and potentially engage in the workplace.

The possibility of a seizure affecting work performance was similarly concerning for the unemployed (less so for the employed, but still significant). All the fears were greater in those presently not working and the impression that epilepsy made it more difficult to secure employment was a common response to those questioned (about one-third of people thought this). This 'self-perception' was more than ten times the actual discriminatory behaviour of employers.[19] Being in employment was therefore a 'myth-busting' exercise and remaining unemployed was reinforcing intrinsic misconceptions. This is not dissimilar to a number of other conditions that prevent an individual seeking work (back pain is a good example) with the misconception that the process of work will simply make things worse.[20]

Does well-controlled epilepsy make a difference, as there is good evidence that employment rates in epilepsy are higher than in other disabilities? A recent systematic review of the employment status of people with epilepsy revealed variable employment rates around the globe[21] although in this study the variability was multifactorial and not always related directly to seizure control. An important confounder though will be that around 50% do not disclose their condition[13] and therefore were excluded from the data. This may indicate an actual higher employment rate than the unadjusted figures, which by definition exclude the non-disclosure population.

Overt extrinsic—predominantly statutory or regulatory

An individual with a diagnosis of epilepsy can undertake the majority of jobs, but not all. The overarching legislation in the UK is the Health and Safety at Work etc. Act 1974 (HSAWA), which is regularly amended to take into account modern working practices and is intended keep everybody safe at and around the workplace. This legislation is effectively 'superior' to the disability provisions of the Equality Act 2010, which applies to the protected characteristics of a disabled person. An individual with epilepsy is protected by this Act, even when they have not suffered a seizure event for years but simply remain on continuous and regular antiseizure medication (ASM). The superiority of the HSAWA, though, means that the safety of the worker and their colleagues is of greater importance than ensuring the individual with epilepsy is employed. An employer may nonetheless be required to defend any decision they make in respect of the employment of an individual at an employment tribunal. The success rate of placing and employing people with epilepsy is far greater if they have fewer than six seizures per year, with focal aware seizures being far less disruptive than convulsive events. Periods of automatism (performance of acts without conscious will) may upset colleagues. Other disadvantageous characteristics are periods of prolonged postictal confusion and atonic and tonic seizures where the potential for injury is considerably higher.[22]

Some jobs present very special hazards and these fall into three distinct groups:

Group 1, jobs in transport—these include vocational drivers, train drivers, drivers of large container-terminal vehicles, crane drivers, aircraft pilots, and seafarers.

Group 2, jobs that involve working at unprotected heights—these include scaffolders, steeplejacks, and firefighters.

Group 3, jobs near unprotected hazards—these include work on and around mainline railways; near high-voltage electricity, hot metal, or dangerous unguarded machinery; or near large open containers of water, slurry, chemical fluids, or grains and mineral dusts.

The working environment and equipment should always be inspected by the occupational health professional and possibly the safety officer. The employee's immediate supervisor should ideally be involved in any decisions. Maintenance of confidentiality must always be observed and permission to disclose epilepsy should be sought from the employee if this would be advantageous to the extended role of the worker. Such permission is usually received, in my experience, but coercion should never occur. The objective is to have a binding agreement with the employee on what activities are allowable and what is completely restricted (there is no room for occasional permission, the employee is either safe performing an activity or they are not). Contravention of the agreement may well in turn contravene the HSAWA and should any personal injury claim result from an accident the personal liability injury insurance of the employer will almost certainly reject the claim.

Lifting of restrictions

A policy should be established for the lifting of restrictions on work practices. This policy should be made known to the affected employee and the conditions should remain unaltered unless the employee's condition changes or, for example, a change in medication regimen is introduced (see Chapter 3). As stated above, there is no place for partial lifting of restrictions as time passes—the employee is either considered safe to undertake the vast majority of activities or they are not. If a particular minor component of the individual's job can be excluded (say, driving a motor vehicle, which is not essential for most work activities), then that particular activity can be specifically excluded.

A difficult situation can arise if an employee changes medication because of possible side effects rather than poor seizure control and it is usual to extend restrictive activities for a further 6 months broadly in keeping with the UK driving regulations for group 1 vehicles (see Chapter 14). Similarly, if an employee wishes to withdraw from medication completely then the guidelines are the same as above. The complication here is that the medication needs to be withdrawn very slowly indeed, usually over a 3-month period. If you then add a further 6 months following full withdrawal, the total restriction period becomes 9 months.

Regardless of the situation, a review date for the withdrawal of restrictions should always be offered, as this will affirm that the employee is still an important part of the workforce and their condition and working practices are being taken very seriously. As a general rule, the UK Department of Transport recommends a restriction of 6 months from driving after a single seizure (unless there is a high risk of seizure recurrence). If the annual risk of recurrence is deemed greater than 20% (high risk in this context) or there has been more than one seizure, a 1-year driving ban is applied. Recurrence rates after a first seizure vary considerably but the risk of recurrence decreases as time elapses after the index initial seizure if there are no further seizures. This is a factor of great importance when considering safety to drive and safety at work where driving may be an important component of the job (see Chapter 14). In the National General Practice study of Epilepsy (in which only 15% of first-seizure patients received any treatment), the 3-year risk of recurrence after a seizure-free period of 6 months was 44%, after a 12-month seizure-free period the recurrence risk was 32%, and after 18 months of freedom from seizures the risk fell to 17% (Figure 13.1).

In addition, randomized studies have shown that the risk of recurrence after a first seizure is reduced by ASM treatment.[21-23] People started on treatment after a first seizure though are no more likely to achieve remission than

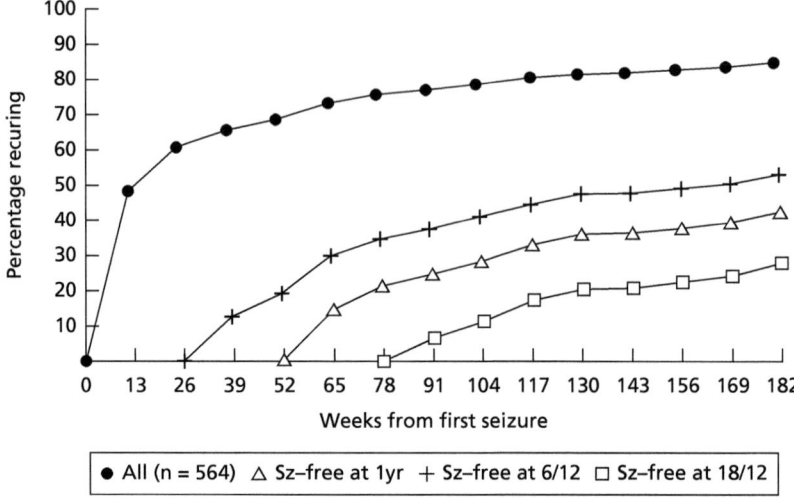

Figure 13.1 Actuarial percentage recurrence rates after a first seizure for those still free of recurrence at 6, 12, and 18 months, and for all patients. Sz, seizure.
Reproduced with permission from Hart, YM et al. National General Practice Study of Epilepsy: recurrence after a first seizure. Lancet. 336(8726), 1272–4. Copyright 1990 Elsevier.

patients where treatment is delayed until after two or more seizures and the MESS study[25] demonstrated that there is little benefit in the immediate treatment of patients at low risk of seizure recurrence (a single-seizure, normal electroencephalogram, and no other neurological comorbidity). A further analysis of the multicentre study of early epilepsy and single seizures[26] concluded that at 6 months after the initial index seizure, for those taking ASMs, the risk of recurrence in the next 12 months was 14% (95% confidence interval (CI) 10–18%) as opposed to those who did not start ASMs, where the 12-month recurrence risk was 18% (95% CI 13–23%). These results and data resulted in a change to the UK Driver and Vehicle Licensing Agency driving restrictions applied after a first seizure.

Overt intrinsic—poor seizure control, cognitive impairment, and low educational achievements

Poor seizure control is possibly the most significant and disturbing overt intrinsic complication of epilepsy, although problems with cognition and mood are also important. The earliest definition and description of epilepsy by the great English neurologist John Hughlings Jackson (1873) stated that 'Epilepsy is the name for occasional, sudden, excessive, rapid, and local discharge of grey matter'[27] and the major problem for all activities, especially work and driving, is the word *sudden*. There is often little or no warning of the event and it is this unpredictability and suddenness that causes many difficulties. The individual may not be able to ensure that they are in a place of safety and from this follows an increase in accident rate and the possibility of mortality (see Chapter 9). The causes of Sudden Unexpected Death in Epilepsy (SUDEP) remain speculative, but are probably related to cardiac, respiratory, or cerebral factors and are far more common in refractory epilepsy.[28] People with epilepsy were 71% more likely to have accidents than a comparable population without the condition.[29] Good seizure control is therefore critical for an uncomplicated and safe working life but this is sometimes not achievable and the individual who still wishes to work may need a more sheltered and protective working environment such as that offered by Remploy[30] in the UK or similar employers in many other countries. The objective of ASMs is to control seizures without significant adverse effects, and in most people this is achievable. For others and those requiring more than one ASM this can be more challenging, and a balance must be achieved between seizure frequency and potential adverse effects. Acute adverse effects are rapidly reversible on drug withdrawal or dose reduction but slowly evolving chronic adverse effects are more difficult and it is often a challenge to disentangle the possible ASM side effects from psychological problems (common in epilepsy; see Chapter 6) and the consequences of the seizures themselves.[31]

Cognitive impairment will adversely affect individuals at the workplace and the effects of ASMs have been examined in this context. There have been a number of studies[32] and this is discussed in greater detail in Chapter 5, but as a generalization, adverse cognitive effects increase with the number of ASMs prescribed and the higher the dose of any individual ASM. The greatest cognitive impairment occurs with phenobarbital. Some of the more recently introduced antiepileptic drugs, such as levetiracetam, have a better cognitive profile although none are without side effects.

People with epilepsy have overall lower educational achievements and the reasons for this are multifactorial. This, though, affects their employment and competitiveness in the job market. The prevalence of epilepsy in adults with learning disability is between 16% and 26% compared with 0.4–1% of the general population[33] (see Chapter 7). The risk of epilepsy increases with increasing learning disability severity and the prevalence of epilepsy increases as the IQ decreases.[34] These statistics do make a connection between learning disability and epilepsy but it is equally important to explore the association between epilepsy and evolving cognitive impairment, which may not have been present before the onset of the condition. There is also a generational effect with evidence of compromise to educational attainment of children born to mothers with epilepsy, which has been associated with *in utero* exposure to antiseizure medications and sodium valproate in particular. A significant decrease in attainment in national educational tests was, for example, found for 7-year-old children who had been exposed to valproate *in utero* compared with both a matched control group and the all-Wales national average.[35] These results give support to the cognitive and developmental effects of *in utero* exposure to sodium valproate as well as certain other ASMs and a balance needs to be achieved between effective seizure control in pregnancy and any cognitive impairment that may occur in the developing fetus.

Cognitive and behavioural impairment is also commonly found in children with epilepsy and this was studied in detail in the CHESS study.[36] The children studied were aged between 4 and 16 years and the results were striking. There were significant problems with academic progress, 40% functioning in the learning disabled range, memory underachievement in 58% in at least one of the four memory tests, 42% underachieving in processing speeds, a high level of underachievement in mathematics and sentence comprehension, and 60% met the criteria for a behavioural or developmental coordination disorder. If such problems continue into adulthood, then the young person's competitiveness in the workplace will be seriously impaired.

It is particularly important to consider what is described as 'state-dependent learning disability', which can seriously impair an individual in the job market yet is reversible. The most common culprits are medication and/or seizures and the first responsibility of the physician is to recognize the condition is occurring and attempt to clinically intervene. Failure to do this will leave the individual with a potentially correctable cognitive problem that will affect their lifestyle and potential employment prospects thereafter. Perhaps the final word on this important facet of employment should come from a recent study[37] which showed that people with epilepsy were significantly more likely to abandon formal education after primary (n = 6; 2.4% compared to none in controls) or secondary school (n = 69; 31.1% compared with controls n = 58; 26.1%). They were also less likely to be currently employed (n = 103; 46.4%) compared with the older same-sex siblings (employed: n = 148; 66.7%; p = 0.0001). In conclusion and notwithstanding the influence of a number of socioeconomic and epilepsy-related variables, childhood-onset epilepsy, particularly if seizures do not rapidly come under control, stands apart in exerting a huge negative impact on educational achievement and employability in adulthood.

The prevention of seizures and epilepsy associated with exposure to risk within the workplace

This really falls into primary and secondary prevention. The avoidance of a serious head injury is of paramount importance. The risk of post-traumatic epilepsy is much higher if the injury is associated with a depressed skull fracture, loss of consciousness, amnesia for more than 24 hours, a dural tear, intracranial haematoma, and/or focal neurological signs. Safety helmets (hard hats) are mandatory on building sites. Under the Personal Protective Equipment Regulations 1992 (UK legislation), employers have to provide workers with a hard hat and the Act also ensures employees are required to wear a hard hat on site where there is a risk of head injuries. This extends to visitors too. Where there are risks of heavy objects falling from a height, a strong netting barrier can be erected beneath the place of work to catch a heavy spanner, wrench, or drill as prevention of a 'striking' injury is much more effective than the personal protective hard hat. A large community study[38] confirmed the findings of a number of earlier studies that the severity of the head injury will dictate the risks of epilepsy over the next decade (standardized incidence ratio 17.0, 95% CI 12.3–23.6). Because of this risk, people with severe head injury are treated similarly to those who have already suffered a seizure, including a 6–12-month driving ban. The risk of post-traumatic epilepsy though is not reduced by the early use of medication although ASMs can reduce the frequency of early seizures.[39]

Shift work

This is now a very common component of working life, especially for the emergency services and where workers are involved in the maintenance of processes or responsibilities that run continuously throughout 24 hours. Does shift work increase the risk of seizure frequency in a well-controlled patient? Studies have been few as people with epilepsy may opt out of shift work[40] although in the experience of the author, many people with well-controlled epilepsy can work on rotating shifts without problems as long as they are well organized and compliant with their medication. Night work is an exception as night workers sleep for shorter periods during their working week and sleep longer on rest days to make up the deficit. Sleep deprivation, even relative sleep deprivation, is an important precipitant of seizures as it causes cortical excitability and is best avoided in all epilepsies, but in particular in those with idiopathic generalized epilepsy.[41]

Stress

People with epilepsy and employers often ask if stress could be a precipitant of seizures. We know that changes in brain arousal, especially excitability, will play a part in affecting neuronal discharge and this may be significant around an epileptic focus.[42,43] Affected individuals often self-report that stress has adversely played a part in their seizure control but this observation may be confounded by other, potentially interrelated seizure-provoking factors such as poor sleep quality and an increase in alcohol consumption. Endogenous stress mediators such as neurosteroids will also contribute to this phenomenon.[43]

Photosensitivity and visual display equipment

Photosensitive epilepsy is a type of reflex epilepsy that can have an impact on the workplace and should be considered where a light source flickers. It has a prevalence of 1 in 10,000 and affects 3 in every 100 people with epilepsy. Photosensitivity is usually recognized before 25 years of age and is more common in women. Photosensitive epilepsy is mostly an age-related, time-limited condition, and is closely associated with juvenile myoclonic epilepsy.[44] Spontaneous seizures may also occur in photosensitive subjects. The diagnosis is supported by performing an electroencephalogram with photic stimulation and eliciting a photoparoxysmal response, which is usually a generalized discharge of spike wave activity that persists until the stimulus ceases. Modern televisions and other display screen equipment (used in virtually every workplace) now present minimal risk to the photosensitive subject because the screens no longer flicker at a rate that can induce seizures.

A flickering source of light does, however, present a seizure-precipitating risk and this may be faulty artificial light in a workplace which should be promptly replaced. Sunlight dappling through the leaves of a tree, light falling between helicopter rotor blades or propellers (the Civil Aviation Authority test for this), light off a rippling water surface, and, as observed in one of the people I have seen, walking quickly past railings with the sun behind can all trigger a photosensitive response. Advising people with photosensitivity to cover one eye when exposed to a potentially photosensitive stimulus can be helpful, as can screen guards on certain flickering screens.

Summary and personal reflections

I have written about epilepsy and employment for more than 30 years[45] and have found an increasing body of clinical research and evidence providing a solid basis for risk assessment in those who wish to work and drive a motor vehicle, perhaps as part of their employment or simply to get to work. The majority of employees with epilepsy maintain excellent seizure control but about 35% have less good control, usually taking a number of ASMs and with more challenging employment prospects. Around half of all people with epilepsy do not disclose the diagnosis to their employer and I can underst and the reluctance because of potential discrimination and stigma (one employee who disclosed her condition to her employer discovered on returning to work after a seizure that the walls of her office had been covered with posters on what to do if an employee has a seizure at work!). Non-disclosure is fine in some circumstances (well-controlled epilepsy) but the employee must not breech the provisions of the HSAWA in the UK or any other national statutory prevailing legislation in all the work-related activities they undertake.

I remain optimistic though, with more effective medication, the possibility of increasingly innovative surgical intervention, the outstanding epilepsy medical services in many countries, and even some evidence of changing attitudes among a number of employers.

Epilepsy is a very common chronic condition and there is still a long way to go in establishing best work and employment practices but I have seen attitudinal changes over the past 30 years in many areas of the globe. Fear, stigma, and discrimination remain and there is considerably more work to do, especially in the education of all sectors of the wider community.

References

1. **Elwes RD, Marshall J, Beattie A, Newman PK.** Epilepsy and employment. A community based survey in an area of high unemployment. J Neurol Neurosurg Psychiatry. 1991;**54**(3):200–203.

2. **Aylward M, Cohen DA, Sawney PE.** Support, rehabilitation and interventions in restoring fitness for work. In: **Palmer K, Brown I, Hobson J,** eds. Fitness for work. Oxford: Oxford University Press; 2013:69–87.

3. American Epilepsy Society. Available at: https://aesnet.org/

4. **Jacoby A, Buck D, Baker G, McNamee P, Graham-Jones S, Chadwick D.** Uptake and costs of care for epilepsy: findings from a UK regional study. Epilepsia. 1998;**39**(7):776–86.

5. **Fisher RS.** Epilepsy from the patient's perspective: review of the results from a community-based survey. Epilepsy Behav. 2001;**1**(4):S9–14.

6. **Chaplin JE, Wester A, Tomson T.** Factors associated with the employment problems of people with established epilepsy. Seizure. 1998;**7**:299–303.

7. **Jacoby A.** Impact of epilepsy on employment status: findings from a UK study of people with well-controlled epilepsy. Epilepsy Res. 1995;**21**(2):125–32.

8. **Holland P, Lane S, Whitehead M, Marson AG, Jacoby A.** Labour market participation following onset of seizures and early epilepsy: findings from a UK cohort. Epilepsia. 2009;**50**(5):1030–39.

9. Jalava M, Sillanpaa M, Camfield C, Camfield P. Social adjustment and competence 35 years after the onset of childhood epilepsy: a prospective controlled study. Epilepsia. 1997;**38**(6):708–15.

10. Wadsworth MEJ. MRC National Survey of Health & Development. Paper presented at a symposium of the International Bureau for Epilepsy 2nd Commission on Epilepsy Risks and Insurability, 24th International Epilepsy Congress, Buenos Aires, 2001.

11. Craig A, Oxley J. Social aspects of epilepsy. In: Laidlaw J, Richens A, Oxley J, eds. A textbook of epilepsy. Edinburgh: Churchill Livingstone; 1993:566–610.

12. Jacoby A, Gorry J, Baker GA. Employers' attitude to employment of people with epilepsy: Still the same old story? Epilepsia. 2005;**46**(12):1978–87.

13. Scambler G, Hopkins AP. Social class, epileptic activity and disadvantage at work. J Epidemiol Community Health. 1980,34(2):129–33.

14. Bishop M, Stenhoff BD, Bradley KD, Allen CA. The differential effect of epilepsy labels on employer perceptions: report of a pilot study. Epilepsy Behav. 2007;**11**(3):351–56.

15. Lee SA, Han SH, Cho YJ, Kim JE. Does the Korean term for epilepsy reduce the stigma for Korean adults with epilepsy? Epilepsy Behav. 2020;**102**:106719.

16. Parfene C, Stewart TL, King TZ. Epilepsy stigma and stigma by association in the workplace. Epilepy Behav. 2009;**15**(4):461–66.

17. Brown I, Prevett M. Epilepsy. In: Palmer K, Brown I, Hobson J, eds. Fitness for work, 5th ed. Oxford: Oxford University Press; 2013:155–73.

18. Mogil JS. Social modulation of and by pain in humans and rodents. Pain. 2015;**156**(Suppl):S35–41.

19. Jacoby A. Epilepsy and the quality of everyday life: findings from a study of people with well-controlled epilepsy. Soc Sci Med. 1992;**34**(6):657–66.

20. Palmer KT, Greenough C. Spinal disorders. In: Palmer K, Brown I, Hobson J, eds. Fitness for work, 5th ed. Oxford: Oxford University Press; 2013:207–32.

21. Wo MC, Lim KS, Choo WY, Tan CT. Employability in people with epilepsy: a systematic review. Epilepsy Res. 2015;**116**:67–78.

22. Bishop M. Determinants of employment status among a community-based sample of people with epilepsy: implications for rehabilitation interventions. Rehabil Counselling Bull. 2004;**47**(2):112–21.

23. First Seizure Trial Group. Randomised clinical trial on the efficacy of antiepileptic drugs in reducing the risk of relapse after a first unprovoked tonic-clonic seizure. Neurology. 1993;**43**(3 Pt 1):478–83.

24. Marson A, Jacoby A, Johnson A, et al. Immediate versus deferred antiepileptic drug treatment for early epilepsy and single seizures: a randomised controlled trial. Lancet. 2005;**36**(9476):2007–13.

25. Kim LG, Johnson TL, Marson AG, Chadwick DW. Prediction of risk of seizure recurrence after a single seizure and early epilepsy: further results from the MESS trial, on behalf of the MRC MESS Study group. Lancet Neurol. 2006;**5**(4):317–22.

26. Bonnett LJ, Tudur-Smith C, Williamson PR, et al. Risk of recurrence after a first seizure and implications for driving: further analysis of the Multicentre study of Early epilepsy and Single seizures. BMJ. 2010;**341**:c6477.

27. Hughlings Jackson J. On the anatomical, physiological, and pathological investigations of epilepsies. West Riding Lunatic Asylum Med Rep. 1873;**3**:315–49.

28. **Devinsky O.** Sudden, unexpected death in epilepsy. N Engl J Med. 2011;**365**(19):1801–11.

29. **Mahler B, Carlsson S, Andersson T, Tomson T.** Risk for injuries and accidents in epilepsy; a prospective population-based cohort study. Neurology. 2018;**90**(9):e779–89.

30. **Remploy.** Available at: https://www.remploy.co.uk/

31. **Kwan P, Brodie MJ.** Neuropsychological effects of epilepsy and antiepileptic drugs. Lancet. 2001;**357**(9251):216–22.

32. **Eddy CM, Rickards HE, Cavanna AE.** The cognitive impact of antiepileptic drugs. Ther Adv Neurol Disord. 2011;**4**(6):385–407.

33. **McGrother CW, Bhaumic S, Thorp CF, Hauck A, Branford D, Watson JM.** Epilepsy in adults with intellectual disabilities: prevalence associations and service implications. Seizure. 2006;**15**(6):376–86.

34. **Fastenau PS, Shen J, Dunn DW, Austin JK.** Academic underachievement among children with epilepsy: proportion exceeding psychometric criteria for learning disability and associated risk. J Learn Disabil. 2008;**41**(3):195–207.

35. **Lacey AS, Pickrell WO, Thomas RH,** et al. Educational attainment of children born to mothers with epilepsy. J Neurol Neurosurg Psychiatry. 2018;**89**(7):736–40.

36. **Young Epilepsy.** The identification of educational problems in childhood epilepsy: the Children with Epilepsy in Sussex Schools (CHESS) study. 2014. Available at: https://www.youngepilepsy.org.uk/sites/default/files/dmdocuments/ChessReport-2014.pdf

37. **Kaur J, Paul BS, Goel P, Singh G.** Educational achievement, employment, marriage, and driving in adults with childhood-onset epilepsy. Epilepsy Behav. 2019;**97**:149–53.

38. **Annegers JF, Hauser WA, Coan SP,** et al. A population based study of seizures after traumatic brain injuries. N Engl J Med. 1998;**338**(1):20–24.

39. **Tempkin NR, Dikmen SS, Wilensky AJ,** et al. A randomised double blind study of phenytoin for the prevention of post-traumatic seizures. N Engl J Med. 1990;**323**(8):497–502.

40. **Dasgupta AK, Saunders M, Dick DJ.** Epilepsy in the British Steel Corporation: an evaluation of sickness, absence and work records. Br J Ind Med. 1982;**39**(2):146–48.

41. **Badawy RAB, Curatolo JM, Newton M, Berkovic SF, Macdonell RAF.** Sleep deprivation increases cortical excitability in epilepsy. Neurology. 2006;**67**(6):1018–22.

42. **Joels M.** Stress, the hippocampus and epilepsy. Epilepsia. 2009;**50**(4):587–97.

43. **Wang Y, Tan B, Wang Y, Chen Z.** Cholinergic signalling, neural excitability, and epilepsy. Molecules. 2021;**26**(8):22.

44. **Martins da Silva A, Leal B.** Photosensitivity and epilepsy: current concepts and perspectives—narrative review. Seizure. 2017;**50**:208–18.

45. **Brown I, Prevett M.** Epilepsy. In: **Hobson J, Smedley J,** eds. Fitness for work, 6th ed. Oxford: Oxford University Press, 2019:540–61 [and the 'Epilepsy' chapter in all previous five Oxford University Press editions, 1988–2013].

Chapter 14

Epilepsy and driving

Ernest Somerville

Introduction

In the 21st century, learning to drive has become a routine element of a young person's development. This applies not just in wealthy countries but also in low- and middle-income countries, where motorcycle riding is the norm. For older adolescents, acquisition of a driving licence is viewed as a rite of passage. In reality, it does facilitate the independence sought by young people, who are now able to go wherever and whenever they want, without being dependent on their parents for transport. There may be considerable social pressure on young people to the extent that there is some stigma attached to not possessing a driving licence. For people of working age, being able to drive may be a requirement of their job (e.g. driving to call on customers or deliver goods) or it may be necessary to be able to travel to work if public transport is unavailable at an appropriate time of day. Professional drivers, of course, are totally dependent on having a driving licence. As well as for leisure, many people depend on driving to fulfil specific social needs, such as childcare. Inability to drive may lead to social isolation, particularly in areas without public transport. In some rural areas, driving may be the only means of transport and a driving licence is essential for at least one member of the household. Studies in the US and Australia have shown that loss of the driving licence is more important to many people with epilepsy than work restrictions, lifestyle restrictions, stigma, medication side effects, and the risk of seizures.[1,2]

Driving by a person with epilepsy carries a risk that a seizure will occur, causing them to lose control of the vehicle and crash. This is usually associated with impairment of awareness, as occurs in focal impaired awareness seizures, absence seizures, generalized onset tonic–clonic seizures, and focal to bilateral tonic–clonic seizures. In focal impaired awareness seizures, people, will sometimes be able to continue driving for some distance, but in this state, they are unlikely to be able to respond to an emergency. More commonly, the individual simply stops controlling the vehicle. However, tonic contraction of the lower limbs in focal impaired awareness seizures or in the tonic phase of a tonic–clonic seizure frequently results in acceleration of the vehicle because in normal driving, the foot rests on the accelerator pedal rather than the brake pedal. This may result in a higher-velocity crash than might otherwise have occurred. The crash may also be more severe because the patient is unable to take any evasive action, such as braking. In the public discussion that often occurs in the media following seizure-related crashes, the risk to the community is often the only consideration. In fact, the risk to the person with epilepsy is far greater because of the duration of their exposure to the risk. The magnitude of the risk has been addressed in several studies, some showing a mildly elevated risk compared to the general driving community and some even showing a reduced risk, possibly due to less time spent behind the wheel.[3–5]

How to ensure safe driving in people with epilepsy

A number of approaches by government authorities have been tried.

The simplest approach is to ban driving for all people who have experienced a seizure. This has been tried in many countries and still applies in some, including India and China. The disadvantages are that many people with epilepsy who are safe to drive, are unnecessarily prevented from doing so. Furthermore, if a driver with epilepsy knows that divulging their diagnosis will result in a lifetime driving ban, they are less likely to accurately report seizures to their doctor. This impedes optimal seizure control, resulting in a paradoxical increase in the risk of a seizure-related crash. The most widely adopted approach is one of harm minimization, in which the community accepts that allowing people to drive who have had seizures will result in some seizure-related crashes but that if that risk can be kept to an acceptable level, allowing people to drive whose risk falls at or below that level, will result in the greatest reduction in risk to the community (and to drivers with seizures). This is the same approach widely employed to manage the risk of alcohol-related crashes. The community accepts that the very slight increase in risk posed by drivers with a blood alcohol concentration of 0.05% is acceptable.

This strategy can be implemented in several ways. In some jurisdictions, individual risk assessment by the driver licensing authority is performed,[6] while in others, the treating doctor or a government-appointed doctor is the decision-maker.[7] Another approach is to develop a set of criteria or standards that a person with seizures must meet before they may drive. This last method forms the basis of the European Union (EU) driving laws[8] and will be discussed in some detail.

If such a system is to be employed, the level of risk that might be acceptable to the community needs to be determined and then, a set of standards needs to be drawn up to identify drivers whose risk falls at or below that level. Both of these tasks are challenging.

Acceptable risk

What is acceptable as a statistical measure applying to an entire community may be completely unacceptable to victims, their families, the media, and the courts. The approach taken by the EU has been to set the level of acceptable risk at a point comparable to or below some other risk factors for a crash.[9] Examples of factors that elevate the crash risk, but are considered acceptable and are legally permitted, include a concentration of alcohol in the blood of 0.05% or less, old age, and, especially, youth. Many such factors result in a doubling or worse of the crash risk, so the reasoning has been that if a person's risk of a crash due to a seizure is no more than double the risk of a person without seizures (i.e. a relative risk of 2), that person should be allowed to drive. The Driving Licence Committee of the EU noted that the crash risk of young drivers is far higher than double the risk of the general driving population and therefore far higher than the risk of a person whose crash risk due to a seizure is at the maximum acceptable level of twofold.[8]

To determine relative risk, the absolute risk in the non-affected population needs to be known. The crash risk of people without seizures is readily obtainable from databases maintained by driving regulators. For example, in the Australian state of New South Wales, the risk of involvement in a crash that involves the death or injury of a person or the need for a vehicle to be towed away is approximately 1% per year. The maximum acceptable crash risk in a person with seizures would therefore be double this figure (half of this risk being the background risk of all drivers and the other half being the risk of a crash being caused by a seizure). Thus, the maximum acceptable crash risk due to a seizure would be 1% per year. However, not all seizures that occur at the wheel result in a crash. This will depend on the type of seizure and the situation in which it occurs. For example, the car may be stationary at the time, or come to a stop of its own accord, the person's awareness and responsiveness may be preserved, or a passenger may be able to stop the vehicle.

The chance that a seizure occurring while driving will result in a crash is approximately 50%.[10,11] For a seizure to result in a crash, the patient must be driving at the time. If seizures are randomly distributed through the day and night, the chance that the patient will be driving at the time they have a seizure will equal the fraction of the day and night that the person spends driving. For example, if a seizure occurs in a person who drives for 1 hour every day, the chance that they will be driving when that seizure occurs is 1 in 24 (4%), whereas the chance in a person who drives for 3 hours per day will be 3 in 24 (12%). This is especially relevant for commercial drivers, who may spend almost all their work hours behind the wheel.

The driving time of private drivers is extremely variable between communities and within communities. The figure used by the EU Committee was 60 minutes per day (equating to 4%), while the figure in Australia is more like 90 minutes per day (6% of 24 hours).[12] The risk that a seizure will result in a crash is the risk that a seizure behind the wheel will result in a crash (50%) multiplied by the proportion of time spent driving (6%). This yields a figure of 3%. If each seizure carries a crash risk of 3%, and a maximum acceptable seizure-related crash risk of 1% per year is adopted, a person with a chance of having a seizure of 33% per year or less would satisfy that standard. While the EU Committee used the risk of fatal crashes in their calculations, significant but non-fatal crashes should also be considered (although one might expect that the relative risk of a fatal crash and the relative risk of a non-fatal crash would be the same, seizure-related crashes may have a greater chance of being fatal than crashes unrelated to seizures, for the reasons outlined above).

Identifying drivers with an acceptable risk

Following this reasoning, people with a seizure risk in the next 12 months of less than 30% should be allowed to drive. For some groups of people with seizures, there is sufficient published data to allow them to be confidently placed in this acceptable risk group. A large group of such people is those who have experienced a single seizure. In the early months following a single seizure, the risk of recurrence over the next 12 months greatly exceeds 30% but falls with time. Thus, it may be reasonable to allow such people to resume driving if they have not experienced a further seizure after 6 months. This has been supported by data from first-seizure database studies.[13] The ability to determine seizure risk in other groups of patients is variable and, in some situations, there are few reliable data.

The approach in Australia has been to set a 'default standard' that is satisfied by 12 months of seizure freedom (and adherence to medical advice), with 'discounts' if the patient's situation is one that carries a lower risk. These discounts include the first seizure, acute symptomatic seizures, epilepsy treated for the first time (to allow some time to optimize therapy), seizures occurring only during sleep, seizures that do not impair the ability to drive safely, single seizures occurring after long periods of seizure freedom, provoked seizures (where the provocation can be reliably avoided), and childhood seizures.[14] Auras are, perhaps surprisingly, not protective, probably because drivers may not stop immediately or they may not be in a position to stop because of traffic conditions or the aura may be of insufficient duration.[11,15] Even if a driver does manage to stop the vehicle before they experience a seizure, they could then find themselves in a confused postictal state in the driver's seat of their car and may resume driving before they have recovered sufficiently to safely control the vehicle. Many people believe their awareness is not impaired during seizures or auras, when, in fact, it is. If a person is allowed to drive despite continuing focal aware seizures, it should perhaps be only after normal responsiveness has been demonstrated through testing by a reliable observer or using driving simulators during video electroencephalography. Furthermore, there must be a low likelihood of other seizure types, and this should be demonstrated by the focal aware seizures being the sole seizure type for a sufficient potentially period of time.

Commercial driving is often even more challenging than private driving for several reasons: the financial consequences are likely to be more severe, the risk of injury and death is greater because of increased driving time, and the consequences of a crash are often more serious because of vehicle size and/or number of passengers. Most jurisdictions ban those with epilepsy from commercial driving unless they can demonstrate prolonged freedom from seizures (10 years in the EU, UK, and Australia). In the EU and UK, commercial drivers (group 2 licence holders) would also have to have taken no antiseizure medication for 10 years prior to being restored to driving. This can end the person's professional driving career.

An interesting approach suggested by a Japanese group is to limit the time that a person is allowed to drive, since the risk is proportional to the time spent at wheel[16]; however, it would be very difficult to monitor its enforcement.

Shortcomings

It is important to note that calculations such as those outlined above involve many assumptions and cannot account for the enormous variation in risk that exists between individuals (Table 14.1). This approach, though, does provide some objective theoretical basis and justification of a system that people with seizures may consider unfair and discriminatory.

No licensing system can completely eliminate the risk that seizures pose to road safety. A person may experience their first seizure while driving,[17] they may not report recurring seizures because they genuinely are unaware that they have happened,[18] they may conceal the occurrence of seizures, and they may choose not to comply with licensing regulations.[11,19]

Mandatory reporting by health professionals to licensing authorities of all persons with epilepsy has been employed in a number of jurisdictions in an attempt to prevent non-compliant individuals from driving when unsafe. However, this encourages concealment of the occurrence of seizures, which, in turn, impedes optimal treatment, resulting in a reduction, rather than an increase, in road safety.[20] Non-compliance by doctors with mandatory reporting systems may also be significant. In most jurisdictions, drivers with relevant medical conditions are legally obliged to self-report to the licensing authority.

Simplicity versus complexity

A licensing system based on one or two simple rules is easier to implement and has less potential to be misunderstood. An example might be that all persons who have had one or more seizures cannot drive until they have been free of seizures for at least 12 months. However, drivers with a history of seizures have a very wide range of crash risk and to maximize the number of people permitted to drive safely, the licensing regime must either rely on individual risk assessment or comprise rules that apply to several different clinical situations. A disadvantage of complex systems of rules is that they may not be remembered or correctly applied by treating doctors, who may certify fitness only occasionally.[21]

Roles and responsibilities of driver, doctor, and licensing authority

The method of implementation of driver licensing rules may be just as important as the rules themselves. In some jurisdictions, assessment of fitness to drive according to official standards is left to the treating doctor.[7] This may create a conflict of interest; at the same time as the doctor is acting as the advocate for the person with seizures and trying to build or preserve a trusting and collaborative relationship that is essential for optimal care, the doctor is also cast in the role of agent of the licensing authority and decision-maker. This may seriously damage the doctor–patient relationship and encourage the patient to conceal relevant information necessary not just to determine driving fitness, but also to optimize therapy. The doctor is aware of the patient's individual circumstances and the consequences for that patient of losing their right to drive. The doctor may be perceived as standing between the patient and the patient's financial ruin, their loss of independence, and be blamed for the patient's misfortune. Doctors may feel pressured because of a desire to avoid damage to their relationship with the patient or because of sympathy for the patient's plight, resulting in fitness decisions that are unsafe. An objective assessment of fitness in such circumstances may be impossible. A further disadvantage of fitness assessments by treating doctors is that the doctor may be held legally liable should a crash occur as a result of a seizure in a person they assessed as fit to drive.[7]

The legal responsibility for driver licensing rests with the licensing authority. However, some licensing authorities effectively outsource this function to treating doctors. For the reasons noted above, this is not ideal. A better system is one in which the doctor's role is to provide clinical information about the licence applicant. The licensing authority then uses these data to determine fitness. If the driving standards are based entirely on clinical data rather than opinion, no medical expertise is required to determine whether the applicant meets the licensing standard (Figure 14.1). Such a system exists in some states of Australia and has been demonstrated to improve compliance with the driving standards.[22] However, this system cannot entirely replace individual assessment and opinion because it cannot cope with exceptional cases in which the rules may be inappropriately lenient or inappropriately restrictive. An expert review panel should be available to review such cases, usually at the request of the treating doctor, who is in a position to judge if their patient's situation is appropriately managed by the driving standards.

Non-compliance

Non-compliance with driving rules may occur for several reasons. The driver may feel under social or financial pressure to continue driving, there may be denial of the risk their driving poses, they may not appreciate the risk, they may believe they can reliably predict or avoid further seizures, or they may believe that their aura will last long enough for them to stop the vehicle before their consciousness is impaired. Non-compliance can be reduced by educating the patient about the risks of seizures while driving and illustration with anecdotes can be helpful. The reasons behind the driving regulations should be explained, emphasizing that the rules are there to protect the patient and the community. Lastly, the legal consequences of non-compliance with the rules, particularly if a seizure at the wheel results in a death, should also be explained. Alternative modes of transport will also reduce the incentive to disobey the rules. Mitigation against this might include improved availability of public transport or fare discounts for taxi services. Employers may also find alternative duties that do not depend on driving. When a doctor becomes aware that a patient is driving when unsafe, their initial step should be to explain the risks of doing so and of the legal penalties that apply. If the individual continues to drive, the doctor is ethically obliged to report the person to the relevant driving licensing authority or police. People who report drivers under such circumstances should be legally protected against action for breaching confidentiality.

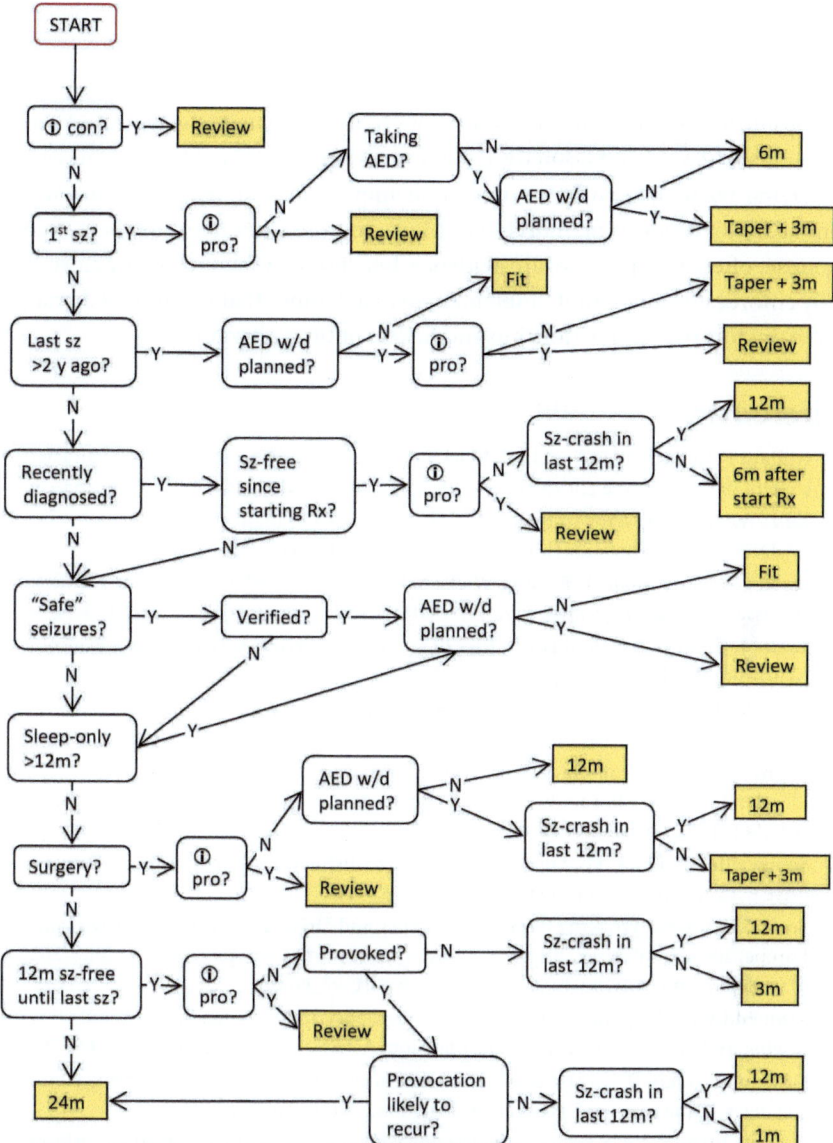

Figure 14.1 Example of a decision tree that aids determination of driving fitness after seizures, using clinical data rather than opinion. This example uses the regulations in force in Australia in 2003 but can be modified to apply to other local driving regulations. Driving fitness recommendations are in yellow boxes, with the applicable non-driving period before reassessment. ① con, additional information provided by treating physician indicating concern that driving may not be safe; ① pro, additional information provided by treating physician indicating that driver may be fit despite not meeting national standard; AED w/d, antiepileptic drug withdrawal; m, months; Rx, treatment; 'Safe' seizures, seizures that do not impair consciousness or driving ability; sz, seizure; Sz-crash, motor vehicle crash due to seizure; Taper + 3m, period of dosage reduction followed by 3 months; Verified, consciousness and responsiveness verified by reliable witness or video-electroencephalography.

Reproduced with permission from Somerville ER, Driving Committee of the Epilepsy Society of Australia. A decision tree to determine fitness to drive in epilepsy: results of a pilot in two Australian states. Epilepsia. 2019;60(7):1445–52.

Any effort to manage driving risk through driver licensing will succeed only if people without a valid licence refrain from driving. This is not always the case.

Driving by people with seizures is an important and sensitive issue with ramifications beyond the individual. Managing the situation must be a compromise, often based on meagre evidence, but should be supported by clear, legally enforceable guidelines, implemented in a manner that minimizes damage to the doctor–patient relationship and fosters optimal therapy.

References

1. **Gilliam F, Kuzniecky R, Faught E, Black L, Carpenter G, Schrodt R.** Patient-validated content of epilepsy-specific quality-of-life measurement. Epilepsia. 1997;**38**(2):233–36.

2. **Xu Z, Ayyappan S, Seneviratne U.** Sudden unexpected death in epilepsy (SUDEP): what do patients think? Epilepsy Behav. 2015;**42**:29–34.

3. **Kwon C, Liu M, Quan H, Thoo V, Wiebe S, Jette N.** Motor vehicle accidents, suicides, and assaults in epilepsy: a population-based study. Neurology. 2011;**76**(9):801–806.

4. **Taylor J, Chadwick D, Johnson T.** Risk of accidents in drivers with epilepsy. J Neurol Neurosurg Psychiatry. 1996;**60**(6):621–27.

5. **Sundelin HEK, Chang Z, Larsson H,** et al. Epilepsy, antiepileptic drugs, and serious transport accidents: a nationwide cohort study. Neurology. 2018;**90**(13):e1111–18.

6. **Ma BB, Bloch J, Krumholz A,** et al. Regulating drivers with epilepsy in Maryland: results of the application of a United States consensus guideline. Epilepsia. 2017;**58**(8):1389–97.

7. **Somerville ER, Black AB, Dunne JW.** Driving to distraction—certification of fitness to drive with epilepsy. Med J Aust. 2010;**192**(6):342–44.

8. **Second European Working Group on Epilepsy and Driving.** Epilepsy and driving in Europe. 2005. Available at: https://road-safety.transport.ec.europa.eu/system/files/2021-07/epilepsy_and_driving_in_europe_final_report_v2_en.pdf

9. **Schmedding E, Belgian Working Group on Epilepsy and Driving.** Epilepsy and driving in Belgium: proposals and justification. Acta Neurol Belg. 2004;**104**(2):68–79.

10. **Gastaut H, Zifkin BG.** The risk of automobile accidents with seizures occurring while driving: relation to seizure type. Neurology. 1987;**37**(10):1613–16.

11. **Guan R, Burbidge A, Somerville E.** Driving with epilepsy: attitudes, behavior, risks in an Australian cohort. 2018. Available at: https://cms.aesnet.org/abstractslisting/driving-with-epilepsy--attitudes--behavior--and-risks-in-an-australian-cohort

12. **Australian Bureau of Statistics.** Australian social trends. Canberra: Australian Bureau of Statistics; 1996.

13. **Bonnett LJ, Marson AG, Johnson A,** et al. External validation of a prognostic model for seizure recurrence following a first unprovoked seizure and implications for driving. PLoS One. 2014;**9**(6):e99063.

14. **Austroads.** Assessing fitness to drive, 5th ed. Sydney: Austroads; 2016.

15. **Punia V, Farooque P, Chen W,** et al. Epileptic auras and their role in driving safety in people with epilepsy. Epilepsia. 2015;**56**(11):e182–85.

16. **Ban T, Kawai K, Nambu K, Iseki H, Masamune K.** Estimating the risk of fatal traffic accidents posed by drivers with epilepsy in Japan: a comparison with traffic accidents caused by sudden death of occupational drivers. Epilepsy Seizure. 2018;**10**(1):1–10.

17. **Pohlmann-Eden B, Hynick N, Legg K.** First seizure while driving (FSWD)—an underestimated phenomenon? Can J Neurol Sci. 2013;**40**(4):540–45.

18. **Elger CE, Hoppe C.** Diagnostic challenges in epilepsy: seizure under-reporting and seizure detection. Lancet Neurol. 2018;**17**(3):279–88.

19. **Dalrymple J, Appleby J.** Cross sectional study of reporting of epileptic seizures to general practitioners. Br Med J. 2000;**320**(7227):94–97.

20. **Bacon D, Fisher RS, Morris JC, Rizzo M, Spanaki MV.** American Academy of Neurology position statement on physician reporting of medical conditions that may affect driving competence. Neurology. 2007;**68**(15):1174–77.

21. **Caruana P, Hughes AR, Lea RA, Lueck CJ.** Australian driving restrictions: how well do neurologists know them? Intern Med J. 2018;**48**(9):1144–49.

22. **Somerville ER, Driving Committee of the Epilepsy Society of Australia.** A decision tree to determine fitness to drive in epilepsy: results of a pilot in two Australian states. Epilepsia. 2019;**60**(7):1445–52.

Chapter 15

Epilepsy, marriage, and other social relationships

Neha Kinariwalla and Arjune Sen

Introduction

Although medically accurate, simply classifying epilepsy as a neurological disorder disregards the many psychosocial aspects of the condition.[1] Epilepsy can significantly affect a person's social experience, emotional functioning, and quality of life (QOL).[2] While the severity and frequency of seizures is, without doubt, an important factor in QOL, studies have shown that a lack of social support can be more indicative of low QOL in the most debilitated people with epilepsy.[3] Social support, in turn, has been defined as 'the commitment, caring advice and aid provided in personal relationships'.[4] Social support provides a number of major functions: emotional support, informational support, appraisal, social companionship, and affectionate support. These are all forms of social support that can greatly improve QOL.[5]

Chronic illness requires readjustments that can repeatedly interfere with day-to-day living and role-related activities. People with less social support are more likely to have both psychological and physical ailments.[6] One study found that 90% of the variance for self-rated, health-related QOL in people with epilepsy was explained by a combination of disease severity, availability of social support, locus of control, and epilepsy self-efficacy.[7] Social support was found to be a mediator between disease severity and the belief that people can control their course of life despite their epilepsy.[7] When social support decreases, so does health-related QOL.[7] Conversely, as social support increases, the person's ability to cope with potential limitations of their condition improves.[7]

As such, social support is tremendously important in the lives of individuals with epilepsy. However, the level of support received can vary, particularly owing to the associated stigma of the disorder. Stigma refers to the loss of status that arises from being in possession of an attribute that is considered to be different in an undesirable way, and therefore 'deeply discrediting'.[8] This chapter aims to additionally discuss the effects of the stigma of epilepsy on social support. First, the chapter briefly examines the historical foundation of stigma in epilepsy and assesses how this, in turn, affects felt and enacted stigma experienced by people with epilepsy today. The body of the chapter will contend that stigma within the social environment may be a primary factor that influences social support for people with epilepsy. We will also explore the effect of epilepsy on various relationships through social, political, and economic factors.

Social perception of epilepsy: a brief history of stigma and discrimination

The history of social perceptions of epilepsy is full of misconceptions ranging from utmost reverence for the disease to the belief that it relates to witchcraft. Showing physical and 'psychic' symptoms, epilepsy has been particularly susceptible to interpretations both that it is a physiological process and that seizures occur as a result of spiritual influences.[9] Accounts of epilepsy date back to that of an epileptic attack in the Mesopotamian civilization.[9] In ancient societies, epilepsy was thought to be associated with demonic possession (Figure 15.1).[10] A biblical account described Jesus as driving out the 'unclean spirit' from a young boy who had seizures in which 'he foameth, and gnasheth with his teeth, and he pineth away'.[9]

In the Middle Ages, epilepsy was considered to be a punishment for sin because of its apparent connection with possession. Even when biomedical explanations for seizures began to be more prominently espoused, this new paradigm brought its own connotations and stigma. Studies began linking epilepsy to aggressive or criminal behaviour, abnormal sexual activity, inherited degeneracy, and an 'epileptic personality'.[11] In the late 19th century, physicians in North America mistook people with epilepsy to have a personality disorder, predisposed towards criminal actions, who therefore qualified for eugenic policies.[12]

Apart from the effects of stigma on policy and perceptions in the medical realm, social influences can have a profound effect on a person's sense of identity. Stigma is not solely the outcome of societal devaluations, but also the acceptance of this devaluation by the individual. People construct identities in material and symbolic contexts especially in relation to health.[13] A diagnosis of epilepsy can appear to be interpreted negatively, leading to an overwhelming sense of shame.[14]

A study conducted by Scambler and Hopkins in 1986 found that almost all participants feared the diagnosis of epilepsy because it transformed them from a 'normal' person to an 'epileptic', and many considered epilepsy to be, first and foremost, a stigmatizing condition.[15] There was, though, little empirical

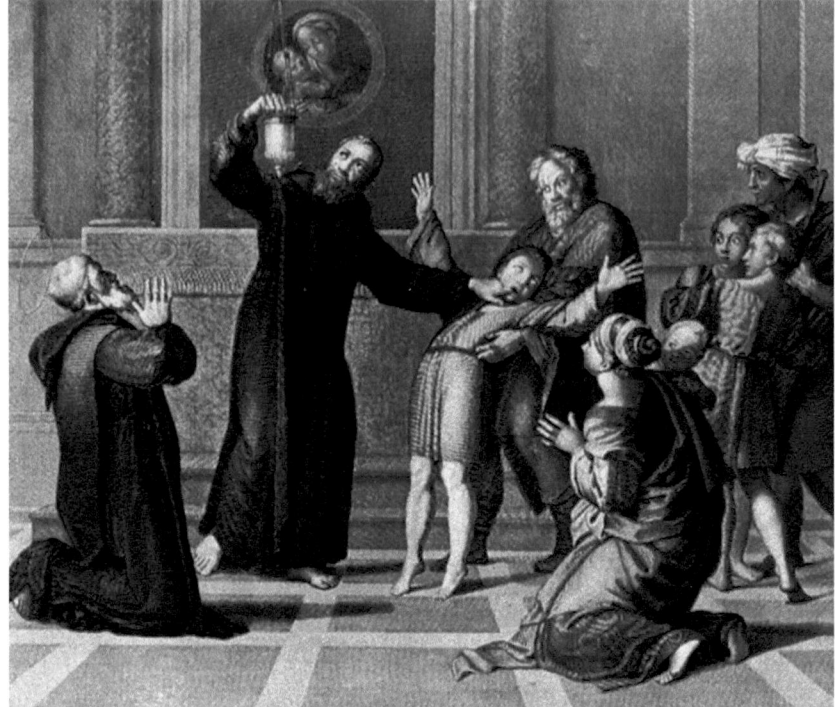

Figure 15.1 St Nilus healing a 'possessed' boy with epilepsy through anointment with lamp oil.
From a painting in the church at Grottaferrata. Engraving by Oskar Rosenthal, published Leipzig, 1925. Wellcome Images reference no. L0005933.

evidence of enacted stigma upon the people who felt stigmatized.[15] Considering this, the authors suggested that the general public is not necessarily as stigmatizing as the people with epilepsy might sometimes fear.[15] They proposed that a distinction in stigma could be drawn from 'felt' and 'enacted' stigma. Enacted stigma refers to episodes of discrimination against people with epilepsy, solely on grounds of negative perceptions; felt stigma is the experience associated with being a person with epilepsy and the apprehension of enacted stigma[16] (see Chapter 13).

The degree to which epilepsy is the central part of identity for the individual varies greatly and can result in marked differences in QOL from one individual to another. In a study of people with epilepsy in remission, for example, only 2% could recall or recount any occasion of unfair treatment at work and only 3% thought they had not been successful with a job application due to their epilepsy.[17] A third, however, felt their epilepsy made it more difficult for them than for others to gain employment and many did not disclose their condition to employers out of fear of discrimination[17] (see Chapter 13).

When people become primarily associated with epilepsy, their behaviour often alters in response. This change in behaviour has been conceptualized through the labelling theory, which describes how the self-identity and behaviour of individuals may be influenced by the term a society may use to classify them. In 1989, Link and colleagues derived predictions from the classic labelling approach for those with mental health difficulties.[18] They assert that 'in the course of being socialised, individuals develop negative conceptions of what it means to be a person with epilepsy and thus form beliefs about how others will view and then treat someone with that status'.[18] People's beliefs about their label, in epilepsy as in other conditions, understandably shapes the nature of their social connectedness.[18] Further, given that seizures are episodic, people may choose to hide epilepsy, owing to concern about how others may view them were the diagnosis to be declared.

Parents, children, and epilepsy: the effects on a family

For most children, parents are the primary mediators of experience.[19] This is certainly the case when children are young and, often, through adolescence. One of the most significant ways parents shape children's lives is by interpreting events that they themselves may not fully understand. Family members' reactions to a diagnosis of epilepsy in the child set the stage for the child's own interpretation of its significance.[20] Parents must face the news of their child's diagnosis as well as the medical risks associated with that diagnosis. When family members, particularly parents, have a negative reaction to the diagnosis, a child may learn to think about epilepsy as something 'shameful'. Similarly, when the parents' attitudes are that epilepsy will attract hostile reactions, the child may learn that epilepsy is not something to disclose.[20] Such attitudes can result in strategies to manage stigma, such as renegotiation of the diagnosis for a more socially benign one, social withdrawal, and reduction of expectations for the future.[20]

It is not just at the onset of epilepsy that there can be difficulties for the family of a person with epilepsy. A number of studies have indicated that childhood chronic illness often impacts the entire family system and continues to impact any progression of the disorder.[21] When examining families of children with epilepsy, it was found that family members reported high levels of depression, anger, guilt, and frequently reported helplessness and frustration.[22] For example, families of children with epilepsy had higher levels of stress and lower levels of self-esteem compared to families of children with asthma.[23] Furthermore, over 20% of mothers who had children with epilepsy had histories of 'nervous breakdowns' and were at risk of psychological morbidity.[24,25] Epilepsy can also appear to a family as a burden with restrictions on family activities as well as anxiety about life expectancy and care of the person with epilepsy being primary concerns. Such restrictions can result in a change in family behaviour and limit recreational activities that serve as stress relief in everyday life.[26]

One novel aspect in this complex milieu is that with the widescale rollout of whole exome/genome sequencing, many children with difficult epilepsy and epileptic encephalopathies will receive a genomic diagnosis for their condition (see Chapter 2). As well as significantly shortening the diagnostic odyssey for these individuals, identifying a genetic cause of the condition can also assuage guilt for parents who now have proof that the epilepsy is not a result of 'something that they did.' A confirmed genetic diagnosis can also allow families to better access appropriate support groups as well as being more enabled to claim benefits and support to which they are entitled. In time, this may reduce, at least partly, some of the adverse impact of epilepsy on parents.

Siblings of children with epilepsy are also at risk of psychosocial difficulties, which may sometimes relate to jealousy caused by attention being paid to the child with epilepsy.[27] Interestingly, in a study by Hoare and Kerley, it was found that parents rated disturbance in siblings less than that rated by teachers.[28] This could be an indication of the fact that poor sibling adjustment is a consequence of the concentrated parental focus on the child with epilepsy, who may consequently be less able to objectively recognize the impact on their other children.[26] In contrast, though, several studies found that siblings of individuals with newly diagnosed epilepsy did not have an increase in rates of psychological disturbance.[23,28] The negative consequences of epilepsy in siblings may also be related to the course and prognosis of the condition, social stigma, and any alteration in family relations.[26]

Epilepsy in the workplace and education

Higher education and occupational attainment have been thought to modify the QOL trajectory in individuals with epilepsy.[10] However, population studies from the US show that persons with a history of epilepsy report lower educational attainment, lower household income, and poorer health status compared to those without epilepsy.[29,30] Epilepsy can affect the ability of an individual's capacity to work because of absenteeism, lower productivity, unemployment, underemployment, and/or premature mortality (see Chapter 13).[31] Even a single seizure has the capacity to impart negative consequences with regard to driving motor vehicles and working in general (see Chapters 13 and 14).[32] More recent data, though, have shown that people with later-onset epilepsy have the same educational attainment as those with earlier-onset seizures—both groups having less scholastic achievement than controls.[33] This suggests that it is not seizures alone that contribute to educational prospects and other factors may play a role. Identifying and mitigating those factors will be crucial going forwards.

Teachers, who can play a pivotal role in disseminating information and a basic knowledge of epilepsy to students, often have a poor knowledge of the condition. In a study conducted in north-western Nigeria, 200 teachers were selected and surveyed regarding their knowledge and attitudes towards students with epilepsy.[34] Over 25% of the teachers would object to having a child with epilepsy in their class and 60% believed that students with epilepsy should be separated from students without epilepsy in the classroom.[34] This could have been because some teachers believed that epilepsy is contagious, a belief that reflects poor understanding of the disorder. A more recent study in Saudi Arabia found that 68% of teachers would not approve of marriage to a person with epilepsy.[35] In Zimbabwe, 22.6% of the responding teachers thought epilepsy was contagious, although a majority of the teachers would still accommodate a student with epilepsy and teach that student in their class.[36] Ensuring that teachers have an accurate understanding of epilepsy is crucial in disseminating that knowledge to future generations (see Chapter 12). As a corollary, if teachers lack this information, or worse have incorrect perceptions about epilepsy, those too can be perpetuated.

Marriage of people with epilepsy: variances around the world

Outside of blood relatives, one of the most important relationships is that with a life partner. Social support, particularly from committed relationships, can serve as a buffer for the negative impact of chronic health conditions. Several theories suggest that social support from marriage works to improve health by providing greater economic resources, fostering a sense of meaning, promoting healthy behaviours, and reducing risk factors such as excess alcohol consumption and substance misuse.[37] A study completed in Tanzania in 2017 evaluated stigma and functional disability in relation to marriage and employment for 84 young people with epilepsy.[38] Younger individuals with seizures were more likely to experience adverse employment, educational, and relationship outcomes in the transition to adult life than the controls.[38] Another study analysing marital status and the social control of

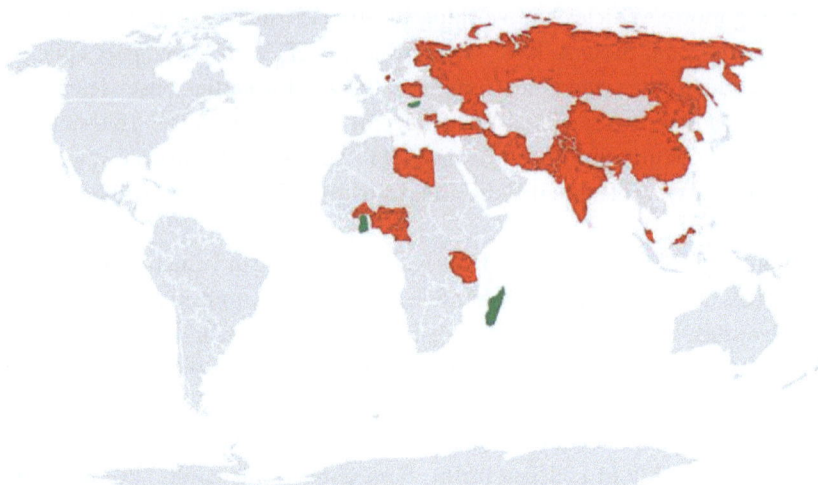

Figure 15.2 Distribution of social attitudes for marriage of people with epilepsy conducted worldwide. Overall positive marriage acceptability is represented as green whereas red represents an overall negative marriage acceptability.

health behaviour theorized that health benefits from marriage can also come from spousal monitoring and attempts to positively influence their partner's health behaviours.[39] Several studies have shown that affectionate support—the sense of being cared about, loved, esteemed, valued as a person, and having someone who cares about you and your problems—is the most important predictor of health outcomes compared with other types of support.[5,40] For those with epilepsy, however, marriage can sometimes constitute as much of a challenge as it offers support.[41] Figure 15.2 depicts the distribution of social attitudes for marriage of those with epilepsy; a majority of the studies found an overall negative marriage acceptability.[38,42–62]

Rates of marriage in people with epilepsy

Individuals with epilepsy are less likely to marry than those without epilepsy.[30] There may be a number of reasons for this ranging from social attitudes towards marriage of those with epilepsy to emotional adjustment. Charyton and colleagues postulated that poor social support for people with epilepsy may also be related to lower rates of marriage.[40]

Lower marriage rates in individuals with epilepsy, as compared with the general population, have been reported in studies from Nigeria, Tanzania, Brazil, Iran, and Pakistan.[62–66] In Ghana, women with epilepsy may not be encouraged to marry because there is a belief that they may give birth to children who will

Table 15.1 Monogamous marriage rates for people with epilepsy and control groups

Reference	Year of publication	Number of controls	Number of people with epilepsy	Number of controls married	Number of people with epilepsy married	Country
Baker et al.[75]	1997	100	100	58	48	European study
Herodes et al.[69]	2001	200	203	–	83	Estonia
Birbeck et al.[73]	2006	169	169	76	47	Zambia
Mushi et al.[71]	2010	41 (carers of people with epilepsy)	41	–	11	Tanzania
Komolafe et al.[70]	2011	69 (women)	63	41	8	Nigeria
Shetty et al.[74]	2011	–	60	–	21	India
Elliott et al.[76]	2011	–	996	–	481	US
Riasi et al.[72]	2015	179,686 (population of Birjand City)	374	163,783	102	Iran

also have seizures.[67] A study by Batzel and Dodrill in 1984 aimed to explore why fewer people with epilepsy are married by testing the emotional adjustment and the mental abilities of 178 individuals with epilepsy (92 males, 86 females) over the age of 25.[68] On all measures, the married and the unmarried independent groups had the best scores, the separated/divorced group was intermediate, and the never-married dependent group had the lowest scores. The study concluded that marital status may, therefore, be more related to emotional adjustment than to mental abilities.[68] For a summary of international studies looking at monogamous marriage rates for people with epilepsy and control groups, see Table 15.1.[69-76]

Sex-based differences and marriage in people with epilepsy

Older studies tend to report that rates of marriage are lower in men with epilepsy than women.[77-79] In the early 1990s in Ireland, only 33% of men with epilepsy aged more than 20 years were married while in the general population the rate was 65%.[79] In women, the rates were 46% and 73%.[79] A study completed in the US found that 37% of men with epilepsy were married, as opposed to 51% of women with epilepsy.[78] These authors also found that those with onset of epilepsy at age 11 or younger were less likely to be married (35%) than people whose epilepsy started after they were 11 years old (51%).[78] When assessed for sex, the findings were only significant for men.[78] A large study from northeast China, however, has shown that age and age of seizure onset independently affected marriage in both men and women with epilepsy. Other recent studies report that it is women with epilepsy who may find it more difficult to find a spouse and that they are at higher risk of abandonment or other marital difficulties.[80–83] The exact reasons for this seeming shift are uncertain and would be worthy of further investigation.

Attitudes to marriage

In a review of social attitudes to marriage for people with epilepsy, 12 of 14 studies within the existing literature indicated negative views within the public for those with epilepsy to marry.[45,46,49,77,84–89] For example, a study of 800 respondents in Iran found that only 28% of respondents were willing to accept the marriage of a family member to someone with epilepsy.[44] Another study administered to 219 students in India found that nearly 67% of the respondents stated that epilepsy was a hindrance to marriage.[90]

There is some suggestion that attitudes towards those with epilepsy may be improving, although much more needs to be done. Mirnics and colleagues, for example, found that there was a significant decrease in prejudice towards people with epilepsy regarding attitudes towards marriage, children, and work when comparing results from 1994 with those obtained in 2001.[50]

Negative perceptions seem more difficult in ethnic minorities. In 2011, non-white people with epilepsy were significantly less likely to report being married (8% vs 22% of total sample size).[30] A recent study from India showed that 93.5% of people, with and without epilepsy, thought that those with epilepsy should be allowed to marry. Only 41.8%, however, would declare that their daughter had epilepsy prior to marriage.[91] One possible explanation may be that people from ethnic minorities with epilepsy face more social stigma within their communities or that, for example, there are more common misperceptions about the heritability of epilepsy in certain settings (Box 15.1).[92]

As would be predicted, attitudes to epilepsy and marriage are very nuanced. For example, within Malaysia the Sabah people have been shown to have better acceptance of marriage in people with epilepsy than West Malaysians.[53] Similarly, words and phrasing are of critical importance. Two groups of college high school students were presented with identical questionnaires except

---

Box 15.1 Case vignette

A 22-year-old male with learning difficulty and of South Asian heritage was admitted to hospital following a bilateral tonic–clonic seizure at home. He had fallen awkwardly during the event and the emergency services had to break down the bathroom door to reach him. In the emergency department, the young man was stable, but as he was almost non-verbal he was not able to provide additional information. Shortly after his arrival, two of his sisters attended, both of whom were highly educated and working in professional capacities. They clearly were very close and caring of their younger sibling. When reviewing the history with them it transpired that their brother had experienced intermittent convulsions for several years, but medical attention had never been sought. On this occasion, they were obliged to seek help owing to how he fell. When asked why his seizures had not been mentioned before, the sisters explained that there was concern within the family that the brother's epilepsy would affect their marriage prospects.

---

that one referred to individuals as either a 'person/child with epilepsy' and the other referred to individuals as 'epileptic/epileptic child.' The group presented with a questionnaire worded with 'epileptic/epileptic child' gave significantly more negative responses, including when asked about marrying an affected individual.

Concealment of epilepsy before and during marriage

Perhaps influenced by all these factors, some people choose not to disclose epilepsy prior to marriage, and this especially applies in cultures where marriages may be arranged.[93] In a Japanese study of 278 people with epilepsy, 29 were divorced and of these, seven listed epilepsy as the cause of that divorce.[94] Analysis of those seven individuals showed that six had not disclosed their epilepsy prior to marriage and discovery of antiseizure medication was thought to have led to the separation. While this may in part relate to stigma relating to epilepsy itself, additional contributing factors may include trust as spouses might wonder what else is being hidden.

In India, concealment of epilepsy in women prior to marriage has also led to high rates of divorce (18% vs 1.3% in the general population).[95] These data, though, can be difficult to interpret. It might, for example, be that if epilepsy had been declared beforehand that the marriage would not proceed at all, particularly as large dowries can be demanded from the parents of daughters with epilepsy, even if their prospective husband has comorbidities.[96] These findings again seem very culturally specific. In Korea, lack of disclosure was not generally cited as a cause for divorce and in Vietnam it has been reported that people with epilepsy and their family members overall favoured disclosing the diagnosis of epilepsy.[97,98]

Difficulties for people with epilepsy within marriage

Relationships with a close partner can be very beneficial whether one member of the couple has epilepsy or not. There is, though, relatively little work on sex-based perceptions of the impact of epilepsy in marriage. People who are married might be less fearful of injury during a seizure, but also more concerned about employment, as there may be more dependants relying on their income. In China, for example, employment status correlated with marriage, but only in men.[99] Somewhat unusually, studies from Kenya have demonstrated that being single was associated with greater adherence to antiseizure medication.[100] One possibility is that those with more active epilepsy are more likely to be single and the severity of seizures results in better adherence. Alternative explanations may include individuals seeking to avoid the adverse effects of antiseizure medications (e.g. on libido) if they are in a relationship—although this is speculative.

Even successful treatment for epilepsy can have a seemingly adverse impact on marriage. A study from the early 1990s showed that 35% of people who reported a significant (>75%) reduction in seizures after epilepsy surgery had family-related difficulties.[101] Six per cent divorced.[101] Other studies have shown similar findings. If people become seizure free postoperatively with all of the associated liberty that this entails, such as being able to drive, then there is more likely to be a change in marital status for that individual. People may newly marry or those who have been married may divorce, the latter being particularly seen in women rendered seizure free by surgical intervention.[78,102]

More recently, a questionnaire-based approach was taken to evaluate whether there were differences in the perceived impact of epilepsy between the person with epilepsy and their spouse in the UK.[103] Sex-based differences were identified with, for example, male spouses' assessment of 'overall health' correlating well to seizure severity in their wives. Psychosocial scores reported by husbands of women with epilepsy were, though, inversely correlated with those that the women themselves gave. Males with epilepsy were particularly affected by not being able to drive. There were also differences depending on when the epilepsy began. If seizure onset was after marriage, then this could associate with a greater sense of stigmatization, low mood, and anxiety—particularly if the person with epilepsy had more severe seizures.

Conclusion

Even in the 21st century, epilepsy can remain a very stigmatizing condition around the world. In addition to testing the resilience of those with the condition, epilepsy can apply additional pressure on parents, siblings, carers, and life partners. An overarching theme is that education is critical and that improved knowledge of the condition within communities will empower people with epilepsy. Attitudes to epilepsy can be culturally specific, perhaps more so than for any other chronic health condition. It is, for example, essential to dispel myths that epilepsy is contagious or universally heritable.

Both men and women can be adversely affected in marriage although current data would suggest that women with epilepsy are particularly disadvantaged. Concealing epilepsy prior to marriage seems hazardous although the reasons for doing this are evident. Better global access to antiseizure medications, with the resulting improvement in seizure control, should enable more people to declare their epilepsy and potentially form secure life partnerships. Within marriage, the impact of epilepsy can be differentially perceived by the person with epilepsy and their spouse suggesting that tailored education for spouses may improve the QOL for both partners.

Additional work is needed to explore the impact of epilepsy on other social relationships, especially in adulthood. For example, people may cohabit, rather than marrying, and non-binary relationships are increasingly common. Studies of the impact of epilepsy on such life partnerships are, therefore, essential. It is apparent that only through positively changing attitudes within society as a whole will people with epilepsy experience improvements in their social relationships and life chances.

References

1. de Boer HM, Mula M, Sander JW. The global burden and stigma of epilepsy. Epilepsy Behav. 2008;**12**(4):540–46.
2. Suurmeijer TPBM, Reuvekamp MF, Aldenkamp BP. Social functioning, psychological functioning, and quality of life in epilepsy. Epilepsia. 2001;**42**(9):1160–68.
3. Droge D, Arntson P, Norton R. The social support function in epilepsy self-help groups. Small Gr Res. 1986;**17**(2):139–63.
4. Ross CE, Mirowsky J, Goldsteen K. The impact of the family on health: the decade in review. Impact Fam Heal Decad Rev. 1990;**52**(4):1059–78.
5. Cohen S. Social relationships and health. Am Psychol. 2004;**59**(8):676–84.

6. **Hills MD, Baker PG.** Relationships among epilepsy, social stigma, self-esteem, and social support. J Epilepsy. 1992;5(4):231–38.

7. **Amir M, Roziner I, Knoll A, Neufeld MY.** Self-efficacy and social support as mediators in the relation between disease severity and quality of life in patients with epilepsy. Epilepsia. 1999;40(2):216–24.

8. **Goffman E.** Stigma: notes on the management of spoiled identity. Englewood Cliffs, NJ: Prentice-Hall; 1963.

9. **Temkin O.** The falling sickness: a history of epilepsy from the Greeks to the beginnings of modern neurology. Med Hist. 1973;17(2):214–15.

10. **Jacoby A, Baker GA.** Quality-of-life trajectories in epilepsy: a review of the literature. Epilepsy Behav. 2008;12(4):557–71.

11. **Jacoby A.** Social stigma of adults with epilepsy. J Neurol Sci. 2009;285:S39.

12. **Dwyer E.** Stories of epilepsy: 1880–1930. In: **Golden J, Rosenberg CE,** eds. Framing disease: studies in cultural history. New Brunswick: Rutgers University Press; 1992:248–72.

13. **Howard JA.** Social psychology of identities. Annu Rev Sociol. 2000;26:367–93.

14. **Conrad P, Schneider JW.** Deviance and medicalization. Philadelphia, PA: Temple University Press; 1992.

15. **Scambler G, Hopkins A.** Being epileptic: coming to terms with stigma. Sociol Health Illn. 1986;8(1):26–43.

16. **Guo W, Wu J, Wang W,** et al. The stigma of people with epilepsy is demonstrated at the internalized, interpersonal and institutional levels in a specific sociocultural context: findings from an ethnographic study in rural China. Epilepsy Behav. 2012;25(2):282–88.

17. **Jacoby A.** Stigma, epilepsy, and quality of life. Epilepsy Behav. 2002;3(6 Suppl 2):10–20.

18. **Link BG, Cullen FT, Struening E, Shrout PE, Dohrenwend BP.** A modified labeling theory approach to mental disorders: an empirical assessment. Am Sociol Rev. 1989;54(3):400.

19. **Ziegler RG.** Impairments of control and competence in epileptic children and their families. Epilepsia. 1981;22(3):339–46.

20. **Jacoby A, Thaper A.** The contribution of seizures to psychosocial ill-health. Epilepsy Behav. 2009;15(2 Suppl 1):S41–45.

21. **Kazak AE.** Families of chronically ill children: a systems and social-ecological model of adaptation and challenge. J Consult Clin Psychol. 1989;57(1):25–30.

22. **Thomas SV, Bindu VB.** Psychosocial and economic problems of parents of children with epilepsy. Seizure. 1999;8(1):66–69.

23. **Austin JK, Dunn DW, Perkins SM, Shen J.** Youth with epilepsy: development of a model of children's attitudes toward their condition. Child Health Care. 2006;35(2):123–40.

24. **Rutter M, Graham P, Yule W.** A neuropsychiatry study in childhood (Clinics in Developmental Medicine No. 35/36). London: Spastics International Medical Publications; 1970.

25. **Ferrari M, Matthews WS, Barabas G.** The family and the child with epilepsy. Fam Process. 1983;22(1):53–59.

26. **Ellis N, Upton D, Thompson P.** Epilepsy and the family: a review of current literature. Seizure. 2000;9(1):22–30.

27. **Devinsky O, Westbrook L, Cramer J, Glassman M, Perrine K, Camfield C.** Risk factors for poor health-related quality of life in adolescents with epilepsy. Epilepsia. 1999;40(12):1715–20.

28. **Hoare P, Kerley S.** Psychosocial adjustment of children with chronic epilepsy and their families. Dev Med Child Neurol. 1991;33(3):201–15.

29. **Kobau R, Zahran H, Grant D, Thurman DJ, Price PH, Zack MM.** Prevalence of active epilepsy and health-related quality of life among adults with self-reported epilepsy in California: California Health Interview Survey, 2003. Epilepsia. 2007;48(10):1904–13.

30. **Elliott JO, Charyton C, McAuley JW, Shneker BF.** The impact of marital status on epilepsy-related health concerns. Epilepsy Res. 2011;95(3):200–206.

31. **Heaney D.** Epilepsy at work: evaluating the cost of epilepsy in the workplace. Epilepsia. 1999;40(s8):44–47.

32. **Krumholz A.** Driving issues in epilepsy: past, present, and future. Epilepsy Curr. 2009;9(2):31–35.

33. **Kaestner et al. (2021).**

34. **Owolabi LF, Shehu NM, Owolabi SD.** Epilepsy and education in developing countries: a survey of school teachers' knowledge about epilepsy and their attitude towards students with epilepsy in Northwestern Nigeria. Pan Afr Med J. 2014;18:255.

35. **Alamri S, Al Thobaity A.** Teachers and epilepsy: what they know, do not know, and need to know: a cross-sectional study of Taif City. J Fam Med Prim Care. 2020;9(6):2704.

36. **Mielke J, Adamolekun B, Ball D, Mundanda T.** Knowledge and attitudes of teachers towards epilepsy in Zimbabwe. Acta Neurol Scand. 2009;96(3):133–37.

37. **House J, Landis K, Umberson D.** Social relationships and health. Science. 1988;241(4865):540–45.

38. **Goodall J, Salem S, Walker RW,** et al. Stigma and functional disability in relation to marriage and employment in young people with epilepsy in rural Tanzania. Seizure. 2018;54:27–32.

39. **Umberson D.** Gender, marital status and the social control of health behavior. Soc Sci Med. 1992;34(8):907–17.

40. **Charyton C, Elliott JO, Lu B, Moore JL.** The impact of social support on health related quality of life in persons with epilepsy. Epilepsy Behav. 2009;16(4):640–45.

41. **Kinariwalla N, Sen A.** The psychosocial impact of epilepsy on marriage: a narrative review. Epilepsy Behav. 2016;63:34–41.

42. **Ratsimbazafy V, Andrianabelina R, Randrianarisona S, Preux P-M, Odermatt P.** Treatment gap for people living with epilepsy in Madagascar. Trop Doct. 2011;41(1):38–39.

43. **Choi-Kwon S, Park KA, Lee HJ,** et al. Familiarity with, knowledge of, and attitudes toward epilepsy in residents of Seoul, South Korea. Acta Neurol Scand. 2004;110(1):39–45.

44. **Demirci S, Dönmez CM, Gündoğar D, Baydar ÇL.** Public awareness of, attitudes toward, and understanding of epilepsy in Isparta, Turkey. Epilepsy Behav. 2007;11(3):427–33.

45. **Kartal A, Akyıldız A.** Public awareness, knowledge, and practice relating to epilepsy among adults in Konya. Epilepsy Behav. 2016;59:137–41.

46. **Ghanean H, Nojomi M, Jacobsson L.** Public awareness and attitudes towards epilepsy in Tehran, Iran. Glob Health Action. 2013;6(1):21618.

47. **Kolahi A-A, Abbasi-Kangevari M, Bakhshaei P, Mahvelati-Shamsabadi F, Tonekaboni S-H, Farsar A-R.** Knowledge, attitudes, and practices among mothers of children with epilepsy: a study in a teaching hospital. Epilepsy Behav. 2017;69:147–52.

48. **Riasi H, Rajabpour Sanati A, Ghaemi K.** The stigma of epilepsy and its effects on marital status. Springerplus. 2014;3(1):762.

49. **Lai C-W, Huang X, Lai Y-HC, Zhang Z, Liu G, Yang M-Z.** Survey of public awareness, understanding, and attitudes toward epilepsy in Henan Province, China. Epilepsia. 1990;31(2):182–87.

50. **Mirnics Z, Békés J, Rózsa S, Halász P.** Adjustment and coping in epilepsy. Seizure. 2001;10(3):181–87.

51. **Njamnshi AK, Tabah EN, Yepnjio FN,** et al. General public awareness, perceptions, and attitudes with respect to epilepsy in the Akwaya Health District, South-West Region, Cameroon. Epilepsy Behav. 2009;15(2):179–85.

52. **Aziz H, Akhtar SW, Hasan KZ.** Epilepsy in Pakistan: stigma and psychosocial problems. A population-based epidemiologic study. Epilepsia. 1997;38(10):1069–73.

53. **Chia Z-J, Lim K-S, Fong S-L,** et al. Attitudes toward epilepsy in East Malaysia using the Public Attitudes Toward Epilepsy (PATE) scale. Epilepsy Behav. 2020;110:107158.

54. **Antimov P, Tournev I, Sander JW.** A community-based door-to-door study of epilepsy among children in the Roma district of Kyustendil, Bulgaria. J Neurol. 2011;258:S139–40.

55. **Millogo A, Ngowi AH, Carabin H, Ganaba R, Da A, Preux P-M.** Knowledge, attitudes, and practices related to epilepsy in rural Burkina Faso. Epilepsy Behav. 2019;95:70–74.

56. **Alhagamhmad MH, Shembesh NM.** Investigating the awareness, behavior, and attitude toward epilepsy among university students in Benghazi, Libya. Epilepsy Behav. 2018;83:22–27.

57. **Guekht A, Hauser WA, Milchakova L, Churillin Y, Shpak A, Gusev E.** The epidemiology of epilepsy in the Russian Federation. Epilepsy Res. 2010;92(2–3):209–18.

58. **Staniszewska A, Religioni U, Dąbrowska-Bender M.** Acceptance of disease and lifestyle modification after diagnosis among young adults with epilepsy. Patient Prefer Adherence. 2017;11:165–74.

59. **Adoukonou T, Tognon-Tchegnonsi F, Gnonlonfoun D,** et al. Aspects socioculturels de l'épilepsie dans une communauté rurale au nord Bénin en 2011. Bull Société Pathol Exot. 2015;108(2):133–38.

60. **Seo J-G, Kim J-M, Park S-P.** Perceived stigma is a critical factor for interictal aggression in people with epilepsy. Seizure. 2015;26:26–31.

61. **Dugbartey AT, Barimah KB.** Traditional beliefs and knowledge base about epilepsy among university students in Ghana. Ethn Dis. 2013;23(1):1–5.

62. **Komolafe MA, Sunmonu TA, Afolabi OT,** et al. The social and economic impacts of epilepsy on women in Nigeria. Epilepsy Behav. 2012;24(1):97–101.

63. **Mushi D, Hunter E, Mtuya C, Mshana G, Aris E, Walker R.** Social-cultural aspects of epilepsy in Kilimanjaro Region, Tanzania: knowledge and experience among patients and carers. Epilepsy Behav. 2011;20(2):338–43.

64. **Muthaffar OY, Jan MM.** Public awareness and attitudes toward epilepsy in Saudi Arabia is improving. Neurosciences (Riyadh). 2014;19(2):124–26.

65. **Tedrus GM, Fonseca LC, Carvalho RM.** Epilepsy and quality of life: socio-demographic and clinical aspects, and psychiatric co-morbidity. Arq Neuropsiquiatr. 2013;71(6):385–91.

66. Njamnshi AK, Bissek A-C, Yepnjio FN, et al. A community survey of knowledge, perceptions, and practice with respect to epilepsy among traditional healers in the Batibo Health District, Cameroon. Epilepsy Behav. 2010;**17**(1):95–102.

67. Adjei P, Akpalu A, Laryea R, et al. Beliefs on epilepsy in Northern Ghana. Epilepsy Behav. 2013;**29**(2):316–21.

68. Batzel LW, Dodrill CB. Neuropsychological and emotional correlates of marital status and ability to live independently in individuals with Epilepsy. Epilepsia. 1984;**25**(5):594–98.

69. Herodes M, Õun A, Haldre S, Kaasik A-E. Epilepsy in Estonia: a quality-of-life study. Epilepsia. 2001;**42**(8):1061–73.

70. Komolafe MA, Sunmonu TA, Afolabi OT, et al. The social and economic impacts of epilepsy on women in Nigeria. Epilepsy Behav. 2012;**24**(1):97–101.

71. Mushi D, Hunter E, Mtuya C, Mshana G, Aris E, Walker R. Social-cultural aspects of epilepsy in Kilimanjaro Region, Tanzania: knowledge and experience among patients and carers. Epilepsy Behav. 2011;**20**(2):338–43.

72. Riasi H, Sanati AR, Ghaemi K. The stigma of epilepsy and its effects on marital status. Springerplus. 2015;**3**:762.

73. Birbeck G, Chomba E, Atadzhanov M, Mbewe E, Haworth A. The social and economic impact of epilepsy in Zambia: a cross-sectional study. Lancet Neurol. 2007;**6**(1):39–44.

74. Shetty PH, Punith K, Naik RK, Saroja A. Quality of life in patients with epilepsy in India. J Neurosci Rural Pract. 2011;**2**(1):33–38.

75. Baker GA, Jacoby A, Buck D, Stalgis C, Monnet D. Quality of life of people with epilepsy: a European study. Epilepsia. 1997;**38**(3):353–62.

76. Elliott JO, Charyton C, Sprangers P, Lu B, Moore JL. The impact of marriage and social support on persons with active epilepsy. Epilepsy Behav. 2011;**20**(3):533–38.

77. Dansky LV, Andermann E, Andermann F. Marriage and fertility in epileptic patients. Epilepsia. 1980;**21**(3):261–71.

78. Carran MA, Kohler CG, O'Connor MJ, Cloud B, Sperling MR. Marital status after epilepsy surgery. Epilepsia. 1999;**40**(12):1755–60.

79. Callaghan N, Crowley M, Goggin T. Epilepsy and employment, marital, education and social status. Ir Med J. 1992;**85**(1):17–19.

80. Zhao T, Zhong R, Chen Q, et al. Sex differences in marital status of people with epilepsy in Northeast China: an observational study. Epilepsy Behav. 2020;**113**:107571.

81. Chatterjee A, Nair R, Gandeti R, et al. Socioeconomic consequences of drug-resistant epilepsy in an adult cohort from southern India. Epilepsy Behav. 2020;**110**:107173.

82. Antimov P, Tournev I, Zhelyazkova S, Sander JW. Traditional practices and perceptions of epilepsy among people in Roma communities in Bulgaria. Epilepsy Behav. 2020;**108**:107086.

83. Gopinath M, Sarma PS, Thomas SV. Gender-specific psychosocial outcome for women with epilepsy. Epilepsy Behav. 2011;**20**(1):44–47.

84. Aziz H, Ali SM, Frances P, Khan MI, Hasan KZ. Epilepsy in Pakistan: a population-based epidemiologic study. Epilepsia. 1994;**35**(5):950–58.

85. Chen B, Choi H, Hirsch LJ, et al. Psychiatric and behavioral side effects of antiepileptic drugs in adults with epilepsy. Epilepsy Behav. 2017;**76**:24–31.

86. Choi-Kwon S, Park KA, Lee HJ, et al. Familiarity with, knowledge of, and attitudes toward epilepsy in residents of Seoul, South Korea. Acta Neurol Scand. 2004;**110**(1):39–45.

87. Goel D, Agarwal A, Saxena V, Dhanai J, Mehlotra V. Knowledge, attitude and practice of epilepsy in Uttarakhand, India. Ann Indian Acad Neurol. 2011;**14**(2):116.

88. Njamnshi AK, Angwafor SA, Jallon P, Muna WFT. Secondary school students' knowledge, attitudes, and practice toward epilepsy in the Batibo Health District-Cameroon. Epilepsia. 2009;**50**(5):1262–65.

89. Gambhir SK, Kumar V, Singhi PD, Goel RC. Public awareness, understanding & attitudes toward epilepsy. Indian J Med Res. 1995;**102**:34–38.

90. Goel D, Dhani J, Agarwal A, Mehlotra V, Saxena V. Knowledge, attitude and practice of epilepsy in Uttarakhand, India. Ann Indian Acad Neurol. 2011;**14**(2):116–19.

91. Sethi AK, Singh V, Chaurasia RN, et al. Study of knowledge, attitude, and practice among epilepsy patients in North India. J Neurosci Rural Pract. 2020;**11**(2):278–85.

92. Chen Z, Brodie MJ, Liew D, Kwan P. Treatment outcomes in patients with newly diagnosed epilepsy treated with established and new antiepileptic drugs: a 30-year longitudinal cohort study. JAMA Neurol. 2018;**75**(3):279–86.

93. Singh GK, Ganguly K, Banerji M, et al. Marriage in people with epilepsy: a compelling theme for psycho-behavioral research. Seizure. 2018;**62**:127–30.

94. Tsuji S. [Social aspects of epilepsy: marriage, pregnancy, driving, antiepileptic drug withdrawal and against social stigma]. Rinsho Shinkeigaku. 2004;**44**(11):865–67.

95. Santosh D, Kumar TS, Sarma PS, Radhakrishnan K. Women with onset of epilepsy prior to marriage: disclose or conceal? Epilepsia. 2007;**48**(5):1007–10.

96. Nag D. Gender and epilepsy: a clinician's experience. Neurol India. 2000;**48**(2):99–104.

97. Kim M-K, Kwon O-Y, Cho Y-W, et al. Marital status of people with epilepsy in Korea. Seizure. 2010;**19**(9):573–79.

98. Aydemir N, Trung DV, Snape D, Baker GA, Jacoby A. Multiple impacts of epilepsy and contributing factors: findings from an ethnographic study in Vietnam. Epilepsy Behav. 2009;**16**(3):512–20.

99. Li S, Chen J, Abdulaziz ATA, et al. Epilepsy in China: factors influencing marriage status and fertility. Seizure. 2019;**71**:179–84.

100. Kariuki SM, Kakooza-Mwesige A, Wagner RG, et al. Prevalence and factors associated with convulsive status epilepticus in Africans with epilepsy. Neurology. 2015;**84**(18):1838–45.

101. Bladin PF. Psychosocial aspects of epilepsy and of epilepsy surgery. Clin Exp Neurol. 1992;**29**:49–61.

102. Alonso NB, Mazetto L, de Araújo Filho GM, Vidal-Dourado M, Yacubian EMT, Centeno RS. Psychosocial factors associated with in postsurgical prognosis of temporal lobe epilepsy related to hippocampal sclerosis. Epilepsy Behav. 2015;**53**:66–72.

103. Deli A, Kinariwalla N, Calvello C, et al. An evaluation of the psychosocial impact of epilepsy on marriage in the United Kingdom. Epilepsy Behav. 2019;**94**:204–208.

Index

For the benefit of digital users, indexed terms that span two pages (e.g., 52–53) may, on occasion, appear on only one of those pages.